Extracranial Carotid and Vertebral Artery Disease

Sachinder Singh Hans

Editor

Extracranial Carotid and Vertebral Artery Disease

Contemporary Management

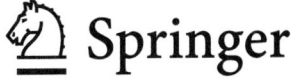 Springer

Editor
Sachinder Singh Hans
Wayne State University School of Medicine
Detroit, MI
USA

ISBN 978-3-030-08268-0   ISBN 978-3-319-91533-3   (eBook)
https://doi.org/10.1007/978-3-319-91533-3

This book is dedicated to the memory of the late Dr. Herbert J. Robb—a pioneering vascular surgeon who guided me through my vascular surgery training in the late 1970s, a time when vascular surgery was just becoming established as an independent specialty.

Foreword

I thank my colleague Dr. Sachinder Singh Hans for inviting me to write this foreword. It is a pleasure to welcome a book dealing with the carotid and vertebral arteries.

In the cerebrovascular field, most of what is published today deals with the new endovascular techniques. This makes this book timely because it reminds us of the prominent role that surgery continues to have in the management of these conditions. The many endovascular procedures being done in the carotid and vertebral arteries have decreased the training we can offer to the newer generations of vascular surgeons in the operative techniques described here. And these are procedures that require refined technique and, indeed, repetition if they are to be done with the levels of safety that patients deserve.

Another positive effect of this multiauthored text is to reflect the different criteria and also the conflicting opinions that different specialties have about how to manage the diseases that affect the supra-aortic trunks, the carotid, and the vertebral arteries.

One view with which I disagree is the tendency to lump vertebral and carotid disease in the neurological studies where a comparison is made between medical and interventional/surgical treatments. My disagreement is founded on a single fact: these two pathologies are apples and oranges that should not be combined in clinical studies. Mixing two different pathologies blurs the validity of any conclusion drawn from the study. The mechanism of brain damage is different: 75% of hemispheric infarcts are embolic while only 30% of those in the posterior brain have this mechanism. In terms of brain infarction, those in the vertebrobasilar territory are three times more likely to result in death.

In the carotid population the laterality of the lesion is easily inferred by the side of the brain that has been injured. In vertebral pathology, particularly when dealing with microembolization, the side originating the embolus can only be presumed by some appearance of the arterial lesion. Furthermore, it has been shown that in a large number of normal people one vertebral artery occluded temporarily with neck rotation, leaving the other vertebral artery as the only temporary supply to the posterior brain. There are patients in whom this temporary occlusion of a dominant vertebral with neck rotation/extension will result in physical impairment and occasionally in severe trauma (from severe dizziness or syncope); their outcome will not be accounted for in the usual categories of death and stroke. Symptomatic vertebral occlusion caused by rotation/extension of the head can only be positively identified when, as we elicit the symptom in the angiogram table by rotating/extending the head, we can see simultaneously the occlusion of the vertebral artery on the angiography screen. This finding is a common indication for distal vertebral reconstruction at the level of C2 or C1. I am aware of how reluctant angiographers are about this maneuver, but I nevertheless missed an entry for this dynamic vertebral arteriography in the corresponding chapter.

Neurology, as a medical specialty, inherited an all-consuming interest in the cerebral hemispheres from the revolutionary work of Hughlings Jackson at the end of the nineteenth century. As a result, the understanding of disease of the posterior brain has lagged two decades behind that in the anterior brain. And in terms of their surgical treatment, the first reconstructions of the vertebral (proximal) artery took place in 1979, a quarter of a century after the first carotid endarterectomy.

I enjoyed the historical summary that precedes most chapters; it enriches our comprehension and enlightens our appreciation for the many individuals in various specialties that contributed to what we can offer to our patients.

Ramon Berguer, MD, PhD
Emeritus Professor of Vascular Surgery
University of Michigan
Ann Arbor, MI, USA

Preface

Carotid and vertebral artery disease affects a large segment of population with the potential of causing severe disability from a major stroke. Although successful internal carotid surgery dates from 1954, vertebral artery surgery has lagged behind carotid surgery by almost twenty years and this delay was due in large part to the difficulty in establishing accurate clinical and radiographic diagnosis of vertebral-basilar insufficiency. In this book emphasis is placed on the medical, endovascular, and surgical approaches in managing patients with extracranial carotid and vertebral artery disease following pertinent diagnostic studies. Besides surgical anatomy, physiology, and pathology, strong emphasis was placed on the imaging techniques such as duplex ultrasound, computed tomography head, CTA neck and brain, MRI brain, MRA neck and brain, and diagnostic arteriography. In contrast to similar book publications on this topic, this book reflects the contributions of many interrelated specialties: cerebrovascular physiology, pathology, neuro-radiology, neuro-interventions, stroke neurology, and, more importantly, vascular surgery whose varying perspectives have significantly enhanced our knowledge of carotid and vertebral artery disease. It is my sincere hope that the reader will find the scholarship of their contributions not only informative but of a great practical value. In addition, multiple-choice questions have been added at the end of each chapter in order to improve the comprehension of the material.

Our intent has been to provide a comprehensive text and publish it in a timely fashion so as to anticipate the rapid pace of progress in this field.

Warren, MI, USA   Sachinder Singh Hans

Acknowledgements

The editor wishes to acknowledge the contributions of all the authors who gave up valuable time from their busy schedules to assist with this endeavor and their help is highly appreciated. I also wish to acknowledge the unflinching support of my wife Dr. Bijoya Hans, MD-Interventional Radiologist, in providing practical and sage advice in challenging times encountered during publication. Last but not least, my sincere thanks and gratitude to Springer Publishing, particularly executive editor Richard Hruska, editorial assistant clinical medicine Lillie Mae Gaurano, and Connie Walsh, developmental editor, for providing the guidance and professional support in getting this project completed.

Contents

Contributors

Ziad Al Adas, MD Division of Vascular Surgery, Henry Ford Hospital, Detroit, MI, USA

Surgery, Wayne State University School of Medicine, Detroit, MI, USA

Moayd M. Alkhalifah, MBBS Vascular Neurology, University of Miami Miller School of Medicine, Miami, FL, USA

Mitual Amin, MD Department of Anatomic Pathology, Beaumont Health System, Royal Oak, MI, USA

Robert A. Augustyniak, PhD Biomedical Sciences, Edward Via College of Osteopathic Medicine–Carolinas Campus, Spartanburg, SC, USA

Praveen C. Balraj, MD Division of Vascular Surgery, Henry Ford Hospital, Detroit, MI, USA

Surgery, Wayne State University School of Medicine, Detroit, MI, USA

Seemant Chaturvedi, MD, FAHA, FAAN Vice-Chair for VA Programs, University of Miami Miller School of Medicine, Miami, FL, USA

Frank M. Davis, MD Vascular Surgery, University of Michigan, Ann Arbor, MI, USA

Stephen E. DiCarlo, PhD Physiology, College of Osteopathic Medicine, Michigan State University, East Lansing, MI, USA

Muneer Eesa, MBBS, MD Department of Radiology, Foothills Medical Center, University of Calgary, Calgary, AB, Canada

Richard D. Fessler, MD Department of Surgery, St. John Hospital and Medical Centers, Detroit, MI, USA

Paul M. Gadient, MD Vascular Neurology, University of Miami Miller School of Medicine, Miami, FL, USA

Brent Griffith, MD Radiology, Henry Ford Health System, Detroit, MI, USA

Sachinder Singh Hans, MD Medical Director of Vascular and Endovascular Services, Henry Ford Macomb Hospital, Clinton Township, MI, USA

Chief of Vascular Surgery, St. John Macomb Hospital, Warren, MI, USA

Department of Surgery, Wayne State University School of Medicine, Detroit, MI, USA

Melanie Hoehn, MD Department of Surgery, Division of Vascular Surgery, University of Maryland Medical Center, Baltimore, MD, USA

Vishal B. Jani, MD Neurology in Stroke, Department of Neurology, Creighton University School of Medicine/CHI Health, Omaha, NE, USA

Ahmed Kayssi, MD, MSc, MPH Vascular Surgery, University of Toronto, Toronto, ON, Canada

Brendan P. Kelley, MD, MSc Radiology, Henry Ford Health System, Detroit, MI, USA

Judith C. Lin, MD, MBA, FACS Department of Surgery, Division of Vascular Surgery, Henry Ford Hospital, Detroit, MI, USA

Heidi L. Lujan, PhD Physiology, College of Osteopathic Medicine, Michigan State University, East Lansing, MI, USA

Nitin G. Malhotra, MD Division of Vascular Surgery, Michigan Vascular Center, McLaren Regional Medical Center, Michigan State University, Flint, MI, USA

Horia Marin, MD Radiology, Henry Ford Health System, Detroit, MI, USA

Robert G. Molnar, MD, MS Division of Vascular Surgery, Michigan Vascular Center, McLaren Regional Medical Center, Michigan State University, Flint, MI, USA

Mark D. Morasch, MD, FACS Division of Vascular and Endovascular Surgery, Department of Cardiac, Thoracic and Vascular Surgery, Billings Clinic, Billings, MT, USA

Nicolas J. Mouawad, MD, MPH, MBA, RPVI McLaren Bay Region Hospital, Bay City, MI, USA

Dipankar Mukherjee, MD, FACS, RPVI Vascular Surgery, Inova Fairfax Hospital, Falls Church, VA, USA

Andrea Obi, MD Vascular Surgery, University of Michigan, Ann Arbor, MI, USA

Vascular Surgery, Ann Arbor Veterans Medical Center, Ann Arbor, MI, USA

Nicholas Osborne, MD Vascular Surgery, University of Michigan, Ann Arbor, MI, USA

Vascular Surgery, Ann Arbor Veterans Medical Center, Ann Arbor, MI, USA

Suresh C. Patel, MD Radiology, Henry Ford Health System, Detroit, MI, USA

Emily Reardon, MD Department of Surgery, Division of Vascular Surgery, University of Maryland Medical Center, Baltimore, MD, USA

Yevgeniy Rits, MD Vascular Surgery, Detroit Medical Center, Detroit, MI, USA

Jeffrey R. Rubin, MD Vascular Surgery, Detroit Medical Center, Detroit, MI, USA

Rajabrata Sarkar, MD, PhD Department of Surgery, Division of Vascular Surgery, University of Maryland Medical Center, Baltimore, MD, USA

Bhagwan Satiani, MD, MBA, FACS, FACHE, RPVI Department of Surgery, Division of Vascular Surgery and Diseases, The Ohio State University College of Medicine, Columbus, OH, USA

Hosam Farouk El Sayed, MD, PhD, FACS, RVT Department of Surgery, Division of Vascular Surgery and Diseases, The Ohio State University College of Medicine, Columbus, OH, USA

Paola M. P. Seidel, MD Department of Physical Medicine and Rehabilitation, Wayne State University, Detroit, MI, USA

Geoffrey K. Seidel, MD Department of Physical Medicine and Rehabilitation, Wayne State University, Detroit, MI, USA

Michigan State University, Lansing, MI, USA

Alexander D. Shepard, MD Division of Vascular Surgery, Henry Ford Hospital, Detroit, MI, USA

Surgery, Wayne State University School of Medicine, Detroit, MI, USA

Justin G. Thomas, DO Section of Neurosurgery, Department of Surgery, Providence-Providence Park Hospital, Southfield, MI, USA

J. Devin B. Watson, MD Department of Surgery, David Grant Medical Center, Travis AFB, CA, USA

Mitchell R. Weaver, MD Wayne State University College of Medicine, Vascular Surgery, Henry Ford Hospital, Detroit, MI, USA

Wendy N. Wiesend, MD Department of Anatomic Pathology, Beaumont Health System, Royal Oak, MI, USA

Surgical Anatomy of Carotid and Vertebral Arteries

Sachinder Singh Hans

The Arch of Aorta

The main arteries of the head and neck supplying the cerebral arterial bed arise from the arch of the aorta (Fig. 1.1). Three major branches arise from superior aspect of the arch of the aorta:

1. The brachiocephalic trunk (innominate)
2. Left common carotid artery
3. Left subclavian artery

Anatomical Variations

These three major branches may arise from the most proximal segment of the arch or distal portion of the ascending aorta, or their commencements may be quite separate or very close as the left common carotid artery may have a common origin with the brachiocephalic trunk (the bovine aortic arch). This variation can be present in up to 10% of individuals. There can be a "V-shaped origin" of both common carotid arties from a single short trunk before continuing on each side of the neck [1, 2].

S. S. Hans
Medical Director of Vascular and Endovascular Services, Henry Ford Macomb Hospital, Clinton Township, MI, USA

Chief of Vascular Surgery, St. John Macomb Hospital, Warren, MI, USA

Department of Surgery, Wayne State University School of Medicine, Detroit, MI, USA

Aortic Arch Anomalies

Anomalies of aortic arch include aberrant right subclavian artery (1:200) arising lateral to left subclavian artery is the most common arch anomaly. Patients are usually asymptomatic, but it may result in dysphagia lusoria when aneurysmal subclavian artery compresses the esophagus posteriorly [3].

Other anomalies include right aortic arch with aberrant left subclavian artery, which is its last branch or double aortic arch.

Common Carotid and Internal and External Carotid Arteries

The common carotid arteries (CCA) are variable in length and their anatomic origin. The right common carotid artery originates at the bifurcation of the brachiocephalic trunk posterior to the right sternoclavicular joint and continues into the neck. The left CCA arises from the highest portion of the arch of the aorta to the left and posterior to the brachiocephalic trunk and can be divided into the intrathoracic portion and a cervical portion [1].

The cervical portion of each common carotid artery passes obliquely cephalad and slightly laterally to the upper border of the thyroid cartilage where it divides into the external and internal carotid arteries. The common carotid arteries with the internal jugular vein and vagus nerve are

Fig. 1.1 Heart and great vessels with supra-aortic trunks

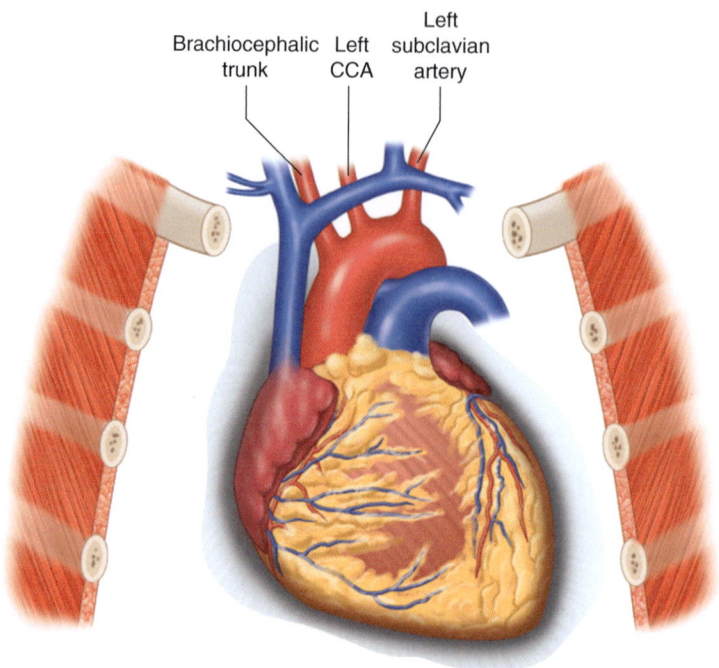

Left
Brachiocephalic Left subclavian
trunk CCA artery

contained in the carotid sheath, the vein coursing lateral to the artery and the vagus nerve lying between the artery and the vein (Fig. 1.2). The upper border of the thyroid cartilage (carotid bifurcation) is usually at the level of the fourth cervical vertebral body. The carotid bifurcation is variable, and bifurcation can be as low as the level of cervical fifth or even cervical sixth vertebral body (48%) or high at the level of cervical third vertebral body (34%). At the point of division of the common carotid artery, internal carotid artery (ICA) is slightly dilated into carotid sinus [1, 2]. The adventitial layer of the internal carotid artery is thicker in the carotid sinus and contains numerous sensory fibers arising from glossopharyngeal nerve [1]. These nerve fibers respond to changes in the arterial blood pressure reflexly. The carotid body, which lies behind the point of division of the common carotid artery, is a small brownish red structure which acts as a chemoreceptor.

In majority of patients (80%), the internal carotid artery is posterior or posterolateral to the external carotid artery.

Anatomic Variations

In about 10–12% of patients, the right common carotid artery arises cephalad to sternoclavicular joint. It may arise separately from the arch of the aorta, or both common carotid arteries could arise as a common trunk from the arch of the aorta. It is extremely uncommon for the common carotid artery to ascend into the neck without its division. Rarely there is agenesis of the common carotid artery on the right side. In persons with agenesis of the right common carotid artery, the right external carotid artery usually arises proximally from the brachiocephalic artery, and internal carotid artery arises distally from the subclavian artery proximal to the origin of the vertebral artery. When agenesis of the CCA occurs on the left side, both the ECA and ICA arise from the aortic arch, with ECA arising proximal to the origin of ICA [1, 2].

The External Carotid Artery

The external carotid artery (ECA) begins opposite to the upper border of the thyroid cartilage between the third and fourth cervical vertebrae and continues cephalad and anteriorly behind the angle of the mandible between the tip of the mastoid process and the angle of the jaw and divides into superficial temporal artery and maxillary arteries in the parotid gland. The external carotid artery branches in order are superior thyroid

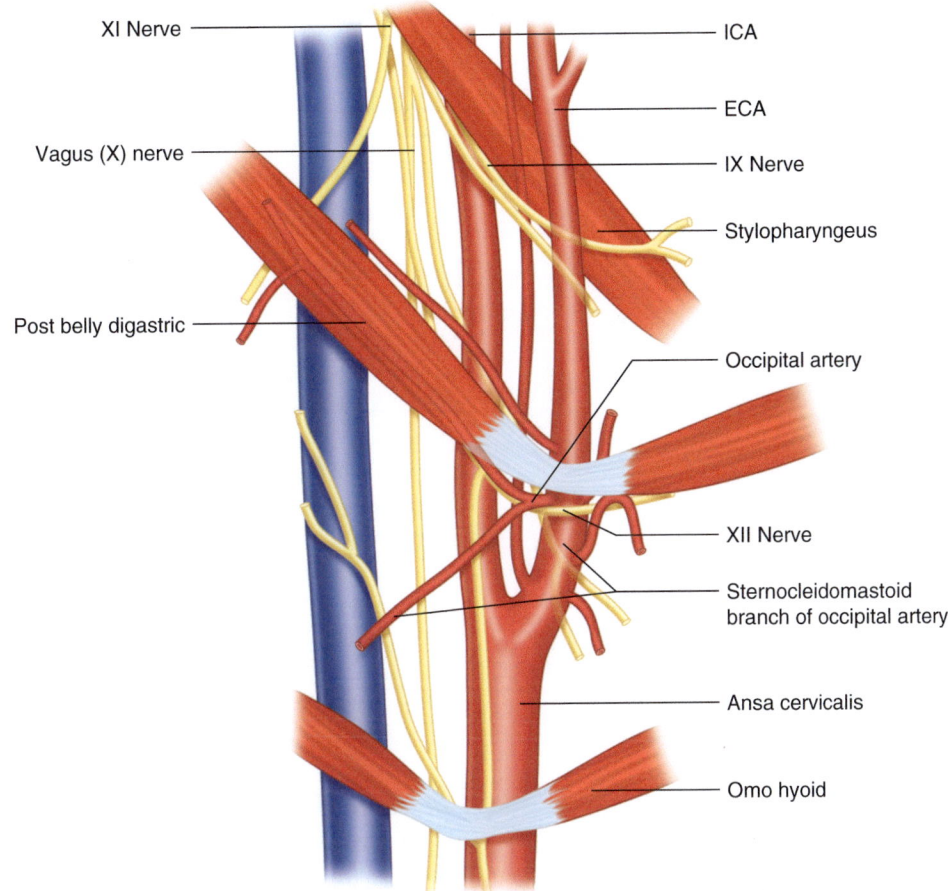

XI Nerve

ICA

ECA

Vagus (X) nerve

IX Nerve

Stylopharyngeus

Post belly digastric

Occipital artery

XII Nerve

Sternocleidomastoid
branch of occipital artery

Ansa cervicalis

Omo hyoid

Fig. 1.2 Relations between carotid arteries and internal jugular vein and nerves of the neck

(which may arise from distal CCA), ascending pharyngeal (which may arise from internal carotid artery), lingual, facial, occipital, posterior auricular, superficial temporal, and maxillary artery [1].

Anatomic Variations

Occasionally, external carotid artery may be absent on one or both sides. Carotid basilar anastomoses are rare arterial anomalies in which embryonic connections between carotid and vertebral arterial system persists (Fig. 1.3) [3].

The persistent trigeminal artery is the most common and most cephalad-located embryological anastomosis between the developing carotid artery and vertebrobasilar system to persist into adulthood. Its incidence ranges from 0.1% to 0.6% by MRA and DSA imaging. The persistent primi-

tive hypoglossal artery (HA) has been reported in 0.03–0.26% on cerebral arteriography. Persistent HA arises from the ICA between c1 and c2 vertebral levels and traverses through the hypoglossal canal to join the vertebrobasilar circulation [3].

The Internal Carotid Artery

The internal carotid artery (ICA) is the primary source of oxygenated blood to anterior portion of the brain and the orbits. The ICA is divided into the following seven segments: cervical ($c1$), petrous ($c2$), lacerum ($c3$), cavernous ($c4$), clinoid ($c5$), ophthalmic ($c6$), and communicating ($c7$). ICA ascends into the skull base and becomes intracranial through the carotid canal of temporal bone. It continues anteriorly through the cavernous sinus and divides into anterior and middle cerebral artery.

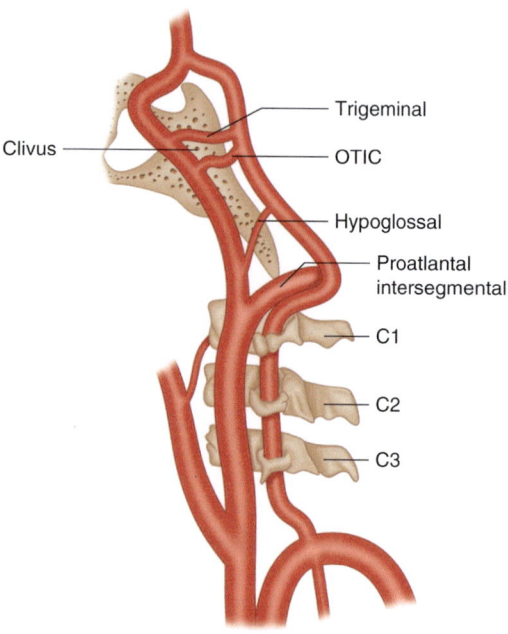

Clivus

Trigeminal

OTIC

Hypoglossal

Proatlantal
intersegmental

C1

C2

C3

Fig. 1.3 Diagrammatic representation of persistent embryological carotid-basilar connections

Anatomic Variations

Instead of ICA being straight, it may be tortuous and may course medially and become retropharyngeal close to tonsil and may appear as a retropharyngeal mass.

Relationship of Nerves in the Neck to Carotid Arteries

The vagus nerve runs vertically down within the carotid sheath lying between the internal jugular vein and the internal carotid artery and inferiorly between the same vein and the common carotid artery. On the right side, it descends posterior to internal jugular vein (IJV) and crosses the first part of the subclavian artery. On the left side, vagus nerve enters the thorax between the common carotid and subclavian arteries and posterior to the left brachiocephalic vein. During the performance of carotid endarterectomy (CEA), the vagus nerve in the lower portion of the neck may course anterolaterally instead of its usual posterior course and thus may be subject to injury.

At the level of second cervical, the vagus nerve gives its superior laryngeal nerve branch which descends along the side of the pharynx first posterior and then medical to the internal carotid artery and divides into the internal and external laryngeal nerve [1].

The Glossopharyngeal Nerve

After its exit from the skull, it courses forward between the internal jugular vein and the ICA and descends anterior to the ICA deep to the styloid process and may get injured during cephalad mobilization of the ICA during CEA for high plaque as it courses deep to the styloid process. Injury to the glossopharyngeal nerve results in loss of sensation to the posterior third of the tongue and difficulty swallowing requiring PEG tube placement.

The Accessory Spinal Nerve

After its exit from the jugular foramina, it runs posterolaterally behind the internal jugular vein in majority of instances but in front of the IJV in about 30% of cases and very rarely passes through the vein. It can be damaged in cases where IJV is more anterior in relation to ICA in the upper portion of the neck.

Ramus Mandibularis

Ramus mandibularis or the marginal mandibular branch of the facial nerve runs anteriorly below the angle of the mandible under cover of the platysma and can be injured during CEA if incision is more anteriorly placed. It can also be injured as a result of overzealous retraction of the tissues (stretch injury).

External Laryngeal Nerve

External laryngeal nerve is smaller than the internal laryngeal nerve and crosses the origin of superior thyroid artery and supplies the cricothyroid muscle. Injury to the external laryngeal nerve results in decreased pitch of the voice.

Hypoglossal Nerve

The hypoglossal nerve is usually posterior or posterosuperior to the common facial vein and is often crossed superiorly by another vein which drains into the internal jugular vein. The hypoglossal nerve curves around the sternocleidomastoid branch of the occipital artery, and its division and ligation aid in mobilization of the ICA during CEA. In a few instances, the hypoglossal nerve may be inferior in its course, close to the carotid bifurcation, and, if not carefully dissected, may result in an inadvertent injury.

Ansa Cervicalis

Ansa cervicalis is formed as a loop from the descending branch of the hypoglossal nerve which contains fibers of the C1. The descending branch is joined by the lower root of ansa cervicalis from second and third cervical nerves, thus forming a loop. The author has encountered anatomic variations in the ansa cervicalis with its superior root arising from the vagus, and its division during CEA can result in hoarseness (Fig. 1.4).

The Vertebral Arteries

The vertebral artery arises from the superior and posterior aspect of the first part of the subclavian artery. It ascends through the foramina in the transverse process of all the cervical vertebra from sixth to the first and then runs laterally entering the skull through the foramen magnum and joins with the opposite vertebral artery at the lower border of the pons to form the basilar artery. A vertebral artery can be divided into four segments. The *first part* runs posteriorly and superiorly between the longus colli and

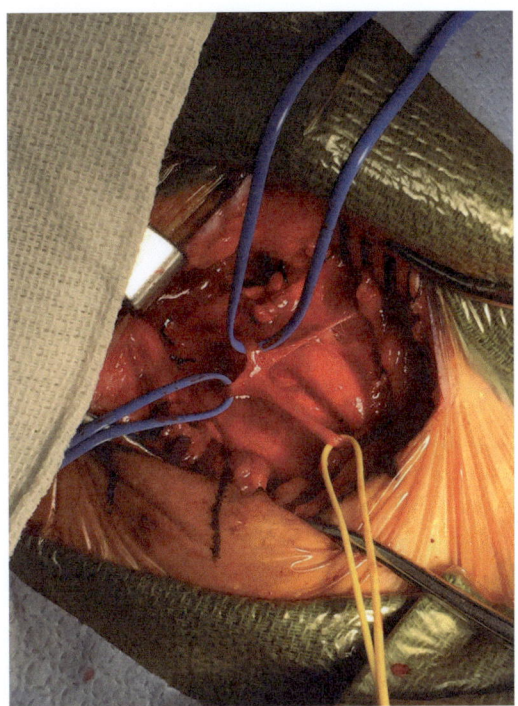

Fig. 1.4 Abnormal nerve connection of ansa cervicalis

the scalenus anticus and posterior to the common carotid artery. The vertebral vein crosses anterior to the artery, and it is crossed interiorly by the inferior thyroid artery. On the left side, the vertebral artery is crossed anteriorly by the thoracic duct. The cervico-dorsal ganglion rests on top of the vertebral artery with medial and lateral rami. The *second part* runs cephalad through the transverse foramina of the upper six cervical vertebrae and runs a straight course. The *third part* exits from the transverse process of the atlas and runs laterally in the suboccipital triangle. The *fourth part* enters the skull by piercing the dura and the arachnoid matter (Fig. 1.5).

Anatomic Variations

Vertebral arteries are usually often variable (80–85%) in their size. One vertebral artery may be large and dominant and contralateral hypoplastic or even absent [2]. The origin of vertebral arteries can also be variable. They can arise as

Fig. 1.5 Left subclavian artery and segments of vertebral artery

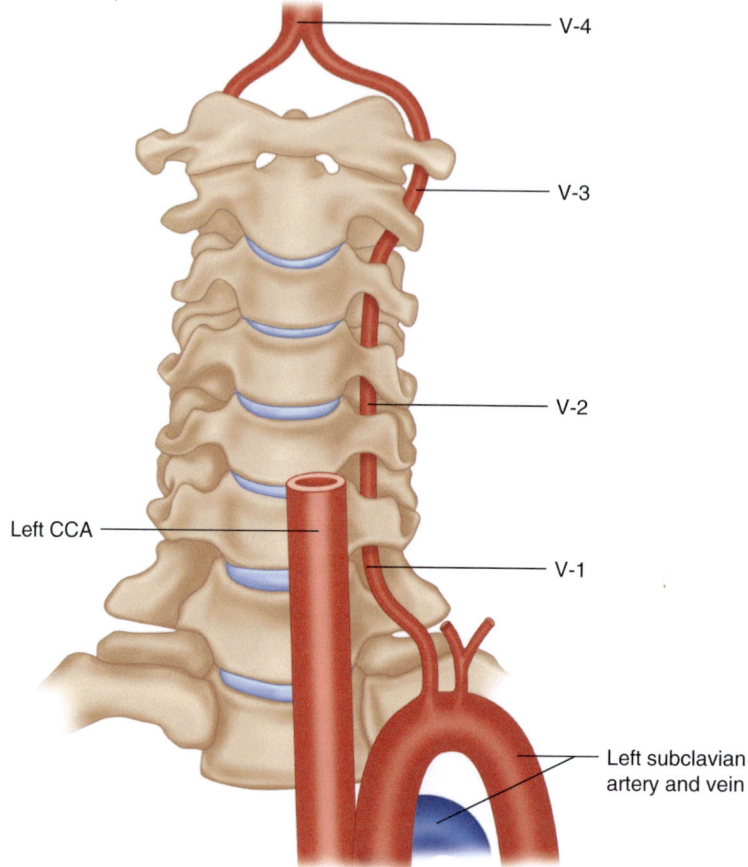

second branch of the subclavian artery and may have duplicate origin [2]. Left vertebral artery may arise from the arch of the aorta between the left common carotid artery and left subclavian artery (5–7%) [4, 5]. Vertebral artery may enter the fifth, fourth, or seventh cervical vertebrae. Occasionally intracranial branches of the vertebral artery such as posterior inferior cerebellar artery may arise at the level of c1–c2 vertebral body. The abnormal course of v2 segment of the vertebral artery has been reported predisposing the patient to iatrogenic vascular injury during anterior spinal surgery [4, 5]. Vertebral artery may enter the transverse foramina of the third cervical vertebrae, fourth cervical vertebrae (1.6%), fifth cervical vertebrae (3.3%), or seventh cervical vertebrae in 0.3% of cases [2, 4, 5].

Review Questions

1. The "bovine aortic arch" (a common origin of the brachiocephalic and left common carotid arteries) is present in:
   A. Under 10% of individuals
   B. 11–20% of individuals
   C. 21–20% of individuals
   D. More than 30% of individuals

   Answer: A

2. Dysphagia lusoria is caused by:
   A. Aberrant aneurysmal left subclavian artery
   B. Aberrant aneurysmal right subclavian artery

C. Double aortic arch

D. Right-sided aortic arch

Answer: B

3. The most common persistent embryo-
    genic connection between the carotid
    and vertebral basilar systems persists in
    the form of a:
    A. Persistent hypoglossal artery
    B. Persistent otic artery
    C. Persistent trigeminal artery
    D. Proatlantal intersegmental artery

Answer: C

4. Injury to the glossopharyngeal nerve
    results in:
    A. Tongue deviation to ipsilateral side
    B. Tongue deviation to contralateral
        side
    C. No significant disability
    D. Loss of sensation in the posterior
        one-third of the tongue and difficulty
        swallowing

Answer: D

5. Left vertebral artery may arise from arch
    of aorta between left CCA and left SCA in:
    A. 0–4% of individuals
    B. 5–7% of individuals
    C. 8–11% of individuals
    D. 12–15% of individuals

Answer: B

References

1. Williams PL, Warwick R. Gray's anatomy. London:
    Churchill Livingstone; 1980.
2. Berguer R. Function and surgery of the carotid and verte-
    bral arteries. Alphen aan den Rijn: Wolters Kluwer; 2013.
3. Meckel S, Spittau B, McAuliffe W. The persis-
    tent trigeminal artery: development, imaging anat-
    omy, variants, and associated vascular pathologies.
    Neuroradiology. 2013;55(1):5–16.
4. Satti SR, Cerniglia CA, Koenigsberg RA. Cervical
    vertebral artery variations: an anatomic study. AJNR.
    2007;28:976–80.
5. Hong JT, Park DK, Lee MJ, Kim SW, Howard
    S. Anatomical variations of the vertebral artery seg-
    ment in the lower cervical spine: analysis by three-
    dimensional computed tomography angiography.
    Spine. 2008;33:2422–6.

Physiology of the Cerebrovascular System

2

Heidi L. Lujan, Robert A. Augustyniak,
and Stephen E. DiCarlo

Introduction

As noted by Carl J. Wiggers in 1905 [1], "Perhaps no other organ of the body is less adapted to an experimental study of its circulation than the brain." Numerous investigators have agreed and been befuddled by the brain's complex and unusual blood supply and multiple arteries and veins, making accurate measurements of blood flow virtually impossible. Even if accurate measurements of blood flow into the brain were valid, differences in mechanisms that regulate flow to extracranial and intracranial compartments and gray and white matter complicate the measurements. Specifically, it is well accepted that blood flow to specific tissues or regions and to the gray and white matter of the brain is heterogeneous and regulated uniquely. These differences may be due to diverse embryonic origins of the extracranial and intracranial vessels [2]. Thus, measurement of total brain blood flow or flow to selected regions may not adequately define the system.

However, despite the brain's unique physiological and anatomical barriers, it is well known that the regulation of the cerebral circulation is similar in many ways to the control of blood flow in other vascular beds in that cerebral vessels are regulated by metabolic and neural factors and by autoregulatory mechanisms induced by changes in arterial blood pressure. The cerebral vasculature, like other vasculature, is also regulated by blood parameters including blood gases and acid-base status.

However, exclusively, the cerebral circulation also has several specialized features that profoundly and uniquely influence its regulation. Among the unique features is the blood-brain barrier that isolates but protects the brain insuring a reduced influence of ionic changes and humoral stimuli on the cerebral circulation. In contrast to the general circulation, large arteries of the cerebral circulation (not just arterioles) account for a greater fraction of vascular resistance in the brain, and these cerebral vessels are exquisitely sensitive to changes in arterial blood pressure producing an enormously effective autoregulatory mechanism. The cerebral circulation is also remarkably responsive to chemical stimuli where hypercapnic acidosis and hypoxia elicit marked vasodilatation. In contrast to the remarkably pronounced autoregulatory and chemical mechanisms controlling cerebral blood flow, the

H. L. Lujan · S. E. DiCarlo (✉)
Physiology, College of Osteopathic Medicine, Michigan State University, East Lansing, MI, USA
e-mail: lujanhei@msu.edu; dicarlos@msu.edu

R. A. Augustyniak
Biomedical Sciences, Edward Via College of Osteopathic Medicine–Carolinas Campus, Spartanburg, SC, USA
e-mail: raugustyniak@carolinas.vcom.edu

© The Editor(s) (if applicable) and The Author(s) 2018
S. S. Hans (ed.), *Extracranial Carotid and Vertebral Artery Disease*,
https://doi.org/10.1007/978-3-319-91533-3_2

cerebral circulation responses to the autonomic nervous system are mainly limited under non-stressed conditions.

The circulation of the brain has evolved these unique regulatory mechanisms and features to match the critical and unusual demands of this exceptional organ. The brain requires a high rate of blood flow to match its impressive metabolic requirements, buffer changing circulating levels of catecholamines and ions, and prevent injury. In this chapter, we briefly discuss the major factors regulating cerebral blood flow including important anatomical features for a functional understanding of the regulation of the cerebral circulation.

Regulation of Cerebral Blood Flow: Anatomical Considerations

Blood flow to the brain is carried by the two internal carotid and two vertebral arteries. The two vertebral arteries merge to form the basilar artery which anastomoses with the two internal carotid arteries to form the circle of Willis. The anterior,

middle, and posterior cerebral arteries extend from the circle of Willis to perfuse the entire cerebral cortex. The pial vessels on the surface of the brain branch to arterioles which divide into the capillaries that supply cortical tissue at all laminar levels. Capillary density is tightly correlated to the number of synapses and local metabolic activity rather than to cell mass [3, 4]. Collateral supply, largely dependent on the circle of Willis, is critical to the maintenance of cerebral blood flow during ischemia. Cerebral blood flow is dependent on arterial blood pressure, venous pressure/intracranial pressure, and the resistance of both large and small cerebral vessels (Fig. 2.1).

The Arterial Pressure Component

The arterial pressure that supplies the cerebral vessels is dependent on factors mainly outside the brain and is the product of cardiac output and total peripheral resistance. Specifically, the heart provides the cardiac output, while the peripheral arterioles provide the total peripheral resistance. In this context, the balance between cerebral vascular

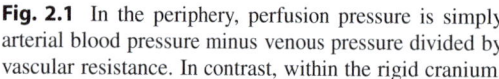

$$\text{Cerebral Blood Flow} = \frac{\text{Arterial Pressure-Venous/Intracranial Pressure}}{\text{Cerebral Vascular Resistance}}$$

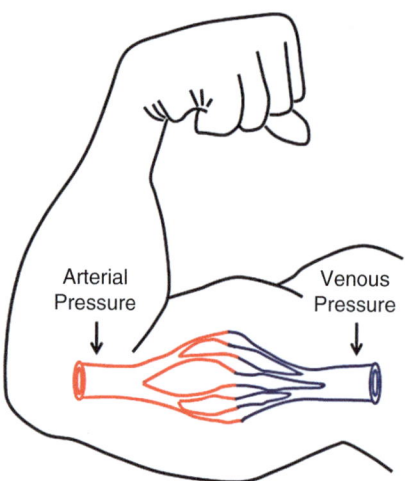
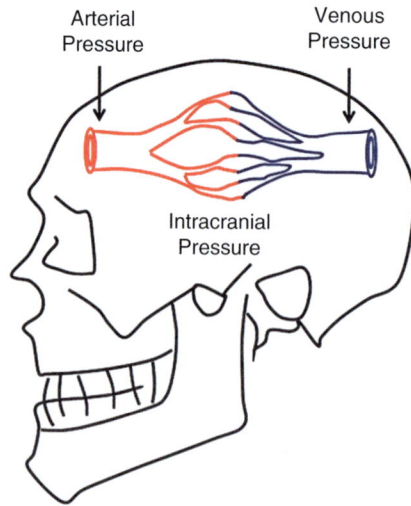

Fig. 2.1 In the periphery, perfusion pressure is simply arterial blood pressure minus venous pressure divided by vascular resistance. In contrast, within the rigid cranium, perfusion pressure is dependent on arterial blood pressure, venous pressure, and intracranial pressure as well as the resistance of both large and small cerebral vessels

resistance and total peripheral resistance determines the proportion of the cardiac output that reaches the brain. However, the relationship between changes in arterial blood pressure and cerebral blood flow is typically nonlinear due to active changes in vascular tone occurring at the level of the cerebral arterioles—a process known as cerebral autoregulation (see below). Despite this mechanism, modulating arterial blood pressure is a therapeutic technique to modulate cerebral blood flow.

Venous Pressure/Intracranial Pressure Component

Cerebral venous pressure provides a back pressure that impedes cerebral blood flow (Fig. 2.1). Importantly, venous pressure is a function of both the venous pressure in the larger cerebral veins and the intracranial pressure. If the intracranial pressure is above the pressure in the lateral lacunae that feed into the large venous sinuses, then these vessels will be compressed leading to a postcapillary venous pressure just above the intracranial pressure [5, 6]. In this situation, an increase in intracranial pressure has the potential to decrease the longitudinal pressure gradient across the vascular bed and impede cerebral blood flow. Specifically, cerebral blood flow is impaired by conditions that impede cerebral venous outflow (such as idiopathic intracranial hypertension or neck position) and by conditions that increase intracranial pressure (such as the edema associated with traumatic brain injury or subarachnoid hemorrhage). The rigid skull promotes an increase in intracranial pressure with any increase in the volume of a brain compartment. Accordingly, increases in volume of the intravascular compartment, the cerebral spinal fluid compartment, or the brain parenchymal compartment can all increase intracranial pressure and therefore decrease cerebral blood flow. These compartmental volume changes could be caused by vascular dilation, hydrocephalus, or cerebral edema. Therapies that alter cerebral blood flow by altering intracranial pressure include mild hyperventilation, cerebral spinal fluid diversion through external ventricular drainage, osmotherapy to reduce the brain tissue volume, or decompressive craniectomy to increase the space available for the brain.

The Cerebrovascular Resistance Component

At the level of the cerebral vessels, cerebral blood flow is regulated by active changes in the diameter of the precapillary arterioles as well as larger arteries modulating cerebral vascular resistance. These arterioles have a pronounced smooth muscle layer and, therefore, the ability for profound dilation and constriction [7, 8]. Larger conduit arteries, capillaries, and venous structures are also important in certain situations [9–12]. For example, relaxation of pericytes surrounding capillaries has been proposed for some proportion of the cerebral blood flow regulation [10]. Cerebral venules and veins exhibit a high compliance [12] which may, in some cases, play a passive role in the regulation of cerebral blood flow. For example, arteriolar dilation leads to an increase in the volume of postcapillary venules that increase cerebral blood volume [13] and by extension could increase intracranial pressure and decrease cerebral blood flow.

Changes in cerebral vascular tone and cerebral vascular resistance are also caused by putative constricting and dilating substances. These vasoactive substances may be supplied to the vessels via the bloodstream [e.g., arterial partial pressure of carbon dioxide ($PaCO_2$)], produced locally (adenosine, nitric oxide, potassium), or reach the vascular smooth muscle through direct autonomic innervation (acetylcholine, norepinephrine). The vasoactive substances produce changes in intracellular calcium concentration, which in turn alters the degree of smooth muscle contraction and vessel constriction.

Cerebral Metabolism and Functional Activity

A very tight coupling between cerebral blood flow and local brain metabolism has been demonstrated in many studies (Fig. 2.2). For exam-

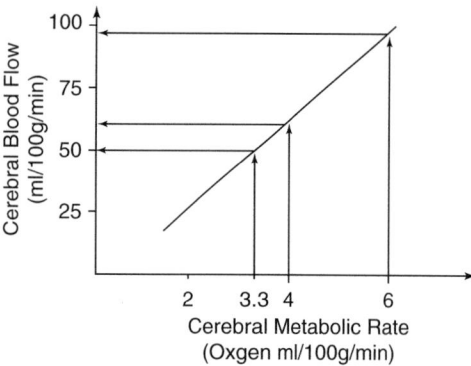

Fig. 2.2 A tight coupling exists between cerebral blood flow and local brain metabolism. The mediator of this close coupling between metabolism and cerebral blood flow is the subject of continuing research

Table 2.1 Local and systemic mediators of cerebral vascular function

Intracerebral	Systemic
Nitric oxide	Vasopressin
Adenosine	Renin-angiotensin system
Prostacyclin	Angiotensin II
Thromboxane A2	Serotonin
Hydrogen ions	–
Potassium	–
Calcium	–

ple, metabolic demand is markedly different between gray and white matter, within the gray matter itself, and between the cerebral cortex and the basal ganglia. Importantly, cerebral blood flow closely matches the regional differences in metabolic rates. Specifically, functional activation varies throughout the brain, and this heterogeneity in metabolic demand is matched by variations in local cerebral blood flow. Thus, there is a rapidly acting and tightly controlled mechanism which ensures that the variations in metabolic demand associated with changes in functional activity are matched by parallel changes in cerebral blood flow. Despite this extremely tight association, it is unclear which chemical products of metabolism mediate the changes in cerebrovascular resistance. The mediator of this close coupling between metabolism and cerebral blood flow is the subject of continuing research, and many potential candidates have been suggested (Table 2.1). Adenosine, nitric oxide, and potassium appear to be the leading candidates. Under physiological conditions, adenosine is a potent vasodilator in the cerebral circulation, and increases in concentration have been recorded in association with systemic arterial hypotension, hypoxia, and hypercapnia. Nitric oxide is also a potent vasodilator on cerebral vessels [14, 15].

Cerebral Autoregulation

Cerebral autoregulation is the response of the cerebral vessels to changes in arterial blood pressure. It is well documented that a decrease in systemic arterial blood pressure causes dilatation of the cerebral vessels and that, conversely, an increase in systemic arterial blood pressure causes vasoconstriction of the cerebral circulation. This autoregulatory response to a change in arterial blood pressure maintains a remarkably stable cerebral blood flow (Fig. 2.3) despite wide fluctuations in systemic arterial blood pressure. This autoregulatory capacity is present in most peripheral vascular beds but not to the same extent as the cerebral circulation. Autoregulation maintains the stability of cerebral blood flow (within certain limits) by varying the diameter of the cerebral blood vessels and, thus, protects the brain from the normal minute-to-minute fluctuations in arterial pressure.

Autoregulation, like all homeostatic control mechanisms, has thresholds and saturation points at systemic arterial blood pressures of approximately 60 mmHg and 150 mmHg, respectively. That is, autoregulation is much less effective at maintaining cerebral blood flow constant at systemic arterial pressures below 60 mmHg or above 150 mmHg (Fig. 2.3). These thresholds and saturation points are not static but are modulated by activity of the autonomic nervous system, by the vessel wall renin-angiotensin system, by the arterial partial pressure of carbon dioxide ($PaCO_2$), by vasoactive agents, and by morphological changes in the vessel walls.

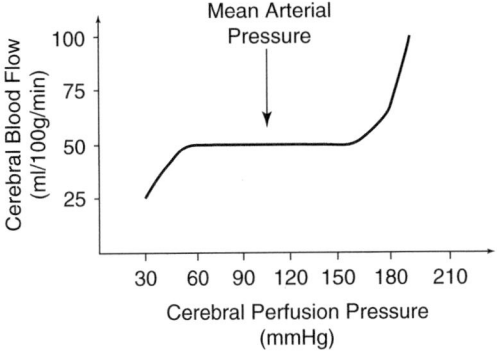

Fig. 2.3 Autoregulatory responses to a change in arterial blood pressure maintain a remarkably stable cerebral blood flow within physiological limits

Below the lower limit or threshold of systemic arterial blood pressure, cerebral blood flow will decrease linearly as arterial blood pressure decreases until the ischemic thresholds [16, 17] are reached provoking a profound increase in sympathetic nerve activity, via the central nervous system (CNS) ischemic response, that dramatically increases systemic arterial pressure. Systemic arterial blood pressure above the saturation point leads to a forced dilatation of the cerebral arterioles, disruption of the blood-brain barrier, and the formation of cerebral edema.

The mechanism mediating autoregulation is incompletely understood and may vary between vascular beds of different organs. Classically, three mechanisms have been documented to explain autoregulation in the cerebral vasculature: (1) myogenic mechanism, (2) metabolic mechanism, and (3) neural mechanism. The myogenic hypothesis proposes that the mechanism mediating autoregulation resides within the intrinsic ability of vascular smooth muscle to respond directly to changes in intraluminal or transluminal pressure. The neurogenic hypothesis suggests that adrenergic and cholinergic nerves from the autonomic nervous system alter cerebral vascular resistance in response to alterations in perfusion pressure. However, this mechanism conflicts with the majority view that autonomic nerve activity has no direct role in the autoregulatory mechanism, although it may modify the autoregulatory responses by limiting the autoregulation.

The metabolic hypothesis suggests that the perivascular accumulation of vasoactive metabolites associated with a decrease in substrate delivery decreases cerebrovascular resistance and increases cerebral blood flow. Conversely, an increase in pressure and thus an increase in substrate delivery increase cerebral vascular resistance to decrease cerebral blood flow and substrate delivery.

Chemical Regulation

Physiological constituents of blood, including oxygen (O_2), carbon dioxide (CO_2), and hydrogen ions (H^+), have a profound influence on the cerebral circulation. Specifically, elevations in CO_2 and H^+ markedly reduce cerebral vascular resistance and dilate the cerebral circulation. In fact, the effect of changes in CO_2 is frequently used to gauge responsiveness of the cerebral circulation. Similarly, low pH relaxes cerebral vascular muscle in vitro, and high pH contracts the muscle [18, 19]. The effect of CO_2 is mediated via a change in extracellular fluid pH because CO_2 does not have a direct vasoactive effect. Thus H^+ but not CO_2 has a direct relaxant effect on the cerebral vasculature. Thus, arterial hypercapnia indirectly increases cerebral blood flow and decreases cerebral vascular resistance via H^+. Interestingly, the magnitude of responses to changes in CO_2 differs in different regions of the brain and is more marked in cerebral gray matter than in white matter [20, 21].

Arterial Partial Pressure of Carbon Dioxide

As noted above, the cerebral vasculature is exquisitely sensitive to changes in the $PaCO_2$. With a decrease in $PaCO_2$, cerebral vessels constrict; and with an increase in $PaCO_2$, cerebral vessels dilate [22]. As noted above, these effects are mediated by changes in extracellular hydrogen-ion concentration. Specifically, carbon dioxide diffuses rapidly across the blood-brain barrier and alters the hydrogen-ion concentration of the cerebral

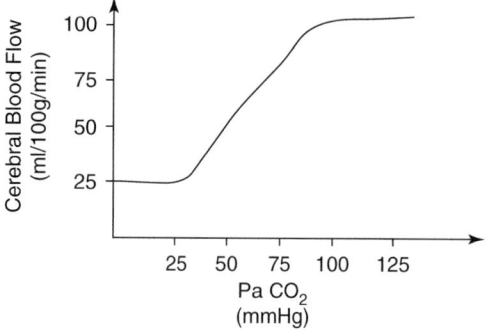

Fig. 2.4 An increase in $PaCO_2$ will increase cerebral blood flow, while, conversely, a decrease in $PaCO_2$ will decrease cerebral blood flow

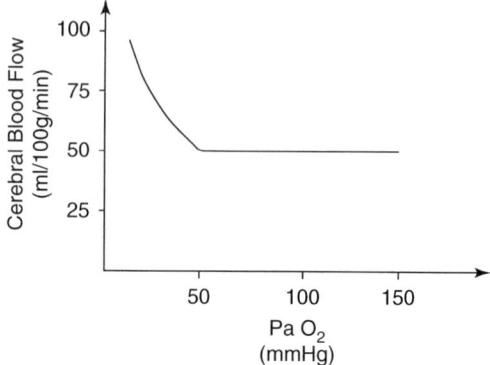

Fig. 2.5 Cerebral blood flow is relatively insensitive to changes in PaO_2 within the normal physiological range. However, large reductions in PaO_2 dramatically increase cerebral blood flow

extracellular fluid. Thus, an increase in $PaCO_2$ will increase cerebral blood flow, while, conversely, a decrease in $PaCO_2$ will decrease cerebral blood flow (Fig. 2.4).

Arterial Partial Pressure of Oxygen

The relationship between changes in the arterial partial pressure of oxygen (PaO_2) and cerebral blood flow is shown in Fig. 2.5. Cerebral blood flow is well documented to be relatively insensitive to changes in PaO_2 within the normal physiological range. For example, increases in PaO_2 cause only a slight decrease in cerebral blood flow such that the administration of 100% oxygen decreases cerebral blood flow by only 10%. Similarly, decreases in PaO_2 have modest effects on cerebral blood flow until PaO_2 values less than 60 mmHg have been achieved. It is important to note that under physiological conditions, the cerebral oxygen extraction or utilization is relatively low, only approximately 25–30%. Accordingly, cerebral blood flow may not increase until the oxygen extraction has been maximized. In this situation, cerebral blood flow may be more closely allied to arterial oxygen content (CaO_2) than to PaO_2. This is suggested because CaO_2 is maintained at near-physiological values until a PaO_2 of approximately 60 mmHg is achieved. Thus, although controversial, CaO_2 may be the principal determinant of cerebral blood flow during hypoxia [23].

Neural Regulation

The autonomic nervous system may also influence cerebral vascular tone and cerebral vascular resistance and thus regulate cerebral blood flow. However, despite studies demonstrating a rich innervation from both parasympathetic and sympathetic innervation, the autonomic control of cerebral blood flow remains controversial [24, 25]. Nevertheless, stimulation of the trigeminal ganglion in humans decreases cerebral blood flow [26], while blockade of the stellate ganglion increases cerebral blood flow [27], documenting a role for the sympathetic nervous system in the regulation of the cerebral circulation in humans.

As noted, it is well accepted that the cerebral vessels receive sympathetic innervation primarily from the superior cervical ganglion [28, 29] and are densely innervated; however the function of sympathetic regulation of cerebral blood flow is controversial and under intense debate [30, 31]. Similarly, parasympathetic nerves supply arteries on the surface of the brain; however its role in the regulation of the cerebral circulation is uncertain. The origin of cholinergic innervation is also uncertain. Uniquely, adrenergic and cholinergic nerve terminals [32] are in close approximation and may interact to control cerebral vessels.

Sympathetic Regulation

Sympathetic regulation of the cerebral vasculature involves a rare receptor-contraction coupling mechanism relative to other vascular beds [33, 34]. This rare mechanism creates a unique situation where the alpha-adrenergic receptors are relatively insensitive to norepinephrine [35], less discriminating, and less sensitive to other agonists than alpha-receptors of the systemic vasculature. Not surprisingly, vasoconstriction of isolated cerebral vessels during electrical stimulation to activate nerves is eliminated by sympathetic denervation [36]. However, surprisingly, the vasoconstriction during electrical stimulation is *not* reduced by alpha-adrenergic antagonists [36]. Moreover, the vasoconstrictor responses to norepinephrine are potentiated by high pH [37]. These results highlight the unconventional neuroeffector mechanisms of the cerebral vasculature.

Importantly, in many studies, it is unclear if the response to agonists is a direct or indirect effect of the catecholamine. For example, intravenous infusion of norepinephrine provokes a profound elevation in systemic arterial blood pressure, and the cerebral vessels constrict. However, it is not clear if the vasoconstriction of the cerebral vasculature is a direct effect of the norepinephrine or an indirect autoregulatory mechanism.

It is always important to remember that the blood-brain barrier limits access of circulating substances to the cerebral vasculature during intravenous administration [38]. However, intracarotid infusion of norepinephrine also has minimal effects on the cerebral vasculature in humans [39] and baboons [40]. However, disruption of the blood-brain barrier increases the effect of intracarotid infusion of norepinephrine on the cerebral vasculature [40]. It is believed that the increase in blood flow is secondary to an increase in cerebral metabolism.

Although, sympathetic nerves do not seem to have a significant effect on cerebral blood flow under normal conditions, there is evidence that sympathetic nerves protect cerebral vessels during sudden increases in arterial pressure [41]. For example, during sudden increases in blood pressure, sympathetic stimulation attenuates the pressor-induced increase in cerebral blood flow [42–45]. The protective effects of sympathetic stimulation during sudden increases in arterial pressure are more pronounced in gray matter than in white matter [43]. Taken together, the major function of sympathetic nerves may be to protect cerebral vessels during sudden increases in arterial pressure.

Nonvascular effects of the sympathetic nervous system have also been documented. As examples, sympathetic nerves modulate the rate of cerebral spinal fluid formation [46], protect the blood-brain barrier during acute hypertension [41, 43, 44, 47], attenuate the increase in permeability to albumin [43], exert a "trophic" effect on cerebral vessels, and promote the development of vascular hypertrophy [48].

Parasympathetic Regulation

The role of cholinergic nerves in regulation of cerebral blood flow is not clear. Similarly, little is known about the effects of vasoactive intestinal peptide, which is also present in nerve terminals on cerebral vessels [49]. Future research is required to determine whether cholinergic, peptidergic, or other parasympathetic transmitters contribute to cerebral vasodilatation.

Summary

In this chapter, we briefly discuss the major factors regulating cerebral blood flow including important anatomical features. The physiological role of the blood-brain barrier may be an area for readers to explore in greater detail as it was beyond the scope of this chapter. In addition to arterioles, the role of large arteries for the regulation of the cerebral vascular resistance was discussed. Specifically, large arteries contribute to the control of cerebral blood flow and protect the brain against marked fluctuations in microvascular pressures.

The role of the autonomic nervous system in the control of cerebral blood flow regulation was also discussed. Sympathetic nerves generally have less pronounced effects on the cerebral circulation than on other vascular beds. However, autonomic activation may be important for its protective effect on cerebral vessels during acute and chronic hypertension. The role of cholinergic and peptidergic neural pathways is controversial, is not well understood, and merits additional exploration.

The role of the partial pressure of carbon dioxide on the cerebral circulation is well understood. The most important mechanism of action of CO_2 is its local effect on blood vessels mediated through changes in extracellular fluid pH. Moreover, an extremely tight coupling between brain metabolism and cerebral blood flow is clearly established. Although intensely investigated, the role of different mediators that provide the link between metabolism and blood flow is not clearly established. Adenosine, nitric oxide, and perhaps potassium seem to be the most promising agents. Clearly, additional research is required to determine the importance of each agent in mediation of the coupling between metabolism and blood flow.

Autoregulation is a critical component in the control of cerebral blood flow and has been carefully characterized. However, the mechanisms underlying autoregulation are incompletely understood. The role of the myogenic mechanism in autoregulation is unclear. Metabolic factors including adenosine and local hypoxia seem important in mediating autoregulatory adjustments.

All of these factors regulating cerebral blood flow should be considered as an understanding of the critical physiological regulators of cerebral blood flow should lead to better understanding of cerebral vascular responses in disease states.

Review Questions

1. A 42-year-old male arrives at the emergency department with complaints of acute and severe abdominal pain in the right lower quadrant. Imaging results reveal an appendicitis. As his doctor describes the necessary surgical procedure, the patient becomes visibly fearful, his respiratory rate increases, and he suffers an episode of syncope. What is the most likely cause of the syncopal episode?
   A. A high PCO_2 leads to cerebral vasoconstriction.
   B. A low PCO_2 leads to cerebral vasoconstriction.
   C. A high PCO_2 leads to cerebral vasodilation.
   D. A low PCO_2 leads to cerebral vasodilation.

   Answer: B

2. A 21-year-old unconscious female arrives at the emergency department 20 minutes after a motor vehicle accident. There is clear head trauma, and the paramedic indicates that the patient was not wearing her seatbelt and was catapulted headfirst into the windshield during the accident. Which of the following sets of hemodynamic changes would be expected in this patient?

	Intracranial pressure	Cerebral vascular resistance	Cerebral blood flow	Cerebral blood vessel diameter
A.	↓	↑	↓	↑
B.	↓	↑	↑	↑
C.	↓	↓	↑	↓
D.	↑	↓	↓	↑
E.	↑	↑	↑	↑
F.	↑	↓	↑	↓

Answer: D

3. A 31-year-old female is seen in the clinic for her annual health screening. All of her laboratory values are within normal range, and her blood pressure is 118/78 mmHg (normal, <120/80 mmHg). As she leaves, she is the victim of a gunshot wound, and she loses a significant amount of blood. When the paramedics arrive, her blood pressure is 105/68 mmHg. Before she receives any fluid replacement therapy, how would the decrease in blood pressure impact her cerebral blood flow and cerebral vascular resistance?

	Cerebral blood flow	Cerebral vascular resistance
A.	↓	↑
B.	↓	↓
C.	↓	Unchanged
D.	Unchanged	↑
E.	Unchanged	↓
F.	Unchanged	Unchanged

Answer: E

4. A 65-year-old male has frequent transient ischemic attacks often leaving him confused and partially paralyzed. All of his laboratory values are within normal range although he suffers from chronic hypotension and often experiences orthostatic hypotension. His cerebral blood flow is most likely regulated by which of the following vasoactive substances?
   A. Adenosine
   B. Norepinephrine
   C. Angiotensin II
   D. Vasopressin
   E. Epinephrine

Answer: A

5. A 16-year-old male with a 2-year history of uncontrollable anger is admitted to a psychiatric unit. The patient is typically normotensive; however, during his fits of rage, his blood pressure increases substantially. What is the mechanism that most likely tries to protect this patient's cerebral blood vessels from the spike in blood pressure?
   A. Sympathetically mediated vasoconstriction
   B. Local release of vasodilating metabolites
   C. Intrinsic vasorelaxation of cerebrovascular smooth muscle
   D. Elevations in local CO_2 levels

Answer: A

References

1. Wiggers C. On the action of adrenaline on cerebral vessels. Am J Phys. 1905;14:452–65.
2. Bevan J. Sites of transition between functional systemic and cerebral arteries or rabbits occur at embryological junctional sites. Science. 1979;204:635–7.
3. Dunning H, Wolff H. The relative vascularity of various parts of the central and peripheral nervous system in the cat and its relation to function. J Comp Neurol. 1937;67:280–6.
4. Sokoloff L, Reivich M, Kennedy C, Des Rosiers MH, Patlak CS, Pettigrew KD, et al. The [14C]deoxyglucose method for the measurement of local cerebral glucose utilization: theory, procedure, and normal values in the conscious and anesthetized albino rat. J Neurochem. 1977;28(5):897–916.
5. Nakagawa Y, Tsuru M, Yada K. Site and mechanism for compression of the venous system during experimental intracranial hypertension. J Neurosurg. 1974;41(4):427–34.
6. Piechnik SK, Czosnyka M, Richards HK, Whitfield PC, Pickard JD. Cerebral venous blood outflow: a theoretical model based on laboratory simulation. Neurosurgery. 2001;49(5):1214–22.
7. Ursino M, Lodi CA. A simple mathematical model of the interaction between intracranial pressure and cerebral hemodynamics. J Appl Physiol. 1997;82(4):1256–69.
8. Czosnyka M, Piechnik S, Richards HK, Kirkpatrick P, Smielewski P, Pickard JD. Contribution of mathematical modelling to the interpretation of bedside tests of cerebrovascular autoregulation. J Neurol Neurosurg Psychiatry. 1997;63(6):721–31.

9. Attwell D, Buchan AM, Charpak S, Lauritzen M, Macvicar BA, Newman EA. Glial and neuronal control of brain blood flow. Nature. 2010;468(7321):232–43.

10. Hall CN, Reynell C, Gesslein B, Hamilton NB, Mishra A, Sutherland BA, et al. Capillary pericytes regulate cerebral blood flow in health and disease. Nature. 2014;508(7494):55–60.

11. Willie CK, Tzeng YC, Fisher JA, Ainslie PN. Integrative regulation of human brain blood flow. J Physiol. 2014;592(5):841–59.

12. Schaller B. Physiology of cerebral venous blood flow: from experimental data in animals to normal function in humans. Brain Res Brain Res Rev. 2004;46(3):243–60.

13. Lee SP, Duong TQ, Yang G, Iadecola C, Kim SG. Relative changes of cerebral arterial and venous blood volumes during increased cerebral blood flow: implications for BOLD fMRI. Magn Reson Med. 2001;45(5):791–800.

14. Rosenblum WI. Endothelium-derived relaxing factor in brain blood vessels is not nitric oxide. Stroke. 1992;23(10):1527–32.

15. Menon D. Cerebral circulation. In: Priebe H-J, Sharvans K, editors. Cardiovascular physiology. London: BMJ Publishing Group; 1995. p. 198–223.

16. Berntman L, Carlsson C, Siesjo BK. Influence of propranolol on cerebral metabolism and blood flow in the rat brain. Brain Res. 1978;151(1):220–4.

17. Berntman L, Carlsson C, Siesjo BK. Cerebral oxygen consumption and blood flow in hypoxia: influence of sympathoadrenal activation. Stroke. 1979;10(1):20–5.

18. Edvinsson L, Sercombe R. Influence of pH and pCO$_2$ on alpha-receptor mediated contraction in brain vessels. Acta Physiol Scand. 1976;97(3):325–31.

19. Pickard J, Simeone F, Vinall P. In: Betsz E, editor. H$^+$, CO$_2$, prostaglndins and cerebrovascular smooth muscle. Berlin: Springer-Verlag; 1976.

20. Busija DW, Heistad DD. Effects of cholinergic nerves on cerebral blood flow in cats. Circ Res. 1981;48(1):62–9.

21. Heistad DD, Marcus ML, Ehrhardt JC, Abboud FM. Effect of stimulation of carotid chemoreceptors on total and regional cerebral blood flow. Circ Res. 1976;38(1):20–5.

22. Ainslie PN, Duffin J. Integration of cerebrovascular CO$_2$ reactivity and chemoreflex control of breathing: mechanisms of regulation, measurement, and interpretation. Am J Physiol Regul Integr Comp Physiol. 2009;296(5):R1473–95.

23. Lassen N. In: Sutton J, Jones N, Houston C, editors. The brain: cerebral blood flow. New York: Thieme-Stratton; 1982.

24. Strandgaard S, Sigurdsson ST. Point: counterpoint: sympathetic activity does/does not influence cerebral blood flow. Counterpoint: sympathetic nerve activity does not influence cerebral blood flow. J Appl Physiol (1985). 2008;105(4):1366–7.

25. van Lieshout JJ, Secher NH. Point: counterpoint: sympathetic activity does/does not influence cerebral blood flow. Point: sympathetic activity does influ-

ence cerebral blood flow. J Appl Physiol (1985). 2008;105(4):1364–6.

26. Visocchi M, Chiappini F, Cioni B, Meglio M. Cerebral blood flow velocities and trigeminal ganglion stimulation. A transcranial Doppler study. Stereotact Funct Neurosurg. 1996;66(4):184–92.

27. Umeyama T, Kugimiya T, Ogawa T, Kandori Y, Ishizuka A, Hanaoka K. Changes in cerebral blood flow estimated after stellate ganglion block by single photon emission computed tomography. J Auton Nerv Syst. 1995;50(3):339–46.

28. Iwayama T, Furness JB, Burnstock G. Dual adrenergic and cholinergic innervation of the cerebral arteries of the rat. An ultrastructural study. Circ Res. 1970;26(5):635–46.

29. Nielsen KC, Owman C. Adrenergic innervation of pial arteries related to the circle of Willis in the cat. Brain Res. 1967;6(4):773–6.

30. Heistad DD, Marcus ML. Evidence that neural mechanisms do not have important effects on cerebral blood flow. Circ Res. 1978;42(3):295–302.

31. Purves MJ. Do vasomotor nerves significantly regulate cerebral blood flow? Circ Res. 1978;43(4):485–93.

32. Owman C, Edvinsson L, Nielsen KC. Autonomic neuroreceptor mechanisms in brain vessels. Blood Vessels. 1974;11(1-2):2–31.

33. Duckles SP, Bevan JA. Pharmacological characterization of adrenergic receptors of a rabbit cerebral artery in vitro. J Pharmacol Exp Ther. 1976;197(2):371–8.

34. Edvinsson L, MacKenzie ET. Amine mechanisms in the cerebral circulation. Pharmacol Rev. 1976;28(4):275–348.

35. Toda N, Fujita Y. Responsiveness of isolated cerebral and peripheral arteries to serotonin, norepinephrine, and transmural electrical stimulation. Circ Res. 1973;33(1):98–104.

36. Lee TJ, Su C, Bevan JA. Neurogenic sympathetic vasoconstriction of the rabbit basilar artery. Circ Res. 1976;39(1):120–6.

37. Navari RM, Wei EP, Kontos HA, Patterson JL Jr. Comparison of the open skull and cranial window preparations in the study of the cerebral microcirculation. Microvasc Res. 1978;16(3):304–15.

38. Oldendorf WH. Brain uptake of radiolabeled amino acids, amines, and hexoses after arterial injection. Am J Phys. 1971;221(6):1629–39.

39. Tindall GT, Greenfield JC Jr. The effects of intra-arterial histamine on blood flow in the internal and external carotid artery of man. Stroke. 1973;4(1):46–9.

40. MacKenzie ET, McCulloch J, O'Kean M, Pickard JD, Harper AM. Cerebral circulation and norepinephrine: relevance of the blood-brain barrier. Am J Phys. 1976;231(2):483–8.

41. Bill A, Linder J. Sympathetic control of cerebral blood flow in acute arterial hypertension. Acta Physiol Scand. 1976;96(1):114–21.

42. Edvinsson L, Owman C, Siesjo B. Physiological role of cerebrovascular sympathetic nerves in the autoregulation of cerebral blood flow. Brain Res. 1976;117(3):519–23.

43. Heistad DD, Marcus ML. Effect of sympathetic stimulation on permeability of the blood-brain barrier to albumin during acute hypertension in cats. Circ Res. 1979;45(3):331–8.

44. Heistad DD, Marcus ML, Gross PM. Effects of sympathetic nerves on cerebral vessels in dog, cat, and monkey. Am J Phys. 1978;235(5):H544–52.

45. MacKenzie ET, McGeorge AP, Graham DI, Fitch W, Edvinsson L, Harper AM. Effects of increasing arterial pressure on cerebral blood flow in the baboon: influence of the sympathetic nervous system. Pflugers Arch. 1979;378(3):189–95.

46. Lindvall M, Edvinsson L, Owman C. Sympathetic nervous control of cerebrospinal fluid production from the choroid plexus. Science. 1978;201(4351):176–8.

47. Johansson B, Li CL, Olsson Y, Klatzo I. The effect of acute arterial hypertension on the blood-brain barrier to protein tracers. Acta Neuropathol. 1970;16(2):117–24.

48. Hart MN, Heistad DD, Brody MJ. Effect of chronic hypertension and sympathetic denervation on wall/lumen ratio of cerebral vessels. Hypertension. 1980;2(4):419–23.

49. Larsson LI, Edvinsson L, Fahrenkrug J, Hakanson R, Owman C, Schaffalitzky de Muckadell O, et al. Immunohistochemical localization of a vasodilatory polypeptide (VIP) in cerebrovascular nerves. Brain Res. 1976;113(2):400–4.

Pathology of the Extracranial Carotid and Vertebral Arteries

3

Wendy N. Wiesend and Mitual Amin

Abbreviations

AIT	Adaptive intimal thickening
ACA	Anterior Cerebral Artery
BA	Basilar artery
CCA	Common carotid artery
CMD	Cystic medial degeneration
COPD	Chronic obstructive pulmonary disease
ECA	External carotid artery
ECCA	Extracranial carotid artery
ECVA	Extracranial vertebral artery
EEL	External elastic lamina
FMD	Fibromuscular dysplasia
FS	Fatty streak
GCA	Giant cell arteritis
ICA	Internal carotid artery
IEL	Internal elastic lamina
LDL	Low-density lipoprotein
PIT	Pathologic intimal thickening
SDHL	Succinate dehydrogenase
TA	Takayasu's arteritis
TIA	Transient ischemic attack
VA	Vertebral artery
VCAM-1	Vascular cell adhesion molecule-1

The original version of the chapter was revised. A correction to this chapter can be found at https://doi.org/10.1007/978-3-319-91533-3_25

W. N. Wiesend (✉) · M. Amin
Department of Anatomic Pathology, Beaumont Health System, Royal Oak, MI, USA
e-mail: Wendy.Wiesend@beaumont.edu

Anatomy and Histology of the Extracranial Carotid and Vertebral Arteries

Understanding the pathogenesis and symptomatology behind diseases involving the extracranial carotid arteries (ECCAs) and extracranial vertebral arteries (ECVAs) requires a basic understanding of the anatomy and histology of these vessels.

Although variations in anatomy exist, the right common carotid artery (CCA) typically originates from the brachiocephalic trunk, and the left CCA originates from the aortic arch [1]. The CCAs divide into two branches (the internal carotid artery (ICA) and external carotid artery (ECA)) at the superior border of the thyroid cartilage. The paired ICAs provide blood to the anterior portion of the brain (anterior cerebral circulation) and meninges. The proximal portion of the ICA has a slight dilation termed the carotid sinus where baroreceptors are present in the vessel wall. These baroreceptors are stretch receptors which are important for blood pressure monitoring. The cervical segment of the ICA is freely mobile and extends through the neck to enter the skull through the carotid canals in the petrous portion of the temporal bone at the skull base. The ICAs give off no branches in the neck. The terminal intracranial branches of the ICAs are the anterior and middle cerebral arteries. The ECAs provide blood supply to the neck, face, and base of the skull and course under the submandibular gland and into the parotid gland. They give off six branches including the superior thyroid artery, lingual artery, facial artery, ascending pharyngeal artery, occipital artery, and posterior auricular artery and terminate in two branches (the maxillary artery and superficial temporal artery).

Although variations in anatomy exist, the vertebral arteries (VAs) typically branch from the subclavian vessels and can be divided into four distinct segments [1]:

- Cervical (V1) segment: Portion of the VA between its origin from the subclavian artery and its entrance into the transverse foramina of the C6 vertebra.
- Vertebral (V2) segment: Portion of the VA that passes vertically through the bony canal of the transverse foramina from the C6 to the C2 vertebra.
- Suboccipital (V3) segment: Portion of the VA that exits the transverse foramina of C2 and ends as the vessel passes through the foramen magnum/posterior atlanto-occipital ligament.
- Cranial (V4) segment: Intracranial portion of the VA. The V4 segments fuse to form the basilar artery (BA) at the inferior border of the pons. The paired vertebral arteries (VAs) via the basilar artery (BA) provide blood to the posterior brain and brainstem (posterior cerebral circulation) and meninges.

Occlusive lesions of the ECVAs only rarely cause a significant decrease in blood flow to the posterior cerebral circulation [2]. As the VAs are paired vessels that join to form a single BA, if one is compromised, the other can typically compensate. Also, even when there is bilateral occlusive disease of the ECVAs, patients typically do not develop posterior circulation stroke. As opposed to the ICAs, the ECVAs give rise to numerous branches in the neck which provide conduits for collateral circulation. For example, the costocervical and thyrocervical branches of the Subclavian Artery can develop collateral circulation between the external carotid and subclavian arteries.

The most common variations of VA anatomy include origin of the left VA from the aortic arch (~5% of people) and entrance of the V1 segment into a vertebral foramen more superior than C6 level. The VAs are often of unequal caliber (only ~25% of people have similar caliber vessels), and the left is commonly larger than the right [3]. One of the two is atretic (<2 mm in diameter) in approximately 15% of the population. The vertebral arteries can also be duplicated or fenestrated.

The circle of Willis connects the anterior and posterior cerebral circulation and is formed by the posterior cerebral arteries (which are the terminal branches of the BA), the posterior communicating arteries (which connect the posterior cerebral arteries to the ICAs), the ICAs, the anterior cerebral arteries (ACAs), and the anterior communicating arteries (which connect the two ACAs). Only ~20% of the population has a complete circle of Willis, with most of the variation attributed to vascular hypoplasias or aplasias [4]. It should be noted that the carotid arteries provide ~80% of the cerebral blood flow while the vertebral arteries supply ~20% [5]. Given the presence of collateral circulation through the circle of Willis, chronic occlusive disease of the extracranial cerebral vasculature is better tolerated than in other vascular beds such as the coronary circulation. Development of symptomatic cerebrovascular ischemia typically requires significant occlusive pathology often involving multiple vessels in both the carotid and vertebrobasilar pathways to overcome this collateral compensation [2, 6].

Arteries in general are composed of three layers (or tunics) histologically [7]:

- Tunica intima: Innermost layer composed of a monolayer of endothelial cells with underlying basement membrane and loose subendothelial connective tissue containing fibroblasts, smooth muscle cells, collagen and elastic fibers, and proteoglycan ground substance.
- Tunica media: Middle layer composed predominantly of varying numbers of smooth muscle and elastic fibers and some collagen fibers.
- Tunica adventitia: Outermost layer composed mainly of connective tissue, nerves, and the vasa vasorum which supplies blood to the vessel wall.

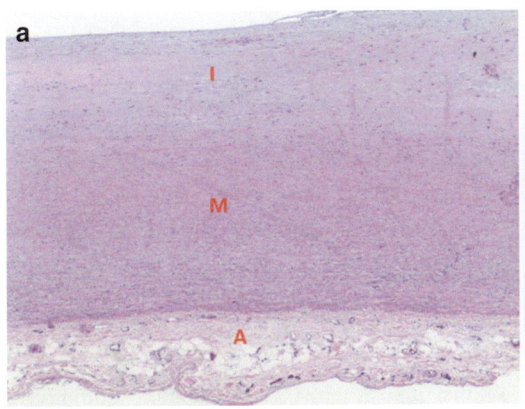
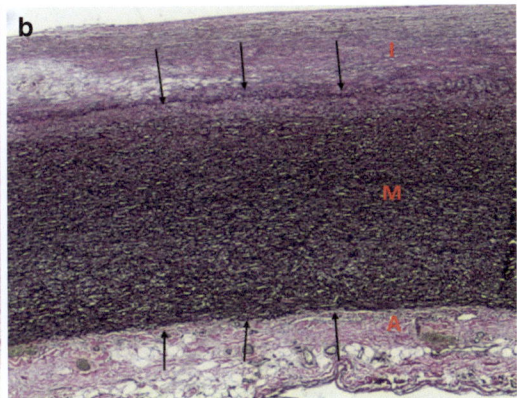

Fig. 3.1 Elastic artery. (**a**) Longitudinal section of the aorta which is an elastic vessel. The vessel intima (I) is the innermost layer and is mildly thickened in this example secondary to atherosclerotic change. The vessel media (M) is thick and composed of numerous concentric elastic fibers. The vessel adventitia (A) is the outermost layer (hematoxylin and eosin, 40×). (**b**) The thick elastic layer (arrows) in the media is best highlighted with an elastic stain (Verhoeff-van Gieson elastic stain, 40×). The vessel intima (I), media (M) and adventitia (A) are also labeled

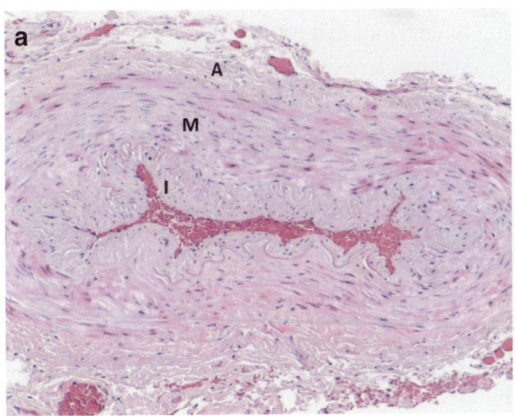
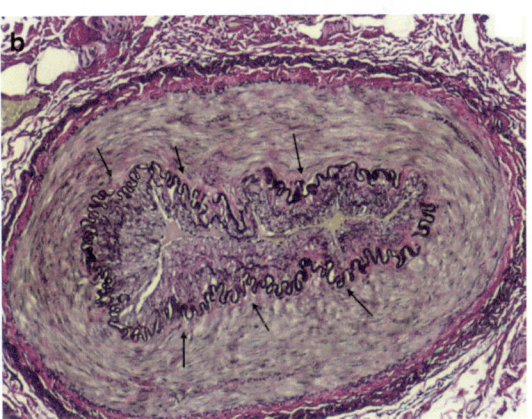

Fig. 3.2 Muscular artery. (**a**) Cross section of the temporal artery which is a muscular vessel. The vessel intima (I) is the innermost layer and is lined by endothelium. The vessel media (M) is composed predominantly of concentric smooth muscle fibers, and the vessel adventitia (A) is the outermost layer which blends into the surrounding connective tissue (hematoxylin and eosin, 40×). (**b**) The internal elastic lamina (arrows) is a layer of concentric elastic fibers which separates the vessel intima from the vessel media and is best highlighted by an elastic stain (Verhoeff-van Gieson elastic stain, 40×)

The internal elastic lamina (IEL) is a thick concentric layer of interwoven elastic fibers, which separates the tunica intima from the tunica media [8]. The external elastic lamina (EEL) is a thinner concentric layer of interwoven elastic fibers which separates the tunica media from the tunica adventitia. The IEL is not well defined universally and may be absent in areas of vessel bifurcation or branching. Fragmentation, duplication, and calcification of the IEL are common changes that occur with aging [9].

Arteries can be subdivided into two major histologic subtypes, elastic (also known as conducting) and muscular (also known as distributing) depending on vessel size and predominant fiber type (elastic or muscular) in the vessel media. Elastic arteries are larger vessels that have a broad tunica media with a higher percentage of concentrically organized elastic fibers (Fig. 3.1). The tunica intima of elastic vessels is often thicker than that of muscular vessels. Muscular arteries are typically medium or small sized vessels which have a higher percentage of concentrically oriented smooth muscle cells within the vessel media (Fig. 3.2). The IEL and EEL are better defined in muscular than they are in elastic vessels. The aorta and its major branches including the CCAs and subclavian arteries with vertebral artery branches are considered elastic arteries [9]. The majority of the remaining grossly identifiable and named arteries are considered muscular vessels. The CAs are considered muscular vessels by some [10] or of "mixed type" by others [9] as they are in a transitional regions between elastic and muscular composition.

Atherosclerotic Disease of the Extracranial Carotid and Vertebral Arteries

The most common pathologic disorder to affect the ECCAs and ECVAs is atherosclerosis [11]. Atherosclerosis is characterized by pathologic thickening of arteries secondary to fibrofatty plaque formation. Atherosclerosis is derived from the Greek "athero" meaning gruel (corresponding to the necrotic core of the plaque) and "sclerosis" meaning hardening (corresponding to the plaque's fibrous cap) [12]. The most detrimental complications of extracranial large vessel atherosclerotic disease include TIA and stroke. Approximately 87% of all strokes are of ischemic etiology, and ECCA and ECVA atherosclerosis accounts for up to 20% of cases of ischemic stroke [13, 14]. Risk factors for ischemic stroke secondary to atherosclerosis of these vessels include advanced age, male gender, race (blacks and Hispanics have higher risk than whites), hypertension, hypercholesterolemia, diabetes mellitus, tobacco smoking, physical inactivity, obesity, prior TIA or stroke, family history of TIA or stroke, or history of significant coronary atherosclerotic disease, among others [13].

The ECCAs are more commonly affected by significant atherosclerotic disease than the ECVAs [2]. In fact, the carotid artery is the fourth most common vessel impacted by atherosclerosis behind the abdominal aorta, coronary, and popliteal artery [15]. In a study of patients aged 60–79 years, 10.5% of men and 5.5% of women had stenosis of their ICA by carotid duplex ultrasound [16]. Around 20% of ischemic strokes involve the posterior circulation, and around 20% of posterior circulation stroke can be attributed to ECVA atherosclerosis [3, 17, 18]. The most common location of extracranial large vessel atherosclerotic disease is at the carotid bifurcation (often with involvement of the proximal portion of the ICA), and the second most common location is in the V1 segment of the vertebral artery (at its origin from the subclavian artery) [2, 18]. It is well known that atherosclerosis is more common at arterial bifurcations and branch points. Studies have shown that disturbed blood flow/blood stagnation and low or oscillatory shear stress on the vessel wall in these regions alters endothelial function by enhancing inflammatory cell activation [19] and release of nitric oxide [20] contributing to development of atherosclerosis.

Atherosclerosis has been most extensively studied in the coronary circulation, which provides insight into other disease loci including the ECCA and ECVA. Elucidation of the pathogenesis of atherosclerosis has relied on gross and microscopic examination of pathologic specimens and clinical and experimental studies (including study of animal models), and multiple theories have developed over time. It is known to be a complex multifactorial process and a chronic inflammatory disease with pathogenesis initiating at formation of a fibrous lipid-rich plaque (known as a fibroatheroma or fibroinflammatory lipid plaque). The components of the plaque include fibrous tissue, smooth muscle cells, lipid, and inflammatory cells in varying proportions. The process of atherosclerosis has traditionally been thought to follow an orderly linear progression [12, 21]; however more recently it has been considered a more variable or dynamic process [22].

Histologic studies have identified precursor lesions which may predispose a region of an artery to develop an atherosclerotic plaque. These precursor lesions include the fatty streak (FS), known by some as the intimal xanthoma and adaptive intimal thickening (AIT). Both develop in childhood and are clinically quiescent as they do not cause significant vessel obstruction. The FS is grossly identifiable as a flat or slightly raised yellow-colored intimal spot, patch, or streak [21]. The FS is present secondary to foam cell (lipid-laden macrophage) accumulation in the subendothelial space. Accumulation of smooth muscle cells and extracellular matrix in the intima leads to AIT [22]. AIT can involve a vessel in a circumferential or eccentric manner. The eccentric form is thought to predispose to atherosclerotic plaque formation [21]. It is common at vessel branch points and has been described in various vessels including the coronary and CAs [8].

The most widely accepted mechanism of atherosclerotic pathogenesis begins when proatherosclerotic conditions (including disturbed blood flow and hyperlipidemia) lead to endothelial dysfunction and stimulate endothelial cells to overexpress adhesion molecules including vascular cell adhesion molecule-1 (VCAM-1) on their surfaces. VCAM-1 participates in the recruitment of monocytes and other inflammatory cells (e.g., T lymphocytes) to the region [23, 24]. LDL particles become entrapped in the intima by proteoglycans and are oxidized by oxygen free radicals that are produced by macrophages and other cells [25]. Monocytes enter the intima via diapedesis having been induced into the subendothelial space by chemoattractants, mature into macrophages and engulf oxidized low-density lipoprotein (LDL) particles via scavenger receptors. Oxidized LDL is degraded in lysosomes in the macrophage, and excess free cholesterol is transferred to the endoplasmic reticulum where it is esterified into cholesterol esters and packaged into cytoplasmic lipid droplets creating the foam cell [26]. Foam cells produce cytokines and reactive oxygen species which further oxidize LDL and recruit modified smooth muscle cells (myointimal cells) and T cells into the intima by chemotaxis. Eventually, the pathways to metabolize excess lipoproteins are overwhelmed, and toxic excess free cholesterol builds up leading to cell death. Myointimal cells proliferate and undergo apoptosis, leading to further inflammatory signaling. As foam cells and myointimal cells undergo apoptosis, necrotic debris and crystalline cholesterol accumulate in small pools (preatheroma) which coalesce to form larger lipid cores (atheroma) typically leading to plaque expansion from the fourth decade of life.

Concurrently, myointimal cells secrete extracellular matrix including proteoglycans which further entrap LDL particles and secrete collagen at the endothelial barrier leading to formation of a fibrous cap (fibroatheroma). Decreased diffusion of oxygen and nutrients from the vessel lumen through the thickened fibrous cap likely contributes to necrosis in the core of the fibroatheroma. Fibroatheroma can involve a vessel in a focal, patchy, or diffuse manner and can be either eccentric or concentric (eccentric growth is more common at vessel branch points). The fibrous cap in a fibroatheroma can be thick or thin [22]. Another poorly defined pathway of plaque formation occurs in areas of pathologic intimal thickening (PIT) and consists of abnormal accumulation of smooth muscle cells and proteoglycan-rich matrix in the vessel intima with very little inflammation or lipid content [22].

Atherosclerosis can lead to end organ ischemia via chronic progressive plaque growth which can lead to narrowing of the vessel lumen over time or a wide range of plaque complications [27]. In the North American Symptomatic Carotid Endarterectomy Trial, there was a correlation between the degree of carotid artery stenosis and risk of stroke in symptomatic patients. Risk of stroke in patients with 70–79% stenosis was 19%, 80–89% stenosis was 28%, 90–99% stenosis was 28%, and 90–99% stenosis was 33% after 18 months of medical therapy without a revascularization procedure [28]. Plaque complications include intraplaque hemorrhage, plaque rupture, plaque erosion, mural thrombosis with or without embolization, plaque calcification, and aneurysm formation. Intraplaque hemorrhage occurs when rupture or leak of thin-walled neovasculature (arising from the vasa vasorum) causes blood pooling/thrombosis within the plaque, plaque expansion, and further luminal obstruction. Rupture of the fibrous cap of a plaque uncovers thrombogenic plaque components which form a nidus for intraluminal thrombosis (which can be occlusive or subocclusive). Intuitively, thin plaque fibroatheroma are more prone to rupture than thick plaque fibroatheroma. The surface of the plaque (including endothelial lining) can erode which can also form a nidus for luminal thrombosis. Plaques that form secondary to PIT are prone to erosion which can form a nidus for intraluminal thrombosis. Repeated plaque rupture or erosion with healing can lead to further luminal narrowing. Portions of luminal thrombus or atherosclerotic debris can break off and travel downstream leading to artery-to-artery thrombo- or atheroembolization. Calcification of atherosclerotic plaques is common, and calcified plaques, also known as fibrocalcific plaques, typically have smaller lipid cores. It is believed that plaque calcification occurs in the process of plaque healing after intraplaque hemorrhage, plaque rupture, or erosion. Large calcium nodules (calcified nodules) can form in some cases which can predispose to cap rupture or erosion and thrombosis [22]. Some plaques undergo osseous metaplasia. Occasionally, atherosclerotic plaque formation can weaken the vessel wall and lead to vascular dilatation or aneurysm formation. This process is more common in larger elastic arteries, including the aorta, than smaller muscular arteries (see section on aneurysm). Morphologic features that contribute to carotid plaque instability include a thin fibrous cap, decreased number of smooth muscle cells, high lipid content, increased numbers of macrophages, increased vascularity, surface irregularity, and presence of plaque erosion [29–32]. Vulnerable carotid plaques have a mean fibrous cap thickness (72 ± 24 μm) thicker than that of vulnerable coronary artery plaques (which have a mean cap thickness of 65 μm or less) [33].

Although the pathophysiology behind formation of an atherosclerotic plaque is similar in the coronary and extracranial cerebral circulation, the mechanism by which acute plaque change leads to ischemic symptomatology typically differs between them [33]. It is well known that atherosclerotic plaque rupture with occlusive thrombosis is the most common cause of acute myocardial infarction. Thrombotic occlusion usually only occurs in the background of severe luminal narrowing in the extracranial cerebral vasculature given the normally high blood flow rate in these vessels [34]. Also given the high flow rate, if acute thrombosis of the ECCA does occur, it often propagates distally [35]. The most common cause of TIA or stroke in patients

with atherosclerosis of the extracranial cerebral vasculature is artery-to-artery embolization. Embolus material (consisting of either atherosclerotic or thrombotic debris) can travel distally to occlude smaller intracranial arteries or arterial branches. Patients with embolization from the ECCA present most commonly with middle cerebral artery territory ischemic symptoms [2, 36]. Embolization from the ECVA typically occludes the V2 segment of the vertebral artery and the intracranial portion of the vertebral or basilar artery and/or its branches and leads to stroke involving the cerebellum, temporal, or occipital lobes.

Endarterectomy is an open surgical procedure which consists of removal of an intimal plaque. As carotid endarterectomy is the most frequently performed surgical intervention to prevent stroke, carotid artery plaques are commonly examined pathologically [33]. It should be noted that not all institutions routinely process endarterectomy specimens histologically. Some may only provide a gross examination of the specimens. Vertebral artery plaques are only rarely examined pathologically as vertebral artery endarterectomy is a rare procedure and specimens are usually not obtained from bypass procedures [3]. Grossly, the carotid endarterectomy specimen consists of a variably fragmented tubular segment of intimal plaque. If performed at the area of carotid bifurcation, the specimen will be bifurcated. A longitudinal surgical excision is typically identified (Fig. 3.3a). When cut in cross section, a noncomplicated intimal plaque appears white to yellow in color (depending on the proportion of fibrous tissue and lipid) and typically has a smooth surface. Plaques with abundant extracellular lipid will have bright yellow cores. Microscopically the intimal plaque has a fibrous cap of varying thickness. The fibrous cap consists predominantly of fibrous tissue with numerous collagen and some elastic fibers. Extracellular matrix, myointimal cells, and inflammatory cells including macrophages, foam cells, and lymphocytes can also be present. The necrotic core is highly variable in size and consists of extracellular lipid, cholesterol clefts, necrotic debris, and various numbers of inflammatory cells including foam cells and T cells. Cholesterol clefts are needle-

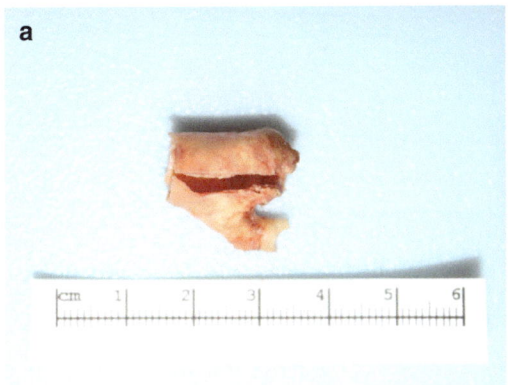
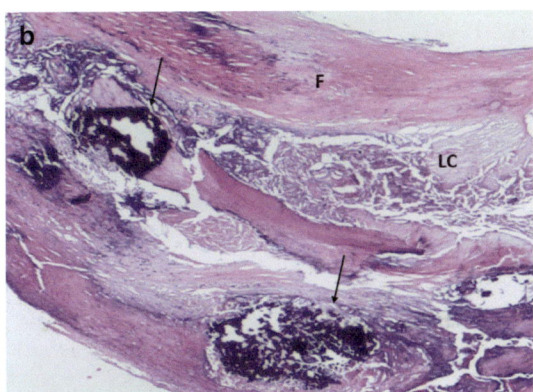

Fig. 3.3 Carotid endarterectomy specimen. (**a**) Gross photograph of a bifurcated intimal atherosclerotic plaque which is white to focally yellow in color and has a longitudinal surgical incision. (**b**) Histologic cross section of the endarterectomy specimen reveals an intimal fibroatheroma with a fibrous cap (F) and lipid core (LC) containing cholesterol clefts (cleft-like spaces). Calcification is also seen (arrows) which is relatively common in atherosclerotic plaques of the carotid artery (hematoxylin and eosin, 20×)

shaped spaces formed when cholesterol crystals are dissolved by the alcohol used in specimen processing/staining (Fig. 3.3b).

Some endarterectomy specimens have plaque complications that can be identified either grossly or microscopically. Calcification is a common finding in an intimal plaque and can be of variable degree. Plaques that are highly calcified must be decalcified before sectioning. Some plaques are ossified. Fibrous cap rupture and erosion with or without luminal thrombus can be seen in some cases. Plaques with intraplaque hemorrhage will appear red-yellow and variegated in color grossly. Hemosiderin-laden macrophages identified within a plaque histologically are evidence of previous intraplaque hemorrhage or healed plaque rupture. Plaque complications that are more common in the extracranial cerebral circulation than the coronary circulation include surface erosion, intraplaque hemorrhage, and calcified nodules [34].

Dissection of the Extracranial Carotid and Vertebral Arteries

Isolated dissection of the ECCA or ECVA is not uncommon and can occur spontaneously, secondary to trauma, or iatrogenically. For example, incidental canalization of the carotid artery during central line placement has been described to cause dissection [37]. These vessels can also be secondarily involved via extension from a thoracic aortic dissection. This section will focus on spontaneous and traumatic dissection.

Spontaneous dissection is the second most common pathology to affect the ECCA or ECVA behind atherosclerosis [38] and accounts for approximately 2% of ischemic strokes overall [39] but 10–25% of ischemic strokes in young and middle-aged patients [40]. Spontaneous dissection of the ECCA occurs more often than the ECVA, and the ICA is most commonly involved. The incidence of spontaneous carotid artery dissection is approximately 2.5–3 per 100,000, and vertebral artery dissection is approximately 1–1.5 per 100,000 [40]. Spontaneous dissection of these vessels can occur at all ages, but there is a distinct peak in the fifth decade [39, 40]. In up to 16% of cases, multiple vessels can be involved [41]. Common traumatic causes of dissection include motor vehicle accidents, assaults, falls, hangings, or sports injuries. Traumatic dissection of the ECCA or ECVA occurs in 1–2% of patients admitted to the hospital with blunt trauma, and 10–20% of these patients develop stroke [42].

The ICA and ECVA are especially sensitive to dissection, even more so than their intracranial portions or other arteries of similar size. This can be attributed to their unique mobility

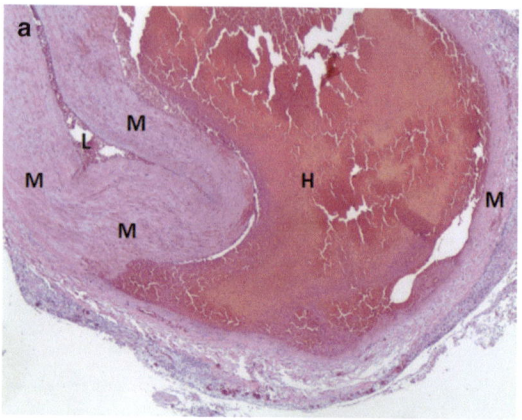
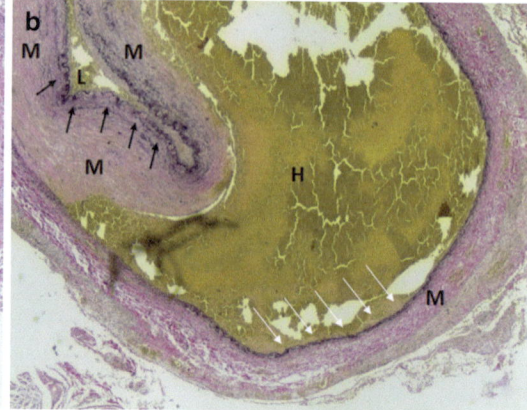

Fig. 3.4 Spontaneous internal carotid artery dissection in a middle-aged man who presented with headache and neck pain. (**a**) Histologic cross section of the internal carotid artery in area of dissection revealing hemorrhage (H) in the outer portion of the vessel media (M). The compressed lumen (L) of the vessel can also be identified (hematoxylin and eosin, 20×). (**b**) An elastic stained cross section of the internal carotid artery in area of dissection highlights the internal (black arrows) and external elastic lamina (white arrows). The vessel lumen (L) and area of dissection/intramural hemorrhage (H) in the outer portion of the vascular media (M) are also labeled (Verhoeff-van Gieson elastic stain, 20×)

during neck movement and their surrounding skeletal anatomy. The entire extracranial ICA and V1 and V3 segments of the ECVA are mobile and prone to stretch injury. The ICA and ECVA are also prone to injury by contact with adjacent bony structures including the cervical vertebrae, styloid process of the temporal bone, and the angle of the mandible [40]. Fracture of a cervical vertebra can lead to ECVA dissection in the V2 segment given the intimate relationship of the vessel with the cervical vertebra including the transverse foramen in this region [42].

Classic clinical symptoms of carotid artery dissection include unilateral pain in the neck, unilateral headache, partial Horner's syndrome (including meiosis and ptosis), cranial nerve palsies and later-onset anterior cerebrovascular ischemic symptoms including TIA or stroke, or, rarely, retinal ischemic symptoms including transient monocular blindness [40]. Classic clinical symptoms of vertebral artery dissection include pain at the back of the neck or occipital headache followed by posterior cerebrovascular ischemic symptoms including TIA or stroke. Clinical diagnosis is typically difficult given the diverse and nonspecific symptomatology and is supported by imaging studies.

As dissection of the ECCA or ECVA is typically treated medically or via minimally invasive surgical techniques, pathologic examination can often only be performed at postmortem examination. Historically, knowledge of the histopathologic features of dissection has helped to elucidate the mechanism of the disorder. Dissection occurs when there is vessel injury leading to intramural hemorrhage into a false lumen between the vessel wall layers (Fig. 3.4). In some cases, blood can dissect back from this false lumen into the true vessel lumen leading to a double channel of blood flow through the vessel (called a double lumen vessel). Dissection typically results from 1 of 2 mechanisms: (1) an intimal tear or (2) rupture of the vasa vasorum [41]. Rarely, the area of intimal disruption that initiated the dissection can be identified histologically. Hemorrhage inward between the vessel intima and media can lead to stenosis or even complete occlusion of the true vascular lumen, while hemorrhage outward between the vessel media and adventitia with associated disruption of the elastic lamina can result in aneurysmal vascular dilatation [40]. Dissection can sometimes extend intracranially which is more common in cases of ECVA than ICA dissection [40]. Dissection which extends intracranially (especially cases with associated aneurysmal vascular dilatation) is more prone to rupture and can result in subarachnoid hemorrhage [38]. The wall of the intracranial portion of the ICA and VA is weaker than the extracranial portion as there is loss of elastic fibers including the external elastic lamina intracranially, and the media and adventitia are thinner [43, 44].

Spontaneous cervical artery dissection is likely a multifactorial disease resulting from a combination of an environmental trigger (such as minor precipitating trauma) superimposed on an underlying vascular abnormality (such as weakness in the vessel wall secondary to an underlying connective tissue disorder) [40, 41, 45, 46]. Patients with spontaneous dissection typically have a history of a minor precipitating event such as a coughing fit, rapid neck rotation, or hyperextension. Other environmental triggers including infection has been suggested [41, 47–49]. Some patients with spontaneous dissection likely have a clinically unapparent undiscovered connective tissue disorder that may be genetic in etiology. A study of dermal connective tissue in patients with spontaneous cervical artery dissection found that 36 of 65 (55%) had ultrastructural connective tissue abnormalities in collagen and elastin, and many of these patients had no other clinical manifestations of connective tissue disease [46]. Up to 20% of patients have a clinically apparent yet unnamed connective tissue disorder. Up to 5% of patients have a known connective tissue disorder (mainly Ehlers-Danlos syndrome type), and an additional 5% of patients have a family history of spontaneous artery dissection in the absence of known connective tissue disease [40]. Histologic findings of cystic medial degeneration (CMD) also called cystic medial necrosis is common in cases of spontaneous carotid artery dissection. CMD is a nonspecific histologic finding that can be seen in dissections or aneurysms from many causes including atherosclerotic disease; however finding significant CMD in a dissection specimen in a younger patient can suggest the possibility of an underlying connective tissue disorder [50]. Microscopically, CMD is characterized by disruption of the elastic lamina in the vessel media (best seen in elastic stained sections) and increased basophilic ground substance.

There may or may not be associated necrosis. Another structural abnormality that may predispose to spontaneous dissection is fibromuscular dysplasia (FMD) [40]. FMD has been reported as the etiology of spontaneous carotid or vertebral artery dissection in ~15–20% of cases [51]. Atherosclerosis as a cause of ICA or ECVA dissection is uncommon.

The intimal injury that results in dissection can form a nidus for luminal thrombosis which can be occlusive or can embolize distally. ICA or ECVA dissection typically result in ischemic stroke by one of two mechanisms: (1) artery-to-artery embolization of intraluminal thrombus from the site of injury downstream or (2) luminal stenosis or obstruction leading to downstream ischemia [38–40, 42]. Ischemic stroke secondary to artery-to-artery embolization is more common and is thought to be the mechanism of stroke in greater than 90% of these cases.

The prognosis of cervical artery dissection is based on many factors including location and severity of the dissection, the number of vessels involved, and the presence or absence of collateral blood flow. Most dissections will heal spontaneously, and the reported death rate is less than 5% [40].

Aneurysm of the Extracranial Carotid and Vertebral Arteries

ECCA or ECVA aneurysms are relatively uncommon [52]. ECCA aneurysms comprise less than 1% of all peripheral aneurysms [53] and represent only 0.1–2% of all carotid artery surgical procedures [54]. Vertebral artery aneurysms comprise ~1% of all vertebral artery lesions. Involvement of the ECVA is very rare as the majority of aneurysms affect the intracranial portion of the vessel [55] (Fig. 3.5).

An aneurysm can be broadly defined as a localized abnormal dilatation of a blood vessel secondary to a congenital or acquired weakness in the vessel wall. To be categorized as an aneurysm, the diameter in the area of vascular dilatation must be at least 50% greater than the normal vessel diameter [56]. As there is normal dilata-

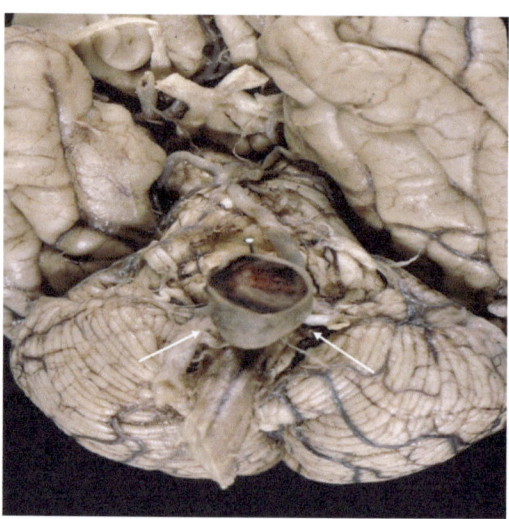

Fig. 3.5 Fusiform aneurysm of intracranial portion of the left vertebral artery with thrombosis (arrows)

tion at the carotid bulb, there has been debate as to what constitutes an aneurysm in this region. The two main subtypes of aneurysms are true aneurysms and false aneurysms (or pseudoaneurysms) [15]. True aneurysms are outpouching that involve all three layers of a vessel wall. A false aneurysm is created when a transmural disruption in a vessel wall leads to formation of an extravascular hematoma which maintains connection with the vessel lumen and is contained by adventitial or extravascular soft tissue. False aneurysms occur most commonly secondary to trauma, in the setting of dissection or iatrogenically (e.g., in areas of suture line disruption). True aneurysms can be subdivided by shape into fusiform or saccular types. Fusiform forms are circumferential outpouchings of the vessel wall (Fig. 3.6a), while saccular aneurysms are localized outpouchings that affect only a portion of the vessel circumference (Fig. 3.6b). Saccular aneurysms are typically more prone to enlarge, rupture and lead to ischemic symptomatology than fusiform types [42].

Aneurysms in general have a wide range of etiologies, many of which are discussed elsewhere in this chapter. Causes of aneurysm include atherosclerosis, trauma, infection, vasculitis, FMD, radiation therapy, and connective tissue disease. They can develop iatrogenically or be

congenital in origin. Aneurysm can develop in the setting of dissection (see previous section) if there is disruption of the elastic lamina and hemorrhage toward the vessel adventitia [42]. The most common cause of ECCA aneurysm is atherosclerosis. Atherosclerotic aneurysms are typically fusiform in shape and most commonly involve the carotid bifurcation or proximal ICA [57]. Histologically, the vessel wall in the region of an atherosclerotic aneurysm will typically have severe atherosclerotic disease with destruction of the internal elastic lamina and thinning of the tunica media. Other common etiologies of ECCA aneurysm include trauma or dissection [58]. Iatrogenic aneurysms of the ECCA are relatively rare but can occur as a complication of carotid endarterectomy. The most common cause of ECVA aneurysm is trauma, and the most common location is the V3 segment [55]. Infection only rarely causes ECCA or ECVA aneurysms and is most commonly bacterial in origin (mycotic aneurysm). Mycotic aneurysms can develop secondary to septic embolization from an infected heart valve or contiguous infection from surrounding structures (such as meningitis or cervical lymphadenitis). Secondary infection can occur after surgical manipulation. Acute inflammation and destruction of the vessel wall predisposes to aneurysm formation in these cases.

Aneurysms can result in significant morbidity, the main complications of which include local symptomatology secondary to compression, thromboembolic events, or rupture [59].

Fibromuscular Dysplasia of the Extracranial Carotid and Vertebral Arteries

Fibromuscular dysplasia (FMD) is a group of nonatherosclerotic, noninflammatory disorders of medium-sized arteries [60]. FMD is characterized by structural abnormalities in the vessel wall which can lead to luminal stenosis/occlusion, dissection, and/or aneurysm formation with or without associated vascular thrombosis or embolization [61, 62]. Clinical manifestations vary

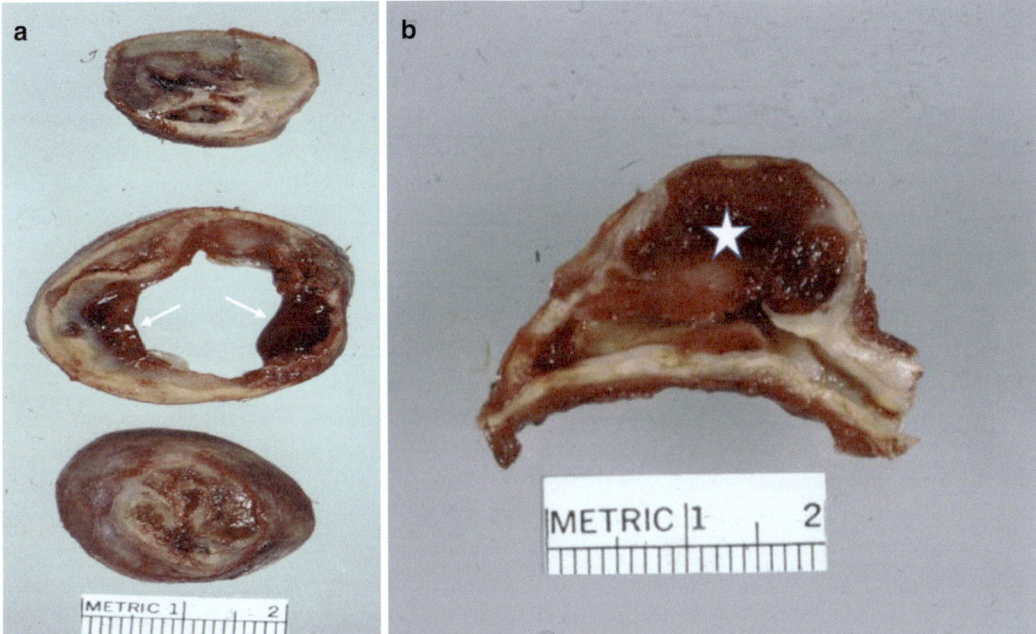

Fig. 3.6 Major subtypes of true aneurysms. (**a**) Fusiform atherosclerotic aneurysm of the right femoral artery cut in cross section revealing circumferential dilatation (middle cross section) and partially occlusive adherent thrombus (arrows). (**b**) Longitudinal section of a saccular atherosclerotic aneurysm of the right popliteal artery revealing a localized outpouching filled with organized thrombus (star)

widely and depend on the vascular bed affected, the histologic type of FMD, and degree of disease, and some patients are asymptomatic. Its prevalence in the general population is unknown and, although historically thought of as a rare disease, may be underdiagnosed [63].

It has been described in nearly every arterial bed but most commonly affects the renal arteries, ICAs and ECVAs [64]. It less commonly affects the ECA and its branches or intracranial vessels [51]. In the US FMD registry, imaging studies demonstrated renal artery involvement in ~80% of patients, carotid artery involvement in ~75% of patients, and ECVA involvement in ~35% of patients [65]. The disease often affects multiple vascular beds. Involvement of the renal artery can result in flank pain and renovascular hypertension. Involvement of the ECCA and ECVA can lead to headache, dizziness, pulsatile tinnitus, neck pain, TIA, or stroke [60]. In the US FMD Registry, ~13% of patients with FMD had a history of TIA, and ~10% of patients had a history of stroke [61]. In FMD, the mid- to distal portion

of a vessel is more commonly affected than the proximal portion. The cervical segment (C1–C2) is the most common location of ICA involvement, and the V2 segment is the most common location of vertebral artery involvement [62].

Although FMD can affect people of all ages, it is most common in the middle-aged and is more common in females than males. In the US FMD registry, the median age at diagnosis was 52 years, and ~90% of patients were females [61]. The etiology of FMD is unknown; however genetic factors or tobacco smoking may play a role [51].

In 1971, Harrison and McCormack developed a detailed histologic classification for FMD in patients with renal artery involvement which can be used to classify lesions in other vascular beds [66]. In this classification system, the disorder is separated into three categories based on the vascular wall layer with the most severe pathology: intimal fibroplasia, medial dysplasia, or adventitial (periarterial) fibroplasia. Intimal fibroplasia is characterized by segmental luminal vascular narrowing secondary to accumulation of collagen in the intima. It can involve a vessel either circumferentially or eccentrically and may cause fragmentation or reduplication of the internal elastic lamina. It is often difficult to distinguish the intimal fibroplasia in FMD histologically from other forms of intimal thickening. The intimal fibroplasia in FMD is noted to lack a lipid or inflammatory component. Although the early study by Harrison and McCormack suggested that intimal fibroplasia was relatively infrequent (1–2% of cases) [66], it is thought to be the second most common subtype today comprising less than 10% of cases overall [67]. Medial dysplasia can be divided into three subcategories: medial fibroplasia, perimedial fibroplasia, or medial hyperplasia. Medial fibroplasia is the most common pattern of FMD and comprises greater than 90% of cases. In medial fibroplasia, involved vessels have alternating areas of luminal stenosis (due to thickened fibroproliferative ridges or webs) and aneurysmal outpouching (secondary to medial thinning and defects in the internal elastic lamina) forming a grossly and radiographically identifiable "string of beads" appearance. In areas with fibromuscular ridges, the smooth muscle of the vessel wall is partly or completely replaced by loose collagenous tissue. Medial hyperplasia is characterized by luminal narrowing secondary to smooth muscle hyperplasia without fibrosis. The internal elastic lamina is unaffected in these cases. Although this early study suggested that medial hyperplasia occurred in 5–15% of cases [66], today it is thought to occur in <1% of cases [51]. Perimedial fibroplasia is characterized by increased collagen deposition in the outer half of the media leading to irregular medial thickening. The external elastic lamina is often replaced by collagen in these cases. Although the early study by Harrison and McCormack suggested it occurred in 15–25% of cases [66], today it is thought to occur in <1% of adult cases [51]. It is the predominant form in children. Adventitial fibroplasia (<1% of cases) is characterized by circumferential adventitial fibrosis, sometimes extending into the periadventitial tissue. The other layers of the artery as well as the elastic laminae remain intact. A mild inflammatory infiltrate (predominantly lymphocytes and plasma cells) may be present in the adventitia.

Diagnosis of FMD used to rely on histologic classification; however pathologic findings can be nonspecific, and the disorder is almost exclusively diagnosed by radiographic methods today. As the disorder is often treated medically or by endovascular procedures which are less invasive, pathologic specimens are only rarely obtained.

Vasculitides of the Extracranial Carotid and Vertebral Arteries

The vasculitides are a heterogenous group of disorders which are characterized by inflammation and damage to blood vessel walls. Vasculitis is considered primary (or idiopathic) when the underlying etiology is unknown and secondary when the etiology is known (e.g., infection or underlying connective tissue disease) [68]. The two primary vasculitides that predominantly affect large vessels and can affect the ECCA and ECVA are giant cell arteritis (GCA) and Takayasu's arteritis (TA). These entities have indistinguishable histologic features and occur predominantly in females. They differ in demographics such as age of onset, ethnic distribution, and vascular predilection [69].

Giant Cell Arteritis

Giant cell arteritis (GCA) is the most common primary systemic vasculitis seen in older adults. It typically affects patients over 50 years of age, and the risk of disease is highest among those 75–85 years of age [70]. It is most common in patients of Scandinavian descent [71, 72] and is 2–4 times more common in women than men [73, 74].

The underlying mechanism regulating GCA pathogenesis has not been fully elucidated; a mixture of genetic and environmental factors appears to be at play. Studies attempting to link GCA to an infectious origin have thus far failed to reach consensus. The most prominent genetic risk factor is HLA-DR4 [75], which has been implicated in various autoimmune syndromes [76]; however co-occurrence of GCA with other autoimmune diseases is rare, indicating pathogenesis may involve unique genetic or environmental triggers. Additional immune-associated genes have been implicated at the genetic and/or epigenetic level [77]. The current understanding of pathogenesis involves progressive immune activation in situ (reviewed in [77]). Dendritic cells (DC) become activated in the adventitia and present tissue-specific antigen to CD4 T cells, recruited by an assortment of chemokines, which in turn break tolerance and become erroneously activated against self-antigen. These autoreactive CD4 T cells are polarized by pro-inflammatory cytokines, including IL-6, toward Th1, Th17, and Th21 in the microenvironment, driving production of IFNγ, IL-17, and IL-21, respectively. These signaling molecules trigger the recruitment of CD8 T cells and monocytes, the latter of which differentiate into macrophages as progenitors of giant cells. This immune infiltrate milieu leads to tissue remodeling in part via PDGF and VEGF production, and cytokines produced by these immune cells contribute to disease symptoms.

GCA typically affects large- and medium-sized arteries in the head and neck (including the aorta and its major branches) and most commonly affects the extracranial branches of the carotid artery [68]. Given its unique predilection for the temporal artery, it is commonly referred to as temporal arteritis. GCA occasionally involves the ECVA or ECCA [78]. Vertebral artery involvement is more common than carotid artery involvement [79, 80]. The disease typically spares intracranial vessels (likely due to lack of the elastic lamina intracranially) [44, 78, 80].

A wide array of symptomatology can be seen in patients with GCA including general manifestations of inflammation such as fever, myalgia, fatigue, malaise, or weight loss [81]. Elevated acute phase reactants are present in over 90% of patients [81]. Ischemic symptoms are dependent on the distribution of arterial involvement and typically result from vessel wall inflammation leading to intimal hyperplasia and associated luminal stenosis/occlusion and/or thrombosis. The classic symptoms of headache, scalp tenderness, and jaw claudication are secondary to involvement of the temporal artery. Involvement of the ECCA or ECVA can result in cerebrovascular ischemic manifestations or pain (carotidynia). Of patients with active GCA, 4% will experience TIA or stroke during their illness [82]. Ophthalmic involvement ranges between 14% and 40% in different studies [83] and can lead to vision loss in as many as 20% of patients [84, 85]. Given the risks of blindness or cerebral infarction, prompt diagnosis and urgent corticosteroid treatment in cases of active disease are required.

The American College of Rheumatology published criteria for distinguishing GCA from other forms of vasculitis in 1990 [86]. Patients who have three of the five following criteria can be classified with GCA with a sensitivity of 93.5% and specificity of 91.2%: (1) age ≥50 at disease onset, (2) new onset of localized headache, (3) temporal artery tenderness or decreased temporal artery pulse, (4) elevated erythrocyte sedimentation rate ≥50 mm/h, and (5) positive temporal artery biopsy. Although the criteria are used by some clinicians to aid in the diagnosis of GCA, they were never intended to differentiate between the presence and absence of vasculitis in any given patient [87].

Given a multitude of factors including high rate of involvement, ease of accessibility, and low complication rate, the superficial temporal artery biopsy remains the gold standard for diagnosis of GCA [88]. A positive temporal artery biopsy has a high specificity for diagnosis (approaching 100%) [7]. Sensitivity of the procedure cannot be formally calculated and widely ranges in the literature. One study calculated the sensitivity of unilateral temporal artery biopsy to be around 87% [89]. Biopsy of the bilateral temporal artery has been shown in some studies to improve the diagnostic yield as much as 5% [90, 91]. It may be beneficial in cases where a unilateral temporal artery biopsy is either negative or has unclear or atypical histologic findings, and there is still a clinical suspicion of GCA. A negative temporal artery biopsy does not rule out the possibility of GCA, and the results must be taken in context of all the available clinical and laboratory findings.

The false negative rate of temporal artery biopsy can be partially contributed to the notoriously focal or patchy nature of the inflammatory process in GCA. Segmental inflammation, also known as skip lesions, has been reported to occur in up to 28% of cases [92]. The length of the temporal artery biopsy is therefore important for diagnostic yield; however the optimal length is still a controversial issue. Many studies recommend an in vivo length of at least 1 or 2 cm [91, 93, 94] with one study reporting minimum length of at least 0.5 cm [95]. The longer the biopsy the better chance of diagnostic sampling and the optimal in vivo length that is typically recommended is 2–3 cm or 3–5 cm [95]. Given the patchy nature of the inflammatory process, it is

also routine for most surgical pathology laboratories to examine the vessel histologically at multiple levels. It is our practice to section the segment of artery at 2–3 mm intervals, embed the whole specimen for histologic examination and serially section each tissue block.

Gross findings in GCA include nodular thickening of the vessel wall with areas of luminal stenosis or occlusion which can be patchy (skip lesions), focal, or diffuse. A spectrum of histologic features can be seen in GCA. Classically, a transmural inflammatory infiltrate consisting predominantly of CD4-positive T cells, histiocytes, and dendritic cells is described (Fig. 3.7). In

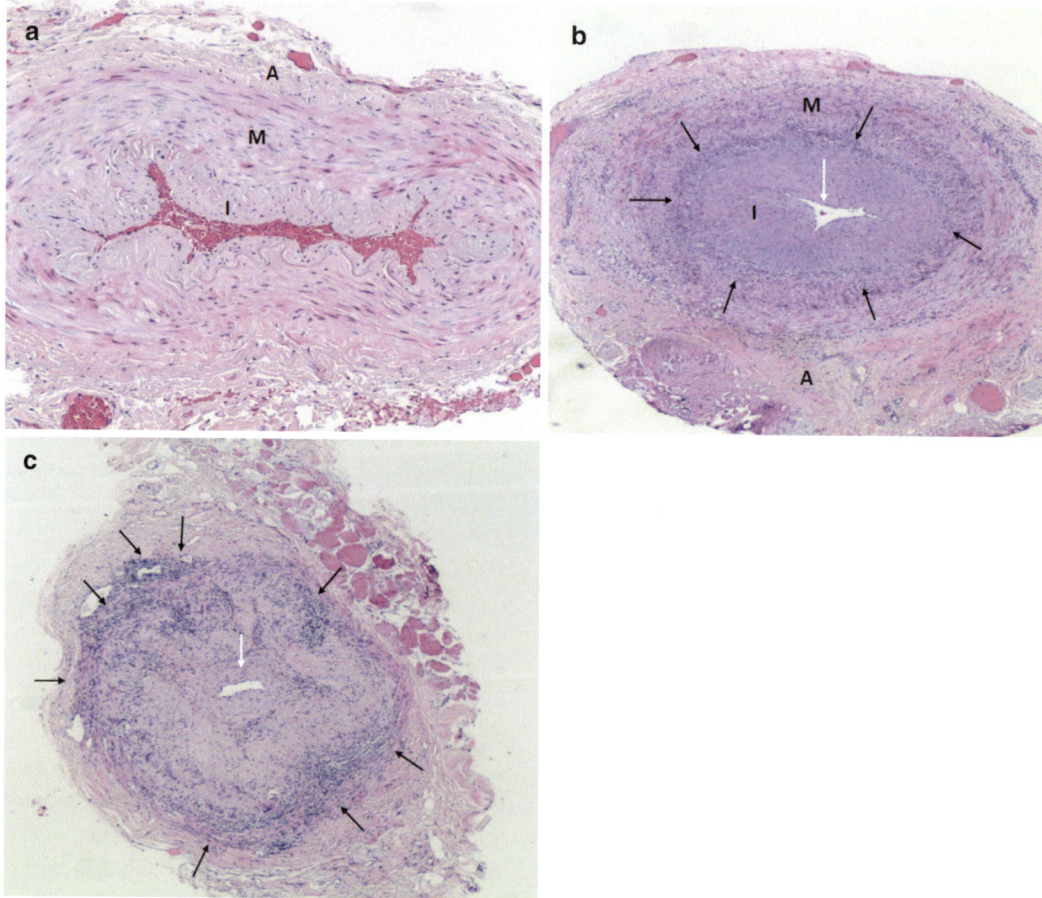

Fig. 3.7 Temporal artery biopsy. (**a**) A temporal artery without arteritis lacks an inflammatory infiltrate. The vessel intima (I), media (M), and adventitia (A) are labeled (hematoxylin and eosin, 4×). (**b**) Temporal artery with giant cell arteritis revealing a markedly thickened intima (I) with a small residual lumen (white arrow). There is a chronic inflammatory infiltrate involving the vessel media

(M) and adventitia (A) with prominent involvement of the internal elastic lamina (arrows). The adventitia (A) is also thickened and fibrotic in this case (hematoxylin and eosin, 4×). (**c**) Another example of giant cell arteritis in a temporal artery revealing a marked inflammatory mural infiltrate (black arrows) and small residual vessel lumen (white arrow) (hematoxylin and eosin, 4×)

some cases, eosinophils or neutrophils can be seen. The inflammatory infiltrate is typically most pronounced along the vessel media and internal elastic lamina (IEL). Multinucleated giant cells can be identified among the inflammatory infiltrate (Fig. 3.8). Although a helpful histologic feature, their presence is not required for diagnosis of GCA. One study reported absence of giant cell in around 25% of cases [96]. The inflammatory infiltrate often causes destruction of the elastic fibers of the IEL which can be better visualized using an elastic stain (Fig. 3.9); however an elastic stain is not required for routine

diagnosis [97]. Giant cells can be visualized engulfing elastic fiber debris and in some cases overt granulomatous inflammation has been described. The presence of necrosis is a relatively rare finding. Continued inflammation results in varying degrees of luminal obstruction, medial scarring, and adventitial fibrosis. Intimal thickening is common. Luminal thrombi can form which can be occlusive. Over time, a completely occluded vessel can recanalize.

Although it is optimal to perform a temporal artery biopsy before initiation of therapy, treatment should not be delayed in patients with a

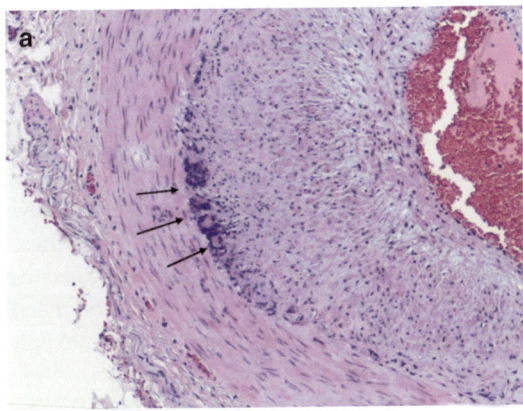
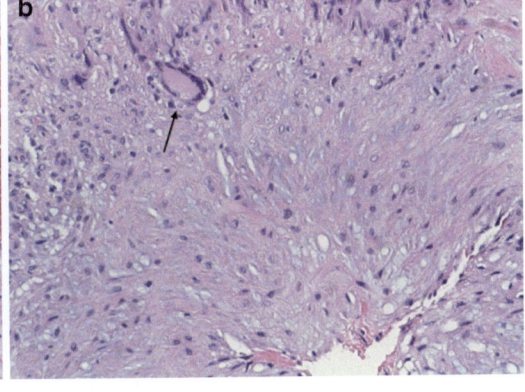

Fig. 3.8 (**a**) When present, giant cells (arrows) in giant cell arteritis are often concentrated along the internal elastic lamina (hematoxylin and eosin, 10×). (**b**) High power view of a multinucleated giant cell (arrow) in the region of the outer intima/internal elastic lamina (hematoxylin and eosin, 40×)

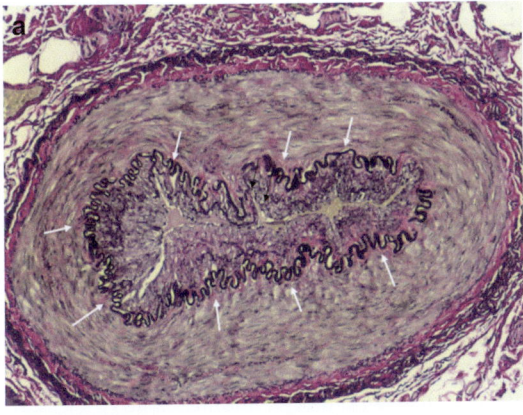
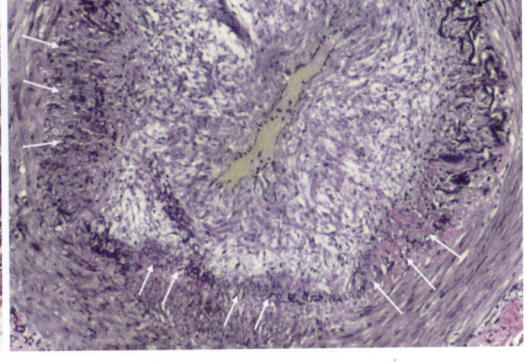

Fig. 3.9 (**a**) Elastic stain of a temporal artery without arteritis revealing a relatively preserved internal elastic lamina (arrows). The focal areas of internal elastic lamina disruption and reduplication seen can be attributed to age-related changes (Verhoeff-van Gieson elastic stain, 4×). (**b**) Temporal artery with arteritis revealing a duplicated (black arrows) and markedly disrupted (white arrows) internal elastic lamina (Verhoeff-van Gieson elastic stain, 10×)

high clinical suspicion for disease given risk of serious complications including blindness. Traditionally it is suggested that temporal artery biopsy be performed within a week of steroid therapy initiation [98]. Although some studies report a drop-off in yield after continued treatment [99], others have reported that the temporal artery biopsy can remain diagnostic at least a month after the start of treatment in some patients [100]. Given more subtle histologic findings in treated cases, the diagnosis is not always straight-forward [101]. Intimal thickening, areas of mural fibrosis, and disruption of the internal elastic lamina can often be identified in treated cases, although the inflammatory infiltrate is often milder. Defects in the IEL are typically substantial involving approximately 40–50% of the vessel circumference [98].

Whether lesser forms of inflammation such as inflammation limited to small periadventitial vessels, vasa vasorum, or adventitia are diagnostic of GCA is a controversial area [96]. Some consider these borderline changes. The concept of "healed" arteritis is also controversial as there are no reliable histologic criteria to diagnose it. Although some regard histologic findings such as IEL disruption and mural scarring as evidence of healed arteritis [102]; others report that in the absence of inflammation, cases with vessel damage secondary to GCA cannot be reliably distinguished from those secondary to arteriosclerosis [103].

Diagnosis of GCA of the ECCA and ECVA typically relies on a combination of clinical findings and imaging studies. Specimens from these arteries are only rarely examined by pathologists.

Takayasu's Arteritis

Takayasu's arteritis (TA) is a relatively rare chronic progressive systemic inflammatory vasculitis syndrome of unknown origin. It typically affects patients younger than 40 years of age [86], with peak incidence occurring during the second or third decade of life [104]. Around 5% of patients are children or adolescents [105]. The reported worldwide incidence is 1–2 per million [104]. It is thought to be more prevalent in Asian countries [104]. There is a striking predominance of the disease in females, and the female to male ratio is 8:1 [106].

TA primarily affects the aorta and its major branches. Given the predilection for the aortic arch, it is also referred to as aortic arch syndrome. Although any of its branches can be involved, the most commonly affected are the subclavian and common carotid arteries [107]. Involvement of the pulmonary or renal arteries is also common. Involvement of the vertebral arteries [108] or intracranial vessels are relatively rare [109]. Vessels can be involved focally, in a patchy manner (skip lesions) or diffusely.

The pathogenesis of TA is uncertain, though multiple factors seem to be involved, namely, genetics and autoimmunity. Specific autoantigens have yet to be elucidated; however a leading hypothesis involves molecular mimicry following prior infection, where mycobacterial heat-shock proteins remain the strongest causative candidates [110, 111]. TA is associated with dendritic cell and T cell infiltration into the adventitia, and the HLA locus has been implicated as a genetic determinant in TA onset [112]. One mechanism of immune activation and tissue destruction is the involvement of cytotoxic, perforin-producing NK and γδ T cells, which may directly induce apoptosis of arterial vascular cells via 4-1BB, Fas, and/or NKG2D signaling pathways [113].

The clinical signs and symptoms of TA are nonspecific and vary from patient to patient. The rarity of the disease and its widely variable symptomatology leads to delayed diagnosis and treatment. The degree of activity tends to wax and wane over time with episodic acute flare-ups. Constitutional symptoms that can occur early in disease include low-grade fever, malaise, arthralgias, and myalgias; however, up to 50% of patients will lack these symptoms [107]. Carotidynia is observed in up to 30% of patients at time of presentation. Laboratory findings early on can include elevation in acute phase reactants [114]. Weeks to months later, patients present with a wide variety of signs and symptoms depending on the vessels affected. Classic signs and symptoms include discrepant blood pressure between the upper extremities (>10 mmHg), absent or weak peripheral pulses (most common at the level of the radial arteries and often asymmetric), limb claudication, and arterial bruits. The term pulseless disease was proposed by Shimizu and Sano in 1951 given the finding of impalpable radial pulse [105]. Hypertension is common (typically secondary to renal artery involvement). Involvement of the aortic root or ascending aorta can lead to aortic valve insufficiency secondary to dilation or aneurysm. Involvement of the pulmonary arteries can result in pulmonary hypertension or thromboembolism. TIA or stroke can occur in up to 20% of patients and is typically due to occlusion of the carotid arteries as the vertebral arteries are only rarely involved [108].

The American College of Rheumatology published diagnostic criteria to distinguish TA from other forms of vasculitis in 1990 [115]. Patients who have three of the six following criteria can be classified with TA with a sensitivity of 92.1% and specificity of 97%: (1) age at onset of disease ≤40 years, (2) claudication of an extremity, (3) decreased brachial artery pulse, (4) difference in systolic blood pressure between arms, (5) a bruit over the subclavian arteries or aorta, and (6) arteriographic evidence of narrowing or occlusion of the entire aorta. Although the criteria are used by some clinicians to aid in the diagnosis of TA, they were never intended to differentiate between the presence and absence of vasculitis in any given patient. As accurate diagnostic criteria are not yet published and a diagnostic laboratory test is not available, clinicians usually rely on a combination of clinical and imaging findings to make a diagnosis of TA. Steroid (glucocorticoid) therapy remains the mainstay of treatment.

Pathologists only rarely encounter TA specimens as the disorder mainly affects large vessels and segments are not typically excised surgically. Therefore, much that is known about the histopathology of the disorder has been elucidated from postmortem examination [105]. The histologic features of TA are often widely variable and nonspecific and can overlap with those seen in GCA. The disease has three phases: active, chronic, and healed. During the active phase, inflammation extends from the adventitia and is most concentrated at the junction between the media and adventitia. It can progress transmurally, and there is often inflammation of the vasa vasorum. The mononuclear infiltrate consists primarily of lymphocytes, plasma cells, histiocytes, and dendritic cells. Giant cells or even granulomatous reaction can be present. The inflammatory infiltrate causes fragmentation and destruction of elastic fibers, and giant cells can be seen engulfing the elastic fibers. In some cases, patchy necrosis of the vessel wall can be seen. In cases with severe inflammation, destruction of elastic fibers and medial smooth muscle cells can lead to weakening of the vessel wall with resulting dilatation or aneurysm formation. Fibroblasts and smooth muscle cells invade the intima and produce excess mucopolysaccharides which contribute to intimal thickening [112]. On gross examination, intimal thickening has a plaque-like appearance [107]. Luminal thrombi can develop which can be occlusive in some cases. In the chronic phase of disease, inflammation (if present) is sparse, and plasma cells are common. Scarring of the vessel wall including the media, adventitia and periadventitial soft tissue can occur and lead to vascular wall thickening. The intimal thickening and mural scar causes stenosis or occlusion of the vascular lumen and thus ischemic symptomatology.

Carotid Body Tumor (Paraganglioma)

Extra-adrenal paragangliomas arise from paraganglia located along the paravertebral sympathetic and parasympathetic chains. Paragangliomas in the head and neck region are neoplasms of uncertain malignant potential of the oxygen-sensing chemoreceptive carotid body and are of neural crest origin [116–118]. The carotid body is the most common site of extra-adrenal paraganglioma, and paragangliomas in this region are also referred to as carotid body tumors. Carotid body tumors comprise as many as 60% of cases of head and neck paragangliomas.

Patients with carotid body tumors often present with a slow-growing, painless, palpable neck mass. The tumors are typically located at the carotid bifurcation, sometimes encasing the ICA or ECA and are nonfunctioning. Surgical resection is the treatment of choice. Upon gross examination, the tumors are typically well circumscribed, round to oval, and solid and rubbery in consistency and may have a surrounding pseudocapsule. The cut surface is often light tan to brown red in color depending on the amount of background vasculature (Fig. 3.10a). Tumor size varies widely, averaging around 4 cm; however some have been described up to 10 cm in greatest dimension. Histologically, the tumor is made up of chief cells (type I cells) which are neuroectodermal in origin and are typically arranged in either a nested "zellballen" or trabecular growth pattern, and there is often prominent background vasculature (Fig. 3.10b). Chief cells are variable in size and have abundant granular cytoplasm that can be eosinophilic, basophilic, or clear. The nuclei vary from round to oval with a dispersed chromatin pattern to large and vesicular. Some cases show nuclear atypia or pleomorphism

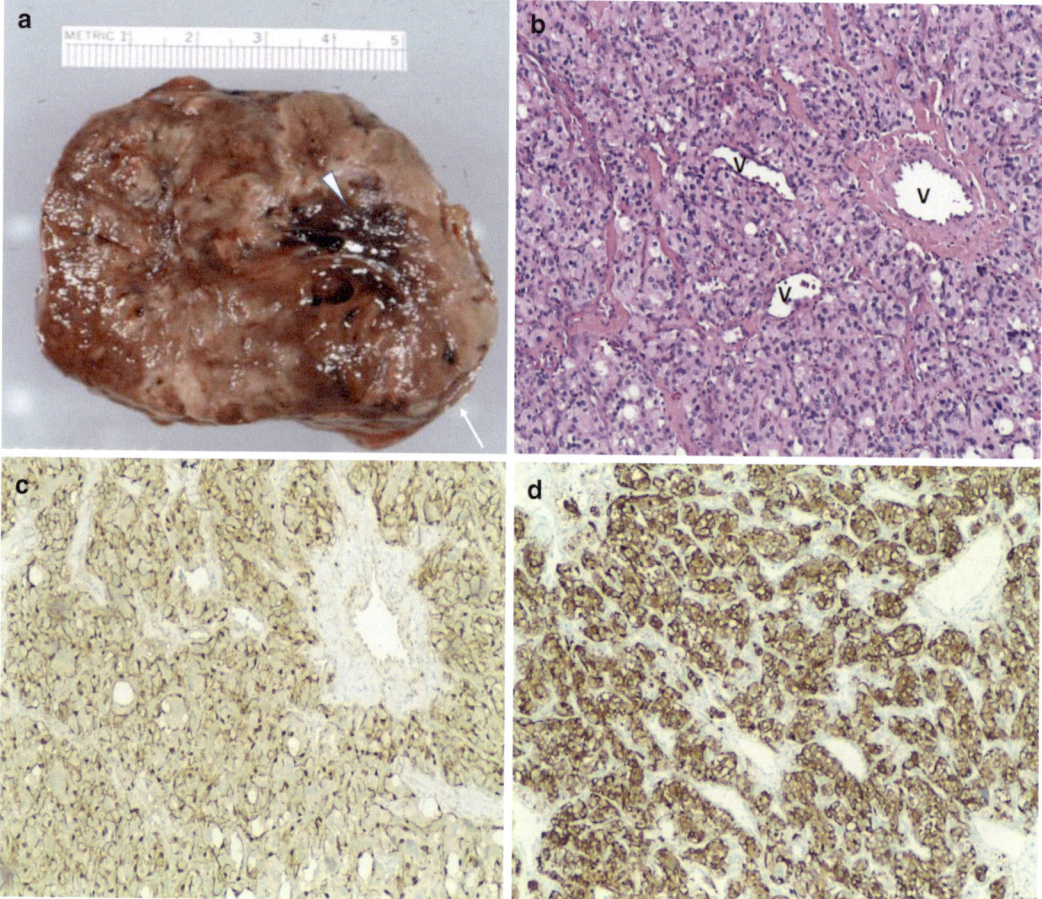

Fig. 3.10 Carotid body tumor (Paraganglioma). (**a**) Cut surface of a carotid body tumor revealing a well-circumscribed ovoid mass with pseudocapsule (arrow) and brown red to tan cut surface with focal hemorrhage (arrowhead). (**b**) Histologic section of a carotid body tumor revealing chief cells arranged in a trabecular and nested growth pattern separated by fibrous septae. Some of the background vessel lumens are labeled (V) (hematoxylin and eosin, 100×). (**c**) Supporting sustentacular cells wrap around the chief cell nests and can be highlighted by an immunohistochemical stain for S100 (S100 immunohistochemical stain, 100×). (**d**) Chief cells can be highlighted immunohistochemically for neuroendocrine markers including synaptophysin (Synaptophysin immunohistochemical stain, 100×)

which is not indicative of malignant potential. Supporting sustentacular (type II) cells wrap around the chief cell nests. Sustentacular cells are typically not morphologically apparent but can be highlighted by immunohistochemical staining for S100 protein (Fig. 3.10c). Immunohistochemically, the chief cells are positive for neuroendocrine markers including synaptophysin and chromogranin and are negative for cytokeratins (Fig. 3.10d).

Worrisome histologic features including necrosis, vascular invasion, increased mitotic rate, or infiltration into surrounding soft tissue do not adequately indicate malignant potential in these tumors. In fact, there is currently no validated histopathologic grading system that can be used to predict malignant behavior in paragangliomas. Malignant potential can only be diagnosed in the presence of local or distant metastasis which occurs in around 4% of cases of carotid body tumors. Patients diagnosed with a paraganglioma require lifetime clinical follow-up to rule out the possibility of recurrence or metastasis.

Carotid body tumors can be sporadic, familial, or hyperplastic (developing in patients with chronic hypoxia such as those with COPD or those living at high altitudes) [119]. As many as 40% of head and neck paragangliomas are familial and commonly have germline mutations in genes that encode subunits of the succinate dehydrogenase (SDH) enzyme complex. The genes SDHD and SDHB are most commonly affected. Patients with Carney triad can also develop head and neck paragangliomas that have mutations in these genes. Other tumors associated with germline mutations of SDH include gastrointestinal stromal tumors, renal cell carcinomas, and pituitary adenomas. The Endocrine Society now recommends that all patients diagnosed with paraganglioma be considered for genetic testing [120]. Loss of immunohistochemical staining for SDHB in paraganglioma can be used to screen patients for mutation in any of the SDH family of genes (SDHA, SDHB, SDHC, or SDHD).

Review Questions

1. What is the most common cause of stroke in patients with atherosclerosis of the extracerebral carotid artery?
   A. Plaque rupture with occlusive thrombosis
   B. Artery-to-artery embolization
   C. Plaque ulceration with occlusive thrombosis
   D. Intraplaque hemorrhage
   E. Ruptured atherosclerotic aneurysm
   Answer: B
      While all the above answers can be causes of stroke, artery-to-artery embolization of thrombotic or atherosclerotic material is the most common cause of stroke in patients with atherosclerosis of the extracerebral carotid or vertebral arteries. Plaque rupture with occlusive thrombosis of a coronary artery is the most common cause of myocardial infarction.

2. Which of the following is the most common cause of extracerebral carotid artery aneurysm?
   A. Connective tissue disease
   B. Trauma
   C. Atherosclerosis
   D. Radiation therapy
   E. Vasculitis
   Answer: C
      While all of the above answers are known causes of aneurysm, atherosclerosis is the most common cause of extracerebral carotid artery aneurysm. Trauma is the most common cause of extracerebral vertebral artery aneurysm.

3. Which of the following is the most common histologic pattern of fibromuscular dysplasia?
   A. Medial fibroplasia
   B. Intimal fibroplasia
   C. Adventitial fibroplasia

D. Medial hyperplasia
E. Perimedial fibroplasia

Answer: A

    While all the above answers are histologic patterns of fibromuscular dysplasia, medial fibroplasia is the most common. In medial fibroplasia, involved vessels have alternating areas of luminal stenosis and aneurysmal outpouching forming a grossly identifiable "beads on a string" appearance.

4. What is the gold standard for diagnosis of giant cell (temporal) arteritis?

    A. Elevated erythrocyte sedimentation rate
    B. Physical exam findings of nodularity and thickening of the temporal artery
    C. Temporal artery tenderness
    D. Imaging studies
    E. Temporal artery biopsy

Answer: E

    Temporal artery biopsy remains the gold standard for diagnosis of giant cell (temporal) arteritis. Diagnosis of giant cell arteritis of the extracerebral carotid or vertebral arteries typically relies on a combination of clinical and imaging studies.

5. Which of the following is indicative of malignant potential in carotid body tumors?

A. High mitotic rate
B. Necrosis
C. Infiltration into surrounding tissue
D. Metastasis
E. Vascular invasion

Answer: D

Although high mitotic rate, necrosis, and infiltration into surrounding tissue, metastasis, and vascular invasion are all worrisome histologic features, malignant potential of a carotid body tumor can only be diagnosed in the presence of local or distant metastasis.

References

1. Moore KL, Dalley AF, Agur AMR. Clinically oriented anatomy, vol. xxviii. 7th ed. Philadelphia: Wolters Kluwer Health/Lippincott Williams & Wilkins; 2014. p. 1134.
2. Caplan LR. Atherosclerotic vertebral artery disease in the neck. Curr Treat Options Cardiovasc Med. 2003;5(3):251–6.
3. Cloud GC, Markus HS. Diagnosis and management of vertebral artery stenosis. QJM. 2003;96(1):27–54.
4. Fabian TC. Blunt cerebrovascular injuries: anatomic and pathologic heterogeneity create management enigmas. J Am Coll Surg. 2013;216(5):873–85.
5. Boyajian RA, Schwend RB, Wolfe MM, Bickerton RE, Otis SM. Measurement of anterior and posterior circulation flow contributions to cerebral blood flow. An ultrasound-derived volumetric flow analysis. J Neuroimaging. 1995;5(1):1–3.
6. Thapar A, Jenkins IH, Mehta A, Davies AH. Diagnosis and management of carotid atherosclerosis. BMJ. 2013;346:f1485.
7. Mills SE. Histology for pathologists, vol. xxi. 4th ed. Philadelphia: Wolters Kluwer Health/Lippincott Williams & Wilkins; 2012. p. 1331.
8. Stary HC, Blankenhorn DH, Chandler AB, Glagov S, Insull W Jr, Richardson M, et al. A definition of the intima of human arteries and of its atherosclerosis-prone regions. A report from the committee on vascular lesions of the council on arteriosclerosis, American Heart Association. Circulation. 1992;85(1):391–405.
9. Buja LM, Butany J. Cardiovascular pathology. Amsterdam: Elsevier/Academic Press; 2016. Available from: http://BN7ZQ5YK2C.search.serialssolutions.com/?V=1.0&L=BN7ZQ5YK2C&S=JCs&C=TC0001587260&T=marc&tab=BOOKS.
10. Berguer R, Gavulic L, Ovid Technologies Inc. Function and surgery of the carotid and vertebral arteries. Philadelphia: Lippincott Williams & Wilkins. Available from: http://libaccess.mcmaster.ca/login?url=http://ovidsp.ovid.com/ovidweb.cgi?T=JS&NEWS=n&CSC=Y&PAGE=booktext&D=books&AN=01787373.
11. Crawley F, Clifton A, Brown MM. Treatable lesions demonstrated on vertebral angiography for posterior circulation ischaemic events. Br J Radiol. 1998;71(852):1266–70.
12. Stary HC, Chandler AB, Dinsmore RE, Fuster V, Glagov S, Insull W Jr, et al. A definition of advanced types of atherosclerotic lesions and a histological classification of atherosclerosis. A report from the committee on vascular lesions of the council on arteriosclerosis, American Heart Association. Circulation. 1995;92(5):1355–74.
13. Soler EP, Ruiz VC. Epidemiology and risk factors of cerebral ischemia and ischemic heart diseases:

similarities and differences. Curr Cardiol Rev. 2010;6(3):138–49.

14. Ooi YC, Gonzalez NR. Management of extracranial carotid artery disease. Cardiol Clin. 2015;33(1):1–35.

15. Robbins SL, Kumar V, Cotran RS, Ellenson LH, Pirog EC. Robbins and Cotran pathologic basis of disease, vol. xiv. 8th ed. Philadelphia: Saunders/Elsevier; 2010. p. 1450.

16. Kiechl S, Willeit J, Rungger G, Egger G, Oberhollenzer F. Quantitative assessment of carotid atherosclerosis in a healthy population. Neuroepidemiology. 1994;13(6):314–7.

17. Savitz SI, Caplan LR. Vertebrobasilar disease. N Engl J Med. 2005;352(25):2618–26.

18. Kocak B, Korkmazer B, Islak C, Kocer N, Kizilkilic O. Endovascular treatment of extracranial vertebral artery stenosis. World J Radiol. 2012;4(9):391–400.

19. Warboys CM, Amini N, de Luca A, Evans PC. The role of blood flow in determining the sites of atherosclerotic plaques. F1000 Med Rep. 2011;3:5.

20. Tsao PS, Buitrago R, Chan JR, Cooke JP. Fluid flow inhibits endothelial adhesiveness. Nitric oxide and transcriptional regulation of VCAM-1. Circulation. 1996;94(7):1682–9.

21. Stary HC, Chandler AB, Glagov S, Guyton JR, Insull W Jr, Rosenfeld ME, et al. A definition of initial, fatty streak, and intermediate lesions of atherosclerosis. A report from the committee on vascular lesions of the council on arteriosclerosis, American Heart Association. Arterioscler Thromb. 1994;14(5):840–56.

22. Virmani R, Kolodgie FD, Burke AP, Farb A, Schwartz SM. Lessons from sudden coronary death: a comprehensive morphological classification scheme for atherosclerotic lesions. Arterioscler Thromb Vasc Biol. 2000;20(5):1262–75.

23. Crowther MA. Pathogenesis of atherosclerosis. Hematology Am Soc Hematol Educ Program. 2005;2005:436–41.

24. Libby P. Inflammation in atherosclerosis. Nature. 2002;420(6917):868–74.

25. O'Brien KD, Olin KL, Alpers CE, Chiu W, Ferguson M, Hudkins K, et al. Comparison of apolipoprotein and proteoglycan deposits in human coronary atherosclerotic plaques: colocalization of biglycan with apolipoproteins. Circulation. 1998;98(6):519–27.

26. Brown MS, Goldstein JL. Lipoprotein metabolism in the macrophage: implications for cholesterol deposition in atherosclerosis. Annu Rev Biochem. 1983;52:223–61.

27. Gonzalez NR, Liebeskind DS, Dusick JR, Mayor F, Saver J. Intracranial arterial stenoses: current viewpoints, novel approaches, and surgical perspectives. Neurosurg Rev. 2013;36(2):175–84.

28. NASCET. Clinical alert: benefit of carotid endarterectomy for patients with high-grade stenosis of the internal carotid artery. National Institute of Neurological Disorders and Stroke stroke and trauma division. North American symptomatic

carotid Endarterectomy trial (NASCET) investigators. Stroke. 1991;22(6):816–7.

29. Redgrave JN, Lovett JK, Gallagher PJ, Rothwell PM. Histological assessment of 526 symptomatic carotid plaques in relation to the nature and timing of ischemic symptoms: the Oxford plaque study. Circulation. 2006;113(19):2320–8.

30. Fisher M, Paganini-Hill A, Martin A, Cosgrove M, Toole JF, Barnett HJ, et al. Carotid plaque pathology: thrombosis, ulceration, and stroke pathogenesis. Stroke. 2005;36(2):253–7.

31. Park AE, McCarthy WJ, Pearce WH, Matsumura JS, Yao JS. Carotid plaque morphology correlates with presenting symptomatology. J Vasc Surg. 1998;27(5):872–8.

32. Ballotta E, Da Giau G, Renon L. Carotid plaque gross morphology and clinical presentation: a prospective study of 457 carotid artery specimens. J Surg Res. 2000;89(1):78–84.

33. Virmani R, Ladich ER, Burke AP, Kolodgie FD. Histopathology of carotid atherosclerotic disease. Neurosurgery. 2006;59(5 Suppl 3):S219–27.

34. Carr S, Farb A, Pearce WH, Virmani R, Yao JS. Atherosclerotic plaque rupture in symptomatic carotid artery stenosis. J Vasc Surg. 1996;23(5):755–65.

35. Golledge J, Greenhalgh RM, Davies AH. The symptomatic carotid plaque. Stroke. 2000;31(3):774–81.

36. Tsiskaridze A, Devuyst G, de Freitas GR, van Melle G, Bogousslavsky J. Stroke with internal carotid artery stenosis. Arch Neurol. 2001;58(4):605–9.

37. Parsons AJ, Alfa J. Carotid dissection: a complication of internal jugular vein cannulation with the use of ultrasound. Anesth Analg. 2009;109(1):135–6.

38. Caplan LR. Dissections of brain-supplying arteries. Nat Clin Pract Neurol. 2008;4(1):34–42.

39. Mohan IV. Current optimal assessment and management of carotid and vertebral spontaneous and traumatic dissection. Angiology. 2014;65(4):274–83.

40. Schievink WI. Spontaneous dissection of the carotid and vertebral arteries. N Engl J Med. 2001;344(12):898–906.

41. Debette S, Leys D. Cervical-artery dissections: predisposing factors, diagnosis, and outcome. Lancet Neurol. 2009;8(7):668–78.

42. Foreman PM, Harrigan MR. Blunt traumatic extracranial cerebrovascular injury and ischemic stroke. Cerebrovasc Dis Extra. 2017;7(1):72–83.

43. Ratinov G. Extradural intracranial portion of carotid artery; a clinicopathologic study. Arch Neurol. 1964;10:66–73.

44. Wilkinson IM. The vertebral artery. Extracranial and intracranial structure. Arch Neurol. 1972;27(5):392–6.

45. Rubinstein SM, Peerdeman SM, van Tulder MW, Riphagen I, Haldeman S. A systematic review of the risk factors for cervical artery dissection. Stroke. 2005;36(7):1575–80.

46. Brandt T, Orberk E, Weber R, Werner I, Busse O, Muller BT, et al. Pathogenesis of cervical artery dissections: association with connective tissue abnormalities. Neurology. 2001;57(1):24–30.

47. Grau AJ, Brandt T, Forsting M, Winter R, Hacke W. Infection-associated cervical artery dissection. Three cases. Stroke. 1997;28(2):453–5.

48. Guillon B, Berthet K, Benslamia L, Bertrand M, Bousser MG, Tzourio C. Infection and the risk of spontaneous cervical artery dissection: a case-control study. Stroke. 2003;34(7):e79–81.

49. Paciaroni M, Georgiadis D, Arnold M, Gandjour J, Keseru B, Fahrni G, et al. Seasonal variability in spontaneous cervical artery dissection. J Neurol Neurosurg Psychiatry. 2006;77(5):677–9.

50. Walker M, Gallagher P. The surgical pathology of large vessel disease. Diagn Histopathol. 2010;16(1):10–6.

51. Olin JW, Gornik HL, Bacharach JM, Biller J, Fine LJ, Gray BH, et al. Fibromuscular dysplasia: state of the science and critical unanswered questions: a scientific statement from the American Heart Association. Circulation. 2014;129(9):1048–78.

52. Skora JP, Kurcz J, Korta K, Szyber P, Dorobisz TA, Dorobisz AT. Surgical management of extracranial carotid artery aneurysms. Vasa. 2016;45(3):223–8.

53. Welling RE, Taha A, Goel T, Cranley J, Krause R, Hafner C, et al. Extracranial carotid artery aneurysms. Surgery. 1983;93(2):319–23.

54. El-Sabrout R, Cooley DA. Extracranial carotid artery aneurysms: Texas heart institute experience. J Vasc Surg. 2000;31(4):702–12.

55. Morasch MD, Phade SV, Naughton P, Garcia-Toca M, Escobar G, Berguer R. Primary extracranial vertebral artery aneurysms. Ann Vasc Surg. 2013;27(4):418–23.

56. Johnston KW, Rutherford RB, Tilson MD, Shah DM, Hollier L, Stanley JC. Suggested standards for reporting on arterial aneurysms. Subcommittee on reporting standards for arterial aneurysms, ad hoc committee on reporting standards, society for vascular surgery and North American chapter, international society for cardiovascular surgery. J Vasc Surg. 1991;13(3):452–8.

57. Reslan OM, Ebaugh JL, Raffetto JD. Bilateral asymptomatic extracranial carotid artery aneurysms. Ann Vasc Surg. 2010;24(5):691.e11-6.

58. Fankhauser GT, Stone WM, Fowl RJ, O'Donnell ME, Bower TC, Meyer FB, et al. Surgical and medical management of extracranial carotid artery aneurysms. J Vasc Surg. 2015;61(2):389–93.

59. McCollum CH, Wheeler WG, Noon GP, DeBakey ME. Aneurysms of the extracranial carotid artery. Twenty-one years' experience. Am J Surg. 1979;137(2):196–200.

60. Slovut DP, Olin JW. Fibromuscular dysplasia. N Engl J Med. 2004;350(18):1862–71.

61. Olin JW, Froehlich J, Gu X, Bacharach JM, Eagle K, Gray BH, et al. The United States registry for fibromuscular dysplasia: results in the first 447 patients. Circulation. 2012;125(25):3182–90.

62. Olin JW, Sealove BA. Diagnosis, management, and future developments of fibromuscular dysplasia. J Vasc Surg. 2011;53(3):826–36 e1.

63. Hendricks NJ, Matsumoto AH, Angle JF, Baheti A, Sabri SS, Park AW, et al. Is fibromuscular dysplasia underdiagnosed? A comparison of the prevalence of FMD seen in CORAL trial participants versus a single institution population of renal donor candidates. Vasc Med. 2014;19(5):363–7.

64. Harriott AM, Zimmerman E, Singhal AB, Jaff MR, Lindsay ME, Rordorf GA. Cerebrovascular fibromuscular dysplasia: the MGH cohort and literature review. Neurol Clin Pract. 2017;7(3):225–36.

65. Sharma AM, Kline B. The United States registry for fibromuscular dysplasia: new findings and breaking myths. Tech Vasc Interv Radiol. 2014;17(4):258–63.

66. Harrison EG Jr, McCormack LJ. Pathologic classification of renal arterial disease in renovascular hypertension. Mayo Clin Proc. 1971;46(3):161–7.

67. Begelman SM, Olin JW. Fibromuscular dysplasia. Curr Opin Rheumatol. 2000;12(1):41–7.

68. Jennette JC, Falk RJ, Bacon PA, Basu N, Cid MC, Ferrario F, et al. 2012 revised international chapel hill consensus conference nomenclature of vasculitides. Arthritis Rheum. 2013;65(1):1–11.

69. Maksimowicz-McKinnon K, Clark TM, Hoffman GS. Takayasu arteritis and giant cell arteritis: a spectrum within the same disease? Medicine (Baltimore). 2009;88(4):221–6.

70. Hunder GG. Epidemiology of giant-cell arteritis. Cleve Clin J Med. 2002;69(Suppl 2):SII79–82.

71. Lee JL, Naguwa SM, Cheema GS, Gershwin ME. The geo-epidemiology of temporal (giant cell) arteritis. Clin Rev Allergy Immunol. 2008;35(1–2):88–95.

72. Salvarani C, Cantini F, Boiardi L, Hunder GG. Polymyalgia rheumatica and giant-cell arteritis. N Engl J Med. 2002;347(4):261–71.

73. Salvarani C, Crowson CS, O'Fallon WM, Hunder GG, Gabriel SE. Reappraisal of the epidemiology of giant cell arteritis in Olmsted County, Minnesota, over a fifty-year period. Arthritis Rheum. 2004;51(2):264–8.

74. Salvarani C, Gabriel SE, O'Fallon WM, Hunder GG. The incidence of giant cell arteritis in Olmsted County, Minnesota: apparent fluctuations in a cyclic pattern. Ann Intern Med. 1995;123(3):192–4.

75. Weyand CM, Hicok KC, Hunder GG, Goronzy JJ. The HLA-DRB1 locus as a genetic component in giant cell arteritis. Mapping of a disease-linked sequence motif to the antigen binding site of the HLA-DR molecule. J Clin Invest. 1992;90(6):2355–61.

76. Fernando MM, Stevens CR, Walsh EC, De Jager PL, Goyette P, Plenge RM, et al. Defining the role of the MHC in autoimmunity: a review and pooled analysis. PLoS Genet. 2008;4(4):e1000024.

77. Samson M, Corbera-Bellalta M, Audia S, Planas-Rigol E, Martin L, Cid MC, et al. Recent advances in our understanding of giant cell arteritis pathogenesis. Autoimmun Rev. 2017;16(8):833–44.

78. Thielen KR, Wijdicks EF, Nichols DA. Giant cell (temporal) arteritis: involvement of the vertebral and internal carotid arteries. Mayo Clin Proc. 1998;73(5):444–6.

79. Husein AM, Haq N. Cerebral arteritis with unusual distribution. Clin Radiol. 1990;41(5):353–4.

80. Wilkinson IM, Russell RW. Arteries of the head and neck in giant cell arteritis. A pathological study to show the pattern of arterial involvement. Arch Neurol. 1972;27(5):378–91.

81. Buttgereit F, Dejaco C, Matteson EL, Dasgupta B. Polymyalgia rheumatica and giant cell arteritis: a systematic review. JAMA. 2016;315(22):2442–58.

82. Caselli RJ, Hunder GG, Whisnant JP. Neurologic disease in biopsy-proven giant cell (temporal) arteritis. Neurology. 1988;38(3):352–9.

83. Varma D, O'Neill D. Quantification of the role of temporal artery biopsy in diagnosing clinically suspected giant cell arteritis. Eye (Lond). 2004;18(4):384–8.

84. Salvarani C, Cimino L, Macchioni P, Consonni D, Cantini F, Bajocchi G, et al. Risk factors for visual loss in an Italian population-based cohort of patients with giant cell arteritis. Arthritis Rheum. 2005;53(2):293–7.

85. Weyand CM, Goronzy JJ. Clinical practice. Giant-cell arteritis and polymyalgia rheumatica. N Engl J Med. 2014;371(1):50–7.

86. Hunder GG, Bloch DA, Michel BA, Stevens MB, Arend WP, Calabrese LH, et al. The American College of Rheumatology 1990 criteria for the classification of giant cell arteritis. Arthritis Rheum. 1990;33(8):1122–8.

87. Danesh-Meyer HV. Temporal artery biopsy: skip it at your patient's peril. Am J Ophthalmol. 2012;154(4):617–9 e1.

88. Hall S, Persellin S, Lie JT, O'Brien PC, Kurland LT, Hunder GG. The therapeutic impact of temporal artery biopsy. Lancet. 1983;2(8361):1217–20.

89. Niederkohr RD, Levin LA. A Bayesian analysis of the true sensitivity of a temporal artery biopsy. Invest Ophthalmol Vis Sci. 2007;48(2):675–80.

90. Niederkohr RD, Levin LA. Management of the patient with suspected temporal arteritis a decision-analytic approach. Ophthalmology. 2005;112(5):744–56.

91. Breuer GS, Nesher G, Nesher R. Rate of discordant findings in bilateral temporal artery biopsy to diagnose giant cell arteritis. J Rheumatol. 2009;36(4):794–6.

92. Klein RG, Campbell RJ, Hunder GG, Carney JA. Skip lesions in temporal arteritis. Mayo Clin Proc. 1976;51(8):504–10.

93. Chong EW, Robertson AJ. Is temporal artery biopsy a worthwhile procedure? ANZ J Surg. 2005;75(6):388–91.

94. Sharma NS, Ooi JL, McGarity BH, Vollmer-Conna U, McCluskey P. The length of superficial temporal artery biopsies. ANZ J Surg. 2007;77(6):437–9.

95. Mahr A, Saba M, Kambouchner M, Polivka M, Baudrimont M, Brocheriou I, et al. Temporal artery biopsy for diagnosing giant cell arteritis: the longer, the better? Ann Rheum Dis. 2006;65(6):826–8.

96. Cavazza A, Muratore F, Boiardi L, Restuccia G, Pipitone N, Pazzola G, et al. Inflamed temporal artery: histologic findings in 354 biopsies, with clinical correlations. Am J Surg Pathol. 2014;38(10):1360–70.

97. Foss F, Brown L. An elastic Van Gieson stain is unnecessary for the histological diagnosis of giant cell temporal arteritis. J Clin Pathol. 2010;63(12):1077–9.

98. Font RL, Prabhakaran VC. Histological parameters helpful in recognising steroid-treated temporal arteritis: an analysis of 35 cases. Br J Ophthalmol. 2007;91(2):204–9.

99. Narvaez J, Bernad B, Roig-Vilaseca D, Garcia-Gomez C, Gomez-Vaquero C, Juanola X, et al. Influence of previous corticosteroid therapy on temporal artery biopsy yield in giant cell arteritis. Semin Arthritis Rheum. 2007;37(1):13–9.

100. Jakobsson K, Jacobsson L, Mohammad AJ, Nilsson JA, Warrington K, Matteson EL, et al. The effect of clinical features and glucocorticoids on biopsy findings in giant cell arteritis. BMC Musculoskelet Disord. 2016;17(1):363.

101. Stacy RC, Rizzo JF, Cestari DM. Subtleties in the histopathology of giant cell arteritis. Semin Ophthalmol. 2011;26(4-5):342–8.

102. Seidman MA, Mitchell RN. Surgical pathology of small- and medium-sized vessels. Surg Pathol Clin. 2012;5(2):435–51.

103. Cox M, Gilks B. Healed or quiescent temporal arteritis versus senescent changes in temporal artery biopsy specimens. Pathology. 2001;33(2):163–6.

104. Richards BL, March L, Gabriel SE. Epidemiology of large-vessel vasculidities. Best Pract Res Clin Rheumatol. 2010;24(6):871–83.

105. Vaideeswar P, Deshpande JR. Pathology of Takayasu arteritis: a brief review. Ann Pediatr Cardiol. 2013;6(1):52–8.

106. Koide K. Takayasu arteritis in Japan. Heart Vessels Suppl. 1992;7:48–54.

107. Mason JC. Takayasu arteritis–advances in diagnosis and management. Nat Rev Rheumatol. 2010;6(7):406–15.

108. Bartels AL, Zeebregts CJ, Bijl M, Tio RA, Slart RH. Fused FDG-PET and MRI imaging of Takayasu arteritis in vertebral arteries. Ann Nucl Med. 2009;23(8):753–6.

109. Vidhate M, Garg RK, Yadav R, Kohli N, Naphade P, Anuradha HK. An unusual case of Takayasu's arteri-

tis: evaluation by CT angiography. Ann Indian Acad Neurol. 2011;14(4):304–6.

110. Kumar Chauhan S, Kumar Tripathy N, Sinha N, Singh M, Nityanand S. Cellular and humoral immune responses to mycobacterial heat shock protein-65 and its human homologue in Takayasu's arteritis. Clin Exp Immunol. 2004;138(3):547–53.

111. Munoz-Grajales C, Pineda JC. Pathophysiological relationship between infections and systemic vasculitis. Autoimmune Dis. 2015;2015:286783.

112. Johnston SL, Lock RJ, Gompels MM. Takayasu arteritis: a review. J Clin Pathol. 2002;55(7):481–6.

113. Arnaud L, Haroche J, Mathian A, Gorochov G, Amoura Z. Pathogenesis of Takayasu's arteritis: a 2011 update. Autoimmun Rev. 2011;11(1):61–7.

114. Kerr GS, Hallahan CW, Giordano J, Leavitt RY, Fauci AS, Rottem M, et al. Takayasu arteritis. Ann Intern Med. 1994;120(11):919–29.

115. Arend WP, Michel BA, Bloch DA, Hunder GG, Calabrese LH, Edworthy SM, et al. The American college of rheumatology 1990 criteria for the classification of Takayasu arteritis. Arthritis Rheum. 1990;33(8):1129–34.

116. Darouassi Y, Alaoui M, Mliha Touati M, Al Maghraoui O, En-Nouali A, Bouaity B, et al. Carotid body tumors: a case series and review of the literature. Ann Vasc Surg. 2017;43:265–71.

117. Williams MD, Tischler AS. Update from the 4th edition of the world health organization classification of head and neck tumours: paragangliomas. Head Neck Pathol. 2017;11(1):88–95.

118. Wieneke JA, Smith A. Paraganglioma: carotid body tumor. Head Neck Pathol. 2009;3(4):303–6.

119. Sajid MS, Hamilton G, Baker DM, Joint Vascular Research G. A multicenter review of carotid body tumour management. Eur J Vasc Endovasc Surg. 2007;34(2):127–30.

120. Lenders JW, Duh QY, Eisenhofer G, Gimenez-Roqueplo AP, Grebe SK, Murad MH, et al. Pheochromocytoma and paraganglioma: an endocrine society clinical practice guideline. J Clin Endocrinol Metab. 2014;99(6):1915–42.

History of Carotid Artery Surgery

4

Praveen C. Balraj, Ziad Al Adas,
and Alexander D. Shepard

The association of carotid disease and neurologic dysfunction was understood by the ancient Greeks. The word "carotid" is derived from the Greek term "Karótide" or "Karos," meaning to stun or deep sleep; the reason for naming the artery so was that compressing it caused loss of consciousness or "sleep" [1]. The Parthenon in Athens depicts a centaur gripping the neck and compressing the left carotid artery of a Lapith during the legendary Centauromachy battle (Fig. 4.1). In the fourth century BC, Hippocrates not only used the term "apoplexy" ("to strike down") but also gave an accurate description of strokes, prodromal symptoms, and transient ischemic attacks and knew that lesions of the carotid artery resulted in contralateral hemiplegia. Galen (AD 131–201) postulated that loss of consciousness was due to compression of nerves around the carotid artery which now is recognized as carotid sinus syncope [2]. Many centuries passed, however, before the relevant cerebrovascular anatomy was recognized. Johann Jakob Wepfer, a Swiss

physician, was the first to describe the cerebral vessels, including the vertebrobasilar system. In his book on apoplexy in the year 1658, he described the hemispheric supply of the brain by the carotid arteries and made the first known reference to the association of pathological changes in the cerebral vessels and symptoms of cerebral ischemia. In 1664, Thomas Willis, an English physician, published his *Cerebri Anatome* which described the vascular ring at the base of the brain (circle of Willis) that now bears his name [3].

Carotid Artery Disease History

The first carotid operations were ligation procedures for hemorrhage or trauma. In 1809, the noted British surgeon Sir Astley Cooper discussed the possibility of stroke after carotid ligation [4]. In the late 1800s, Themistocles Gluck was the first to replace a segment of the common carotid artery with a vein graft in experimental animals. He was also the first to suggest the possibility of restoring blood supply to the brain in his book *Die moderne Chirurgie des circulations Apparates*, published in Germany in 1898 [5]. Although the clinical picture of internal carotid thrombosis was accurately described as early as 1881 by Franz Penzoldt, the syndrome consisting of hemiparesis, aphasia, and transient loss of consciousness was first tied conclusively to occlusive disease of the carotid arteries by Hans Chiari, of

P. C. Balraj · Z. Al Adas · A. D. Shepard (✉)
Division of Vascular Surgery, Henry Ford Hospital, Detroit, MI, USA

Surgery, Wayne State University School of Medicine, Detroit, MI, USA
e-mail: zaladas1@hfhs.org; ashepar2@hfhs.org

© The Editor(s) (if applicable) and The Author(s) 2018
S. S. Hans (ed.), *Extracranial Carotid and Vertebral Artery Disease*,
https://doi.org/10.1007/978-3-319-91533-3_4

Fig. 4.1 Photograph from the Parthenon in Athens depicting a centaur gripping the neck and compressing the left carotid artery of a Lapith (a legendary people of Greek mythology)

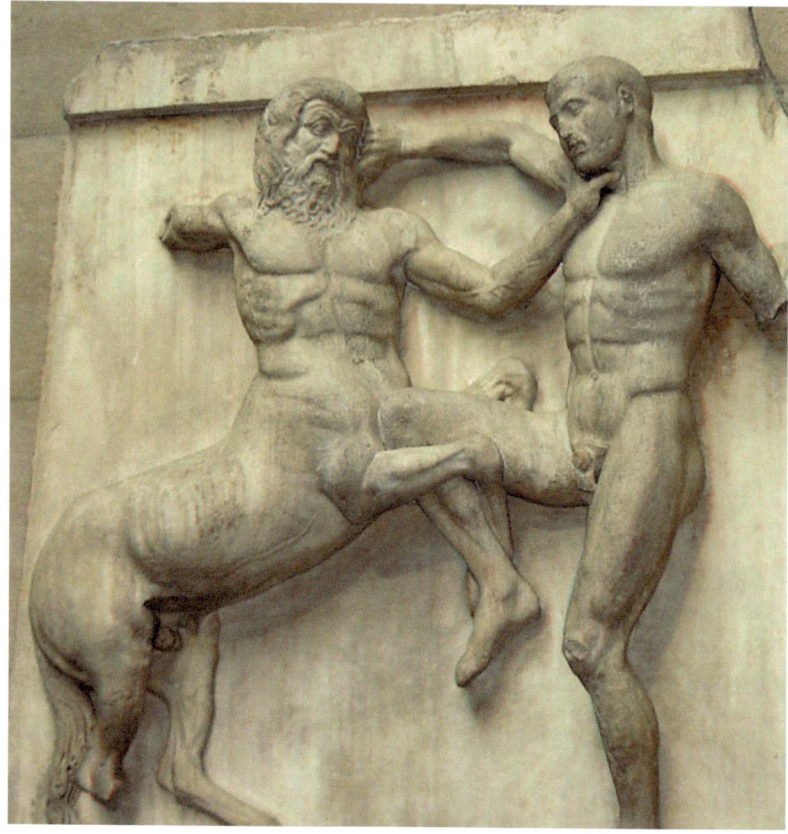

Prague, in 1905 [6]. Ramsey Hunt made one of the first widely recognized descriptions of carotid artery disease and its possible complications. In 1914, he described in detail the clinical syndrome of contralateral hemiplegia and ipsilateral *amaurosis fugax* associated with cervical carotid disease [3]. He presented a strong case connecting extracranial cerebrovascular disease with stroke and urged that "in all cases presenting with cerebral symptoms of vascular origin, the main arteries of the neck should be carefully examined for a possible diminution or absence of pulsation."

In 1927, the first cerebral angiogram was reported by Egas Moniz, a Portuguese neurologist at the Societe de Neurologie in Paris, where he presented his technique using intracarotid injection of strontium bromide and sodium iodide [7]. In 1936, Sjoqvist was the first to diagnose carotid artery occlusion (presumably a thrombosed aneurysm) [8]. A year later, after presenting four patients with internal carotid artery occlusion diagnosed by angiography, Moniz concluded that

cerebral angiography was "the test of choice" to diagnose suspected internal carotid artery occlusion [9].

Perhaps the greatest advances in the understanding of carotid disease and its contribution to stroke came from the seminal work of C. Miller Fisher in the early 1950s [10]. In a series of articles published from 1951 through 1954, Miller reported the occurrence of transient ischemic attacks in relation to carotid artery disease and stroke [11–13]. In his initial paper in 1951, he reported eight cases of internal carotid occlusion resulting in hemiplegia. This article was the first to describe transient hemispheric and retinal attacks, which he called transient unilateral blindness and later transient monocular blindness, today also known as amaurosis fugax. A patient seen by Dr. Fisher in 1950 at Queen Mary Veterans Hospital provided the initial clues that led to his theories on carotid disease: this patient presented with multiple episodes of transient loss of vision in his right eye before he developed left-sided hemiplegia [10]. At that time, it was considered odd that the patient had gone blind in the eye contralateral to his hemiplegia. In the early 1950s, most strokes were still presumed to be secondary to vasospasm, and sympathectomy was the procedure of choice for carotid artery disease. In 1953, Dr. Fisher published one of the first papers that strongly argued against this mechanism [12]. The paper reported a 70-year-old woman who was clinically diagnosed with a basilar artery thrombosis based on presenting symptoms of tetraparesis, vomiting, dizziness, and vision loss. Anticoagulation was started, and her symptoms resolved. When anticoagulation was later stopped, her symptoms recurred, prompting reinitiation of anticoagulation. Years later, an autopsy confirmed basilar artery thrombosis as the cause of her symptoms. This paper is considered one of the earliest pieces of evidence for the thrombotic nature of many cerebrovascular events.

In 1954, Dr. Fisher published another seminal paper describing the various mechanisms underlying carotid disease and plaque "behavior" [13]. This study was based on 432 routine autopsies demonstrating various carotid pathologies: complete occlusion, "pinhole lumens," severe stenosis, and cerebral emboli from ulcerated carotid plaques. In this paper, Fisher made three important observations that contributed to our current understanding of carotid disease: First, he confirmed that stenosis rather than only occlusion could lead to cerebrovascular events. Second, many of the carotid stenoses documented were asymptomatic, suggesting that asymptomatic stenosis is also part of the natural history of carotid disease. And finally, the occurrence of artery to artery embolism as a cause of stroke was highlighted for the first time; this final observation remains the most important finding of the study.

Evolution of Carotid Surgery

Quite naturally, ligation procedures were the first operations performed on the carotid artery. Ambroise Parey in 1552 was the first to report ligating the common carotid artery to control

hemorrhage in a wounded French soldier who unfortunately later developed aphasia and hemiplegia [14]. In 1793, Hebenstreit of Germany also ligated the carotid after it was injured during an elective tumor excision; the patient is reported to have lived [15]. There is a report of carotid artery ligation by John Abernethy in London for carotid trauma in 1798. Abernathy, a pupil of John Hunter, operated on a man whose carotid artery had been gored by the horns of a cow. The patient survived the surgery without immediate consequences but soon thereafter developed hemiplegia and died the following day [16]. The first successful carotid ligation was done by David Fleming in 1803 on a man who attempted suicide by cutting his throat [17]. In the United States, the first successful carotid ligation was performed by Amos Twitchell in 1807 on a cavalry soldier who was accidentally shot [18].

The first operations done for carotid artery aneurysm were proximal carotid artery ligation. Cogswell, in 1803, was the first to perform this procedure followed by Sir Astley Cooper in 1809 [19]. Cooper's first patient died of hemorrhage and his second patient died of infection; however, later, he successfully ligated the carotid for a cervical aneurysm, and the patient survived for 13 years [20]. Ligation remained the operation of choice for carotid aneurysmal disease until the mid-nineteenth century. Benjamin Travers in 1809 and Victor Horsley in 1885 were the first to perform carotid ligation for carotid-cavernous fistula and intracranial aneurysm [21]. Ligation was also employed for carotid involvement by tumor until the complications of ligation were widely recognized.

During the 1930s, excision of the occluded segment was the most frequently performed surgery for carotid artery occlusion because it was believed that removal of the involved segment would reduce reflex spasm in the cerebral vessels. The first such operation was carried out in Peking in 1935 by Chao on a 48-year-old Russian who was afflicted by chronic anxiety and frequent outbursts of tears. The second patient was a 27-year-old student who collapsed suddenly. The "mental condition" of both patients improved following surgery much to the surprise of the surgeons, and it was concluded that excising the diseased segment was a viable treatment for carotid thrombosis [22]. Cervical sympathectomy and carotid sinus denervation were advocated for similar reasons but were later discarded after disappointing results [23]. The age of non-reconstructive surgery for trauma, aneurysms, and thrombosis continued until the 1940s, when Sciaroni introduced the concept of "reversal of circulation of brain" [24]. A side-to-side anastomosis between the common carotid artery and the internal jugular vein was created in an attempt to increase the blood supply to the brain, alleviate the symptoms of stroke, and cure seizures and hypertension. The operation was performed for several years before it was replaced by reconstructive procedures.

Experimental reconstruction of the carotid artery with vein grafts was performed by Gluck in Germany in 1898, by Jaboulay in France in 1902, and by Carrel and Guthrie in the United States that same year [25]. Carotid reconstructions were performed for carotid aneurysms much earlier than occlusive disease because aneurysms were much easier to diagnose. Von Parczewski in 1916 was the first surgeon to restore carotid continuity after resecting an aneurysm by performing an end-to-end anastomosis between the two ends [26]. In 1918, Von Haberer successfully used resection and lateral arteriorrhaphy as well as resection and end-to-end anastomosis on German soldiers wounded during World War I [27]. Carotid reconstruction matured further in the hands of surgeons who operated on neck malignancies. The first repair of an iatrogenic carotid injury by formal reconstruction was reported by Sloan in 1921 [28]. He was operating on a recurrent carcinoma of the lip with cervical metastasis when the ipsilateral common carotid artery was injured. Bleeding was controlled with digital compression proximal and distal to the bleeding site and the artery repaired with resection and end-to-end anastomosis. The patient woke up with no neurological deficit and was noted to have a good temporal pulse postoperatively. In 1952, John J. Conley, a surgical oncologist in New York City, published a series of patients who required resection of their common or internal carotid arteries due to involvement by carotid body tumors or invasive neck tumors. He realized that these patients could die of fatal hemorrhage if left alone. He performed end-to-end anastomosis between the internal and external carotid artery distal stumps, allowing for perfusion through the anastomotic connections of the contralateral external carotid into the external carotid. He proved to be a surgeon "ahead of his time" [3, 29]. In addition, in 1953, he reported the first case of carotid rupture following irradiation which was repaired with a segment of autogenous saphenous vein [29].

Surgery for occlusive disease of the carotid artery was developed after an unnecessarily long interval. Progress was slow as physicians believed that strokes were usually caused by intracranial disease or vasospasm. Massive brain infarcts were recognized commonly at autopsy; however, it was not recognized that extracranial carotid artery disease could be a cause of stroke as the carotid arteries were not routinely examined at autopsy. It was not until the early twentieth century when the landmark papers of Hunt, Moniz, and Fisher suggested that extracranial carotid artery disease was a possible cause of stroke that surgical correction was contemplated [3, 7, 11].

In 1950, Gordon Murray from Toronto was the first to restore blood flow to a left common carotid artery that was occluded at the aortic arch in a 54-year-old syphilitic man with aortitis [30]. The first successful carotid artery reconstruction for stroke was performed in 1951 by the Argentinean neurosurgeon Raul Carrera, who had just read Fisher's landmark paper in the *Archives of Neurology and Psychiatry*. His patient was a 51-year-old man who had suffered right hemiplegia and left eye blindness and was diagnosed with a severe left internal carotid artery "stricture" just above the bifurcation via percutaneous angiography. Dr. Carrera excised the diseased segment and restored flow to the distal internal carotid artery by anastomosing it in end-to-end fashion to the transected end of the external carotid artery; he also performed a concomitant cervical sympathectomy (Fig. 4.2). Postoperatively, the patient's hemiplegia improved though he remained blind in his left eye; he was followed

Fig. 4.2 Dr. Carrera's first carotid artery reconstruction: The segment of diseased internal carotid artery (ICA) was resected, and the distal end of the ICA was sewn end to end to the transected end of the external carotid artery (ECA). The distal end of the ECA was ligated

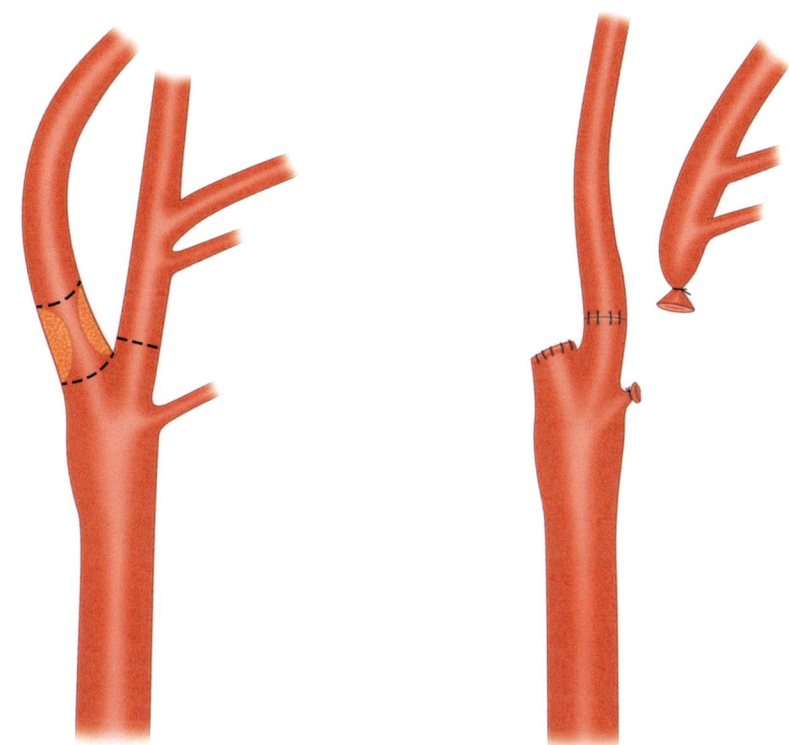

for 27 years. This case report was published in the *Acta Neurologica Latinoamericana* 4 years later in 1955 [31].

The technique of endarterectomy was initially introduced for the treatment of atherosclerotic occlusive disease of the aortoiliac system in the early 1940s by Dos Santos; however, years elapsed before it was utilized for carotid disease [32]. In January 1953, Strully, Blankenberg, and Hurwitt in New York City treated a 52-year-old man who was admitted for headache, right-sided hemiparesis, and aphasia. The initial diagnosis was thrombosis of the left middle cerebral artery. Angiography via a percutaneous left common carotid puncture demonstrated that the left internal carotid artery was occluded 1.5 cm distal to the carotid bifurcation with a patent external carotid artery and retrograde filling of the distal intracranial internal carotid artery from above. Surgical revascularization was attempted by exposing the carotid bifurcation and opening the common carotid artery longitudinally into the internal carotid artery. Thrombus partially

extruded itself through the opening. A 10F catheter was then passed distally into the internal carotid artery and suction applied with removal of additional thrombus. Unfortunately, retrograde blood flow could not be established in the internal carotid artery which was therefore ligated at its origin. The patient's condition remained stable postoperatively with no ill effects from surgery. There was some improvement in his aphasia, but this was attributed to the natural course of the disease [33].

The first successful carotid endarterectomy was performed by Michael DeBakey in August 1953 but went unreported until 1975 [34]. The patient was a 53-year-old school bus driver who had recurring hemispheric transient ischemic attacks and presented with a mild stroke. No abnormalities were detected on his electrocardiogram or X-rays of the chest and abdomen. Electroencephalography showed evidence of a minimal focal abnormality in the left temporal region. A working diagnosis of left internal carotid artery occlusion was made based on phys-

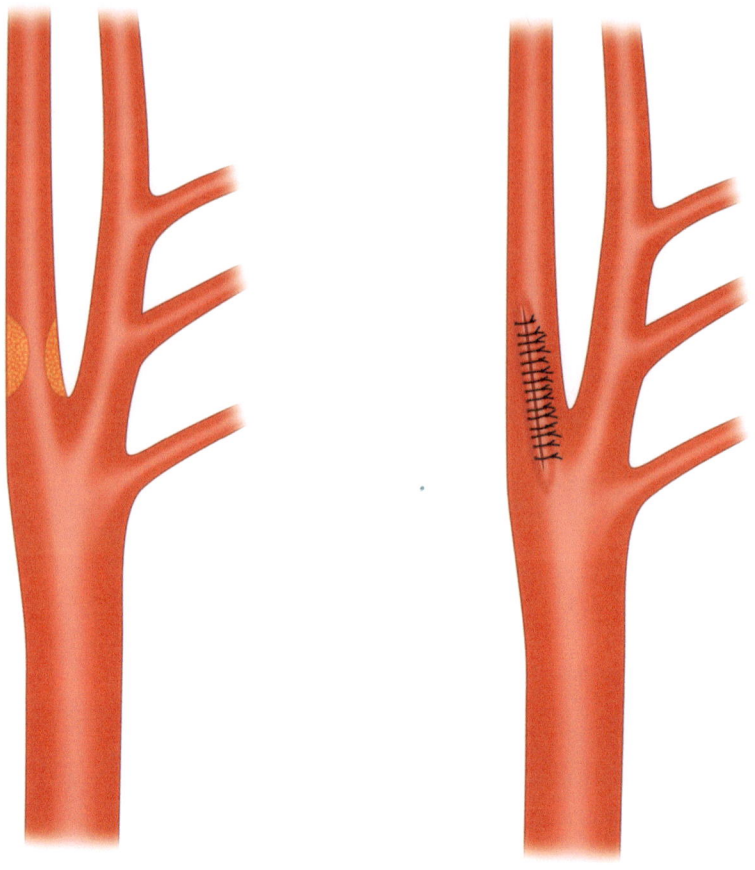

ical exam alone! Because of published reports suggesting that such lesions might well be localized to the carotid bifurcation, it was thought that normal circulation could be reestablished surgically, either by thromboendarterectomy or resection and grafting. At operation, the carotid artery bifurcation was exposed through an incision anterior to the sternocleidomastoid. After an occluding clamp was placed on the common carotid artery, a longitudinal incision was made in the common carotid bulb and extended into the proximal internal carotid. A partially organized but also fresh clot occluding the internal carotid artery was removed followed by endarterectomy of an atheromatous plaque. Brisk retrograde bleeding from the internal carotid artery was established leading DeBakey to close the arteriotomy primarily with fine arterial silk sutures after injecting heparin (Fig. 4.3). Intraoperative arteriography showed radiopaque material extending into the left middle cerebral artery in

an antegrade fashion. The patient recovered without incident and survived for 19 years without any further neurological symptoms. He died of a myocardial infarction in 1972.

The operation which had the greatest impact on carotid reconstructive surgery was performed in 1954 at St. Mary's Hospital in London by Eastcott, Pickering, and Rob [30]. Their patient was a 66-year-old woman who had suffered 33 attacks of aphasia, left transient monocular blindness, and right hemiplegia. Carotid angiography demonstrated delayed filling of the left internal carotid artery from a near-occluding atheromatous lesion at the origin of the vessel. Surgical reconstruction consisted of resection of a 3 cm segment of the diseased proximal internal carotid artery origin with end-to-end anastomosis of the distal internal carotid to the common carotid artery (Fig. 4.4) [35]. Hypothermia to 28 °C was used for cerebral protection. The patient was relieved of her symptoms and lived 20 years, dying in 1974 at age 86.

Fig. 4.4 Drs. Eastcott's, Pickering's, and Robb's carotid artery reconstruction: The diseased segment of internal carotid artery (ICA) was resected, and the distal end of the ICA was sewn end to end to the common carotid artery. The external carotid artery was ligated

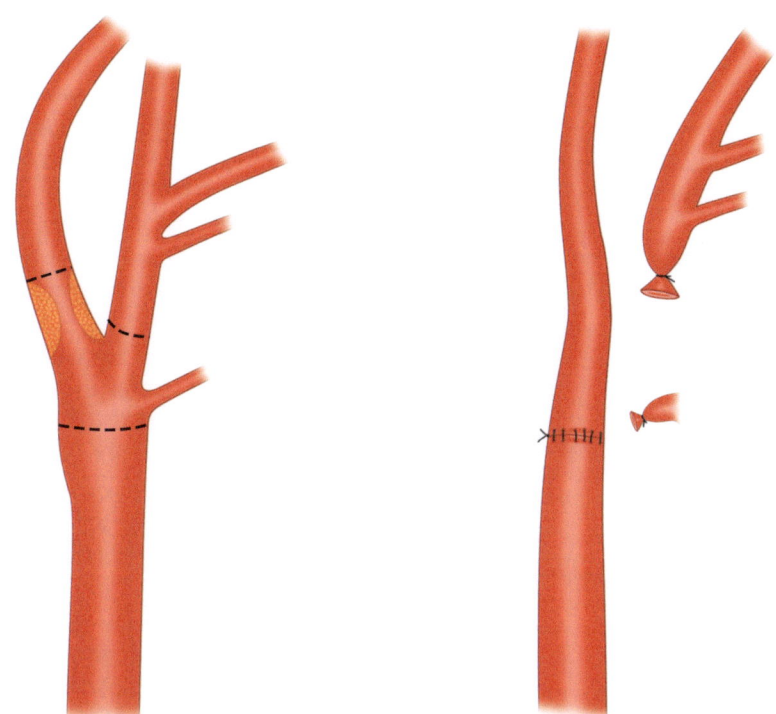

In 1954 Denman, Ehni, and Duty successfully resected a symptomatic internal carotid artery and repaired it with an interposition lyophilized homograft [36]. The first carotid resection and replacement with an interposition autogenous saphenous vein graft for carotid occlusive disease was performed in 1956 by Lin, Javid, and Doyle, at Madigan Army Hospital in Washington State, on a 44-year-old sergeant presenting with recurrent attacks of headache, aphasia, and hemiparesis [37]. In 1956, Lyons and Galbraith used a nylon prosthetic graft to bypass from the left subclavian to the distal internal carotid artery [38]. Bahnson was the first to bypass from the aortic arch to the carotid artery using homologous aorta in 1959 [39]. In 1964, Parrott did the first subclavian to common carotid artery transposition [40].

Development of the Modern Techniques of Carotid Endarterectomy

The technique of modern carotid endarterectomy has slowly evolved since its introduction by DeBakey. Incremental advances over the last 70 years have included a number of steps in the operation that are now considered routine. Early on, cerebral protection was recognized as a major consideration. Hypothermia was used during Eastcott's landmark procedure but did not prove practical or safe because of associated side effects. Induced hypertension with vasopressors (to raise the systolic blood pressure to ≥180 mmHg) is a simple way to augment collateral flow and has been employed since the very first carotid operations. The recognition that certain patients could not tolerate even a short period of temporary carotid occlusion was recognized early on and led to a variety of techniques for cerebral protection. Chief among these was the use of carotid shunting first reported by Cooley, Al-Naaman, and Carton in 1956 [41]. They used a piece of polyvinyl tubing with a 14 G needle attached to one end and a 16 G needle attached to the other to bypass the carotid bifurcation during the period of carotid occlusion (Fig. 4.5). Such external shunts were rapidly supplanted by temporary indwelling shunts used to maintain internal carotid flow. Early shunts consisted of short segments of polyvinyl tubing placed within the lumen of the artery and held in place in the com-

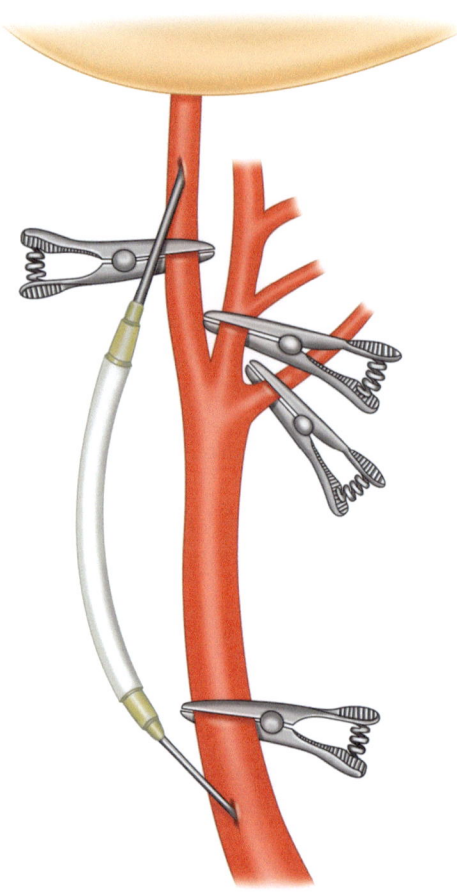

Fig. 4.5 First carotid shunt reported by Drs. Cooley, Al-Naaman, and Carton. A 14 G needle was attached to one end of polyvinyl tubing and a 16 G needle to the opposite end

mon and internal carotid arteries with encircling loops. A variety of commercially available shunts were subsequently developed and have greatly facilitated the use of carotid shunting [42–44].

Because of the reliable cerebral protection afforded by carotid shunting, many authorities advocated its routine use with excellent results [43, 45]. Others, however, found routine shunting cumbersome and associated with its own set of complications and hence advocated selective shunting only for patients who needed it. Operating on an awake patient under locoregional anesthesia was recognized early on as an accurate method for determining the need for shunting and was popularized in the 1970s as the preferred method by some authorities [46,

47]. General anesthesia, however, remained the most popular method of anesthesia because of its obvious advantages in providing a quiet and unhurried environment in which to perform the surgery with better control of the patient's heart rate, blood pressure, and oxygenation. Advocates also promoted the neuroprotective effects of general anesthesia because certain agents (e.g., nitrous oxide) reduce the metabolic demands of the brain.

Several methods to detect the adequacy of cerebral collateral circulation during general anesthesia were developed in the 1960s and 1970s. In 1966, Mical and colleagues introduced the concept of measuring the back or "stump" pressure in the internal carotid artery during temporary occlusion of the common and external carotid arteries as a measure of collateral supply to the affected hemisphere [48]. Moore and Hall in 1969 documented that a stump pressure >25 mmHg was adequate to avoid shunting, though others suggested 50 mmHg as a more accurate value [49, 50]. Later in the 1970s, Sundt and Callow popularized selective shunting based of intraoperative electroencephalographic monitoring [51, 52].

Early on, it was recognized that primary closure of a longitudinal arteriotomy in the internal carotid artery could produce arterial narrowing that could lead to early postoperative obstruction. DeBakey was the first to suggest sewing a patch (knitted Dacron in his case) to the edges of the artery to avoid this problem [53]. Patching was adopted by others particularly when dealing with long arteriotomies in the internal carotid and small caliber internal carotid arteries where the risk of narrowing was thought to be higher. Later, it was felt that restenosis after endarterectomy could be reduced/prevented by routine carotid patching. During the 1990s, a number of studies examined routine patching vs. primary closure with systematic reviews documenting that patch angioplasty was associated with a reduced perioperative risk of ipsilateral stroke, reduced long-term risk of stroke or death, reduced rates of return to surgery, and reduced rates of arterial occlusion compared to primary closure [54, 55]. A variety of patch materials have been used

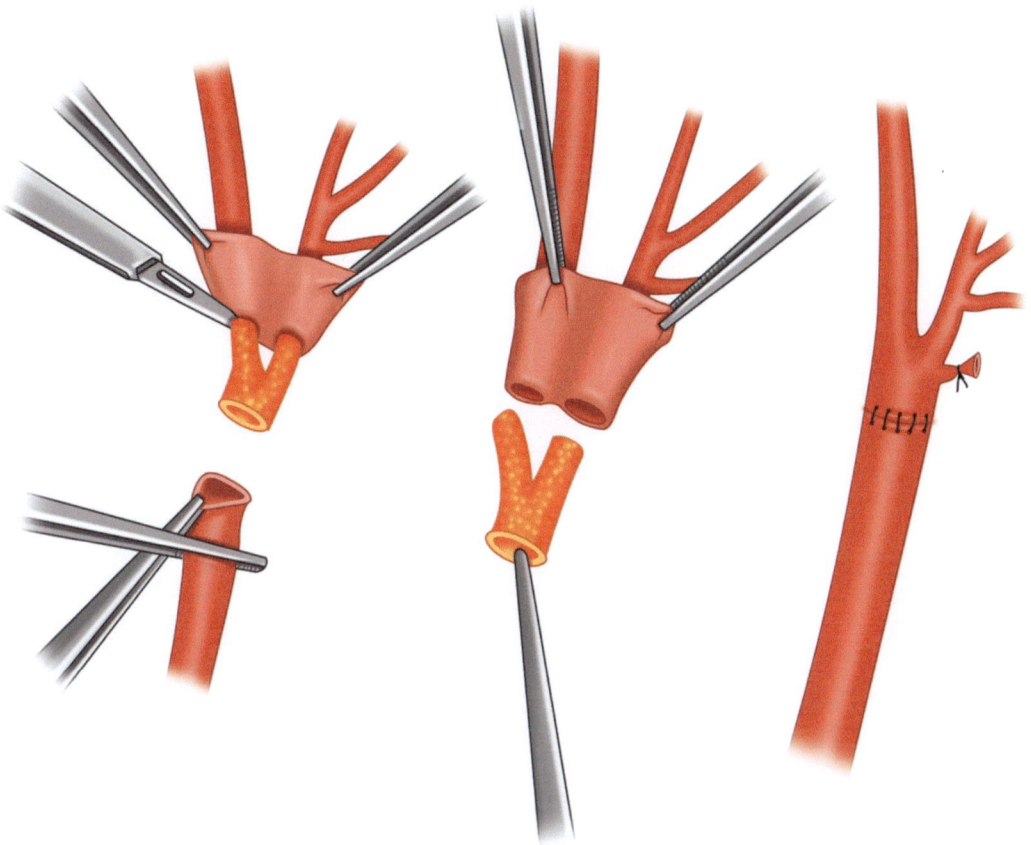

Fig. 4.6 First eversion carotid endarterectomy by Dr. DeBakey involved eversion of both the internal and external carotid arteries after transecting the common carotid just below the bifurcation

including Dacron, saphenous vein, polytetrafluoroethylene (PTFE), and most recently bovine pericardium with no consensus on the best material. Complications of patching are rare and include aneurysm formation and synthetic patch infection [56, 57]. Patching is now considered to be a quality metric for patients undergoing conventional endarterectomy.

The eversion technique of endarterectomy is as old as carotid endarterectomy itself. Some of the first endarterectomies were performed through transverse arteriotomies at the level of the carotid bulb. This obviously required very focal disease to be successful. DeBakey et al. described the first eversion carotid endarterectomy in 1959 [53]. With his approach, the carotid bulb was transected just below the bifurcation and the plaque in the distal bulb and

proximal internal and external carotid arteries removed by peeling away (everting) the outer arterial wall (adventitia and outer media) from the diseased intima and inner media (Fig. 4.6). Samuel Etheredge pioneered this procedure in the 1960s and reported excellent results in over 100 patients [58]. He described transecting the common carotid 5–10 mm below the bifurcation and "endarterectomizing" 2 cm of the distal common carotid before removing plaque from the internal and external carotid arteries. He was also the first to note the utility of this approach when dealing with tortuous, redundant distal vessels. In this situation, approximately 1.5 cm of the common carotid below the transection point is resected prior to reanastomosis to the "endarterectomized" bifurcation, thus straightening out any redundancies in the internal carotid artery.

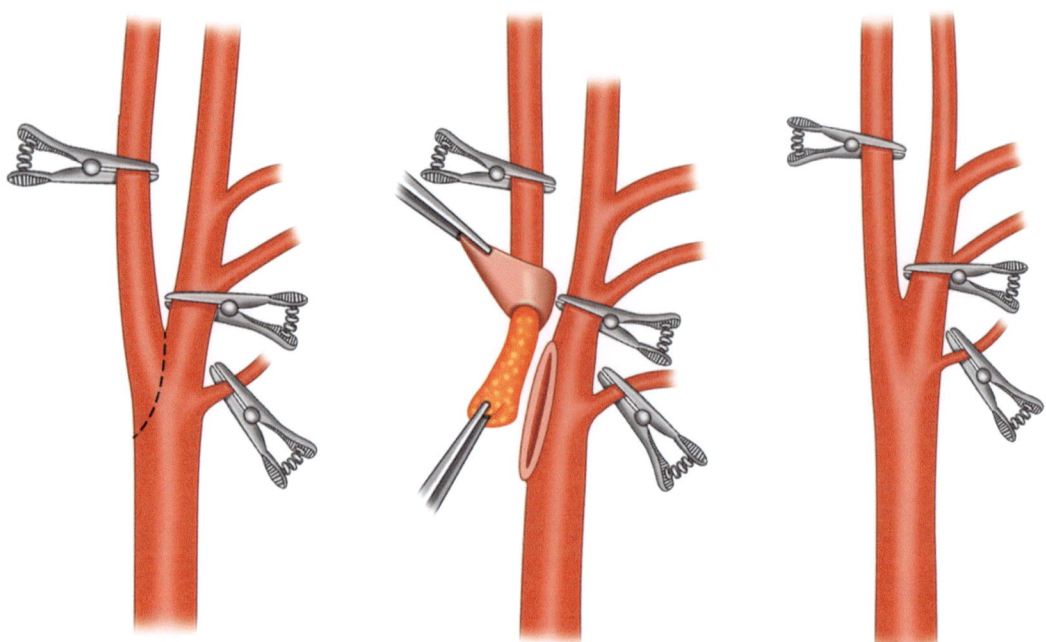

Fig. 4.7 The modern technique of eversion endarterectomy amputates the internal carotid artery off the bulb

The modern technique of eversion endarterectomy involves transecting the internal carotid obliquely at its origin off the carotid bulb (Fig. 4.7). This technique was first described by Kasparzak and Raithel in 1989 and was initially more popular in Europe than the United States [59]. The Albany Group was largely responsible for its adoption in this country [60]. Focusing on the internal carotid artery alone allows more distal mobilization of the artery and extraction of higher plaque with full endpoint visualization. Purported advantages of this eversion technique are a faster operation, lower recurrence rate, and the ability to address concomitant internal carotid redundancy/tortuosity which can lead to postoperative kinking following plaque removal by the conventional endarterectomy technique.

Carotid Angioplasty

Internal carotid artery angioplasty was first described by Morris, Lechter, and DeBakey in 1967 for fibromuscular dysplasia [61]. With this technique, the carotid bifurcation and as much of the internal carotid as is feasible are exposed in the standard fashion. Following heparinization, the internal, external, and common carotid arteries are clamped, and a small transverse arteriotomy is made in the common carotid through which progressively larger biliary dilators are passed distally into the internal carotid to break open the offending webs. Following flushing of the three arteries, the arteriotomy is closed. The use of this dilatation technique preceded the development of the noncompliant balloon catheter dilatation technique of Gruntzig in 1974.

In 1977, Klaus Mathias from Germany introduced percutaneous transluminal balloon angioplasty of the internal carotid artery using animal models [62, 63]. He created carotid stenoses in dogs using cauterization and electric currents. From femoral access, control angiograms were performed to confirm the stenosis followed by balloon catheter dilation. After intervention, the animals were sacrificed and cerebral angiography performed. The carotid arteries were harvested for histopathological evaluation of the vessel wall response to barotrauma. His initial work was met with significant skepticism, but study of carotid angioplasty continued, and in the following decade, Mathias along with other independent physicians including Kerber, Bockenheimer, Wiggli, Gratzl, and Freitag reported successful individual series of carotid artery angioplasty [63].

In 1989, Mathias placed the first stent in a human carotid artery [64]. In 1996, Gary Roubin from Birmingham, Alabama, reported 146 carotid stenting procedures with a total of 210 stents placed in 152 vessels. Technical success was 99% and the stroke and death rate low [63]. In the same year, American surgeon Edward Dietrich published a series of 117 stenting procedures in 110 patients with similar results [63]. The major limitation of carotid artery stenting, compared to endarterectomy, has been the occurrence of procedure-related strokes secondary to embolism of debris from the instrumented artery [65, 66]. In 1987, Theron was the first to introduce the idea of endovascular protection from such debris, and the development of embolic protection techniques followed soon thereafter [67]. Current embolic protection devices include a variety of balloons and filter systems [68]. Reversal of flow within the internal carotid artery was pioneered by Parodi in the late 1990s. With this technique, retrograde internal carotid flow is induced by balloon occluding the common and external carotid arteries and establishing an arteriovenous shunt between a guiding catheter in the common carotid and the common femoral vein. In this fashion, the lesion can be crossed and stented without fear of embolizing debris into the brain [69]. The concept of all these devices is very convincing, and their use is widely disseminated in current clinical practice.

With advancing medical technology and increasing experience, percutaneous carotid interventions have evolved extensively since Mathias' first report. Wire diameters have been reduced from 0.035 in. to 0.014 in., over-the-wire stent platforms are being replaced by monorail systems, a variety of embolic protection devices have been devised, and specialized stents have been developed. Over the past decade, numerous clinical trials, with varying sample sizes and study designs, have investigated the safety and efficacy of carotid stenting starting with the SAPPHIRE trial in 2004 through the ongoing CREST-2 trial [70, 71]. In summary, the data supporting carotid stenting is most robust in high-risk patients, and it encourages the use of embolic protection devices [71–73].

Transcervical Carotid Stenting

It was the French vascular surgeon Patrice Bergeron who first proposed transcervical access for carotid endovascular interventions; however, its use was restricted to exceptional cases where transfemoral access was difficult or impossible [74]. Transcarotid artery revascularization (TCAR) with flow reversal is a new technique developed as an alternative to carotid endarterectomy and transfemoral carotid stenting [75]. This procedure uses direct carotid access through a mini-cutdown low in the neck, with placement of a short sheath. Following proximal common carotid clamping, flow in the internal carotid artery is reversed via an arteriovenous shunt established from the common carotid artery (distal to the clamp) to the common femoral vein. The carotid bifurcation plaque can then be safely traversed and stented without risk of distal embolism. A commercially available system (the ENROUTE Transcarotid Neuroprotection System from Silk Road Medical, Sunnyvale, CA, USA) allows adjustment of the amount of flow reversal with an intervening flow controller combined with an embolic debris filter. The PROOF study was initially a first in-human evaluation of this system that evolved into a phase III/pivotal study. Interim results of the first 44 patients enrolled and treated with the device showed that the technique was feasible, safe, well tolerated, and effective in protecting against embolic events during carotid stenting [76].

Landmark Studies in Carotid Surgery

Of the early landmark papers that led to a better understanding of carotid artery disease and its surgical treatment, those published by the Joint Study of Extracranial Arterial Occlusion certainly stand out [77, 78]. This group was started in 1959 under the leadership of Dr. DeBakey with its original objective being to define the role of arterial reconstructive surgery for surgically accessible cerebrovascular disease. The group consisted of a mix of vascular surgeons, neurologists, and neurosurgeons that started a registry of carotid operations to study carotid disease. This study registry was meticulously directed by the neurologist William Fields and was so successful that it has served as a model for all subsequent studies of cerebrovascular disease. Among the findings of this registry was the importance of arteriography in evaluating patients with transient ischemic attacks and strokes. The classic fourth paper published by this group in 1970 reviewed 2400 carotid operations performed in 24 centers; it described various technical advances, delineated a method for determining the severity of stenosis (identical to that subsequently utilized in NASCET), described the surgically accessible portion of the carotid artery, and defined both the reasonable indications and contraindications to carotid endarterectomy [77]. This paper also highlighted the high risk of operating on patients with acute neurological deficits and the non-benefit of operating on chronically occluded carotid arteries. In their fifth study, the group randomized 316 carotid disease patients with transient ischemic attacks and no neurological deficit into surgical and nonsurgical treatment groups and followed them over a mean of 42 months [78]. The surgically treated patients had a lower risk of transient ischemic attack and stroke over the long term. This study also demonstrated that the perioperative mortality after carotid surgery was low and that myocardial infarction was the principal cause of late death. Although the results of this study were not considered definitive, carotid endarterectomy grew in popularity and became the most commonly performed peripheral arterial procedure by the mid-1980s.

Despite this and other studies, many members of the neurology community remained unconvinced as to the efficacy of carotid endarterectomy particularly as reports of community practice surfaced detailing much higher rates of perioperative stroke and death than described in the academic literature. Calls for randomized trials of carotid endarterectomy grew louder and culminated in the performance of several landmark studies in the late 1980s and 1990s—studies which solidified the role of endarterectomy in the treatment of both symptomatic and asymptomatic carotid stenosis (Table 4.1). With the later

Table 4.1 Clinical trials for carotid endarterectomy vs. medical management

Trial	Year	Study type	No. of patients	Patients enrolled	Assessment time point	Stroke rate for medical treatment arm	Stroke rates for CEA arm
NASCET	1991	Multicenter prospective randomized	1212	TIA within the last 6 months and ≥30% stenosis	3 years for >70% stenosis	9.00%	26.00%
AS	1995	Multicenter prospective randomized	1662	Asymptomatic ≥60% stenosis	5 years	11%	5.10%
ECST	1998	Multicenter prospective randomized	3024	TIA within the last 6 months, any degree of stenosis	3 years for all stenosis groups	Variable in each degree of stenosis	Variable in each degree of stenosis
					3 years for >80% stenosis	2.00%	20.60%
ACST-1	2010	Multicenter prospective randomized	3120	Asymptomatic ≥60% stenosis	5 years	10.00%	4.10%

ACAS [79] Asymptomatic Carotid Atherosclerosis Study, *ACST-1* [80] Asymptomatic Carotid Surgery Trial, *ECST* [81] European Carotid Surgery Trial, *NASCET* [82, 83] North American Symptomatic Carotid Endarterectomy Trial

Table 4.2 Clinical trials for carotid endarterectomy vs. carotid artery stenting

Trial	Year	Study type	No. of patients (CAS/CEA)	Patients enrolled	Assessment time point	Stroke rate for CAS (%)	Stroke rate for CEA (%)
CAVATAS	2001	Multicenter prospective randomized	251/253	Determined by local criteria	3 years (stroke and death)	14.30	13.40
SAPPHIRE	2004	Multicenter prospective randomized	167/167	>50% symptomatic or >80% asymptomatic	3 years (stroke)	6.60	5.40
EVA-3S	2006	Multicenter prospective randomized	265/262	>60% symptomatic	3 years (stroke)	1.26	1.97
SPACE	2006	Multicenter prospective randomized	605/595	>70% symptomatic	2 year (stroke and death)	9.50	8.80
CREST-1	2010	Multicenter prospective randomized	1271/1251	Symptomatic >50% angiography or >70% MRI, CTA, Doppler Asymptomatic >60% angiography or >70% Doppler or >80% MRA, CTA	4 years (stroke, not including periprocedural)	2.00	2.40

CAVATAS [84] Carotid and Vertebral Artery Transluminal Angioplasty Study, *EVA-3S* [85] Endarterectomy Versus Angioplasty in Patients with Symptomatic Severe Carotid Stenosis, *SAPPHIRE* [86] Stenting and Angioplasty with Protection in Patients at High Risk for Endarterectomy, *SPACE* [87] Stent-supported Percutaneous Angioplasty of the Carotid artery versus Endarterectomy, *CREST-1* [88] The Carotid Revascularization Endarterectomy versus Stenting Trial

advent of carotid stenting, similar trials were performed comparing this procedure to both medical management and endarterectomy (Table 4.2). All these trials were performed by dedicated groups of stroke neurologists and carotid surgeons/interventionists committed to determining the best treatment, medical or surgical, for the prevention of strokes from carotid artery disease. The findings of these prospective, randomized clinical trials have weighed heavily on advances in the management of carotid disease and the use of carotid artery interventions. The two accompanying tables present some of the trials that have shaped our current understanding of carotid disease and its current management.

Conclusions

From the first descriptions of carotid artery ligations to the discovery of carotid arteriography and the first operations for stroke, the history of carotid surgery is marked by numerous pioneers and innovators. Over the last 60–70 years, our understanding of and ability to treat carotid artery disease have advanced tremendously from the early work of Dr. C. Miller Fisher to current clinical trials like CREST-2. Our approaches to carotid disease continue to evolve as we seek the best ways to prevent strokes from extracranial cerebrovascular disease.

Review Questions

1. The correlation between carotid artery stenosis and transient ischemic attacks was first reported by:
   A. Hans Chiari
   B. Miller Fisher
   C. Ramsey Hunt
   D. Egas Moniz

   Answer: B

2. The first successful carotid endarterectomy was conducted by:
   A. Michael DeBakey
   B. K.J. Strully
   C. H.H.G. Eastcott
   D. Raul Carrea

   Answer: A

3. The first use of a carotid shunt during carotid endarterectomy was reported by:
   A. Michael DeBakey
   B. Jesse Thompson
   C. Huang Javid
   D. Denton Cooley

   Answer: D

4. The first stent placed in a human carotid artery was performed by:
   A. Gary Roubin
   B. Andreas Gruntzig
   C. Klaus Mathias
   D. Barry Katzen

   Answer: C

5. Reversal of flow for cerebral protection during carotid stenting was pioneered by:
   A. Edward Diethrich
   B. Jay S. Yadav
   C. Klaus Mathias
   D. Juan C. Parodi

   Answer: D

References

1. Thompson JE. Carotid surgery: the past is prologue: the John Homans lecture. J Vasc Surg. 1997;25(1):131–40.
2. Munster AB, Thapar A, Davies AH. History of carotid stroke. Stroke. 2016;47(4):e66–e9.
3. Robicsek F, Roush TS, Cook JW, Reames MK. From hippocrates to Palmaz-Schatz, the history of carotid surgery. Eur J Vasc Endovasc Surg. 2004;27(4):389–97.
4. Cooper A. Account of the first successful operation performed on the common carotid artery for aneurysm in the year 1808, with post-mortem examination in 1821. Guys Hosp Rep. 1836;1:53–9.
5. Gluck T. Die moderne chirurgie des circulations apparates. Berl Klin. 1898;129:1–29.
6. Penzoldt F. Uber thrombose (autochtone oder embolische) der carotis. Dtsch Arch Klin Med. 1881;28:80–93.
7. Moniz E. L'encephalographie arterielle; son importance dans la localization des tumeurs cerebrales. Rev Neurol. 1927;2:72–90.
8. Sjoqvist O. Uber Intrakranielle aneurysmen der arteria carotis und deren beziehung zur ophthalmoplegischen migraine. Nervenarzt. 1936;9:233–41.
9. Fisher C. Clinical syndromes in cerebral arterial occlusion. In: Fields W, editor. Pathogenesis and treatment of cerebrovascular disease. Springfield: Charles C. Thomas; 1961.
10. Estol CJ. Dr C. Miller Fisher and the history of carotid artery disease. Stroke. 1996;27(3):559–66.
11. Fisher M. Occlusion of the internal carotid artery. AMA Arch Neurol Psychiatry. 1951;65(3):346–77.
12. Fisher CMCD. Concerning cerebral vasospasm. Neurol Clin Neurophysiol. 1953;3:468–73.
13. Fisher M. Occlusion of the carotid arteries: further experiences. AMA Arch Neurol Psychiatry. 1954;72(2):187–204.
14. Parey A. The works of that famous chirurgion Ambrose Parey, Translated out of Latin and compared with the French by Thomas Johnson: From the first English edition, London, 1634. Milford House. 1968.
15. Hamby W. Intracranial aneurysms. Springfield: Charles C Thomas; 1952.
16. Abernathy J. Surgical observations on injuries of the head, vol. 2. Philadelphia: Dobson; 1811.
17. Keevil JJ. David Fleming and the operation for ligation of the carotid artery. Br J Surg. 1949;37(145):92–5.
18. Twitchell A. Gunshot wound of the face and neck: ligature of the carotid artery. New Engl Quart J Med Surg. 1842;1(2):188–93.
19. Cooper A. Second case of carotid aneurysm. Me Chir Trans. 1809;1:222–33.
20. Cogswell M. Account of an operation for the extirpation of a tumour, in which a ligature was applied to the carotid artery. N Engl J Med. 1824;12:357–60.

21. Peschillo S, Caporlingua A, Caporlingua F, Guglielmi G, Delfini R. Historical landmarks in the management of aneurysms and arteriovenous malformations of the central nervous system. World Neurosurg. 2016;88(Suppl C):661–71.

22. Chao W, Kwan S, Lyman R, Loucks H. Thrombosis of the left internal carotid artery. Arch Surg. 1938;37:100–11.

23. Denny-Brown D. The treatment of recurrent cerebrovascular symptoms and the question of "vasospasm". Med Clin North Am. 1951;35(5):1457–74.

24. Sciaroni GH. Reversal of circulation of the brain. Am J Surg. 1948;76(2):150–64.

25. Carrel A. Results of transplantation of blood vessels, organs and limbs. JAMA. 1908;51:1662–7.

26. Gurdjian E, Webster J. Thrombosis of the internal carotid artery in the neck and in the cranial cavity: symptoms and signs, diagnosis and treatment. Trans Am Neurol. 1951;241:242–54.

27. Monig S, Walter M, Erasmi H, Pichlmayer H, Haberer HV. A forgotten pioneer in vascular surgery. Ann Vasc Surg. 1997;11:186–8.

28. Sloan H. Successful end-to-end suture of the common carotid artery in man. Surg Gynecol Obstet (Internat Obstet Surg). 1921;33:62–4.

29. Conley JJ, Pack GT. Surgical procedure for lessening the hazard of carotid bulb excision. Surgery. 1952;31(6):845–58.

30. Ross R, McKusick V. Aortic arch syndromes: diminished or absent pulses in arteries arising from the aortic arch. Arch Intern Med. 1953;92:701–40.

31. Carrea R, Molins M, Murphy G. Surgical treatment of spontaneous thrombosis of the internal carotid artery in the neck: carotid carotideal anastomosis. Acta Neurol Latinoamer. 1955;1:71–8.

32. Dos Santos J. Sur la désobstruction des thromboses artérielles anciennes. Mem Acad Chir (Paris). 1947;73:409–11.

33. Strully KJ, Hurwitt ES, Blankenberg HW. Thromboendarterectomy for thrombosis of the internal carotid artery in the neck. J Neurosurg. 1953;10(5):474–82.

34. DeBakey ME. Successful carotid endarterectomy for cerebrovascular insufficiency. Nineteen-year follow-up. JAMA. 1975;233(10):1083–5.

35. Eastcott HHG, Pickering GW, Robb CG. Reconstruction of internal carotid artery in a patient with intermittent attacks of hemiplegia. Lancet Infect Dis. 1954;267:994–6.

36. Denman F, Ehni G, Duty W. Insidious thrombotic occlusion of cervical carotid arteries treated by arterial graft: a case report. Surg Annu. 1955;38:569–77.

37. Doyle EJ, Javid H, Lin PM. Partial internal carotid artery occlusion treated by primary resection and vein graft; report of a case. J Neurosurg. 1956;13(6):650–5.

38. Lyons C, Galbraith G. Surgical treatment of atherosclerotic occlusion of the internal carotid artery. Ann Surg. 1957;146:487–98.

39. Bahnson H, Spencer F, Quattlebaum JJ. Surgical treatment of occlusive disease of the carotid artery. Ann Surg. 1959;149:711–20.

40. Parrott J. The subclavian steel syndrome. Arch Surg. 1964;88:661–5.

41. Cooley DA, Al-Naaman YD, Carton CA. Surgical treatment of arteriosclerotic occlusion of common carotid artery. J Neurosurg. 1956;13(5):500–6.

42. Pruitt C. 1009 consecutive carotid endarterectomies using local anesthesia, EEG, and selective shunting with Pruitt-Inahara carotid shunt. Contemp Surg. 1983;23:49–59.

43. Javid H, Julian OC, Dye WS, Hunter JA, Najafi H, Goldin MD, et al. Seventeen-year experience with routine shunting in carotid artery surgery. World J Surg. 1979;3(2):167–77.

44. Sundt TM Jr. The ischemic tolerance of neural tissue and the need for monitoring and selective shunting during carotid endarterectomy. Stroke. 1983;14(1):93–8.

45. Thompson JE. Complications of carotid endarterectomy and their prevention. World J Surg. 1979;3(2):155–63.

46. Rich NM, Hobson RW 2nd. Carotid endarterectomy under regional anesthesia. Am Surg. 1975;41(4):253–9.

47. Imparato AM, Ramirez A, Riles T, Mintzer R. Cerebral protection in carotid surgery. Arch Surg. 1982;117(8):1073–8.

48. Mical V, Hejnal J, Hejhal L, Firt P. Zeitweilige Shunts in der vaskularen Chirurgie. Thoraxchir Vask Chir. 1966;14:35.

49. Hays RJ, Levinson SA, Wylie EJ. Intraoperative measurement of carotid back pressure as a guide to operative management for carotid endarterectomy. Surgery. 1972;72(6):953–60.

50. Moore WS, Yee JM, Hall AD. Collateral cerebral blood pressure. An index of tolerance to temporary carotid occlusion. Arch Surg. 1973;106(4):521–3.

51. Sundt TM Jr, Sharbrough FW, Anderson RE, Michenfelder JD. Cerebral blood flow measurements and electroencephalograms during carotid endarterectomy. J Neurosurg. 1974;41(3):310–20.

52. Baker JD, Gluecklich B, Watson CW, Marcus E, Kamat V, Callow AD. An evaluation of electroencephalographic monitoring for carotid study. Surgery. 1975;78(6):787–94.

53. DeBakey ME, Crawford ES, Cooley DA, Morris GC Jr. Surgical considerations of occlusive disease of innominate, carotid, subclavian, and vertebral arteries. Ann Surg. 1959;149(5):690–710.

54. Bond R, Rerkasem K, AbuRahma AF, Naylor AR, Rothwell PM. Patch angioplasty versus primary closure for carotid endarterectomy. Cochrane Database Syst Rev. 2004;2:Cd000160.

55. Bond R, Rerkasem K, Naylor AR, Aburahma AF, Rothwell PM. Systematic review of randomized controlled trials of patch angioplasty versus primary closure and different types of patch materials during carotid endarterectomy. J Vasc Surg. 2004;40(6):1126–35.

56. Borazjani BH, Wilson SE, Fujitani RM, Gordon I, Mueller M, Williams RA. Postoperative complications of carotid patching: pseudoaneurysm and infection. Ann Vasc Surg. 2003;17(2):156–61.

57. Krishnan S, Clowes AW. Dacron patch infection after carotid endarterectomy: case report and review of the literature. Ann Vasc Surg. 2006;20(5):672–7.

58. Etheredge SN. A simple technique for carotid endarterectomy. Am J Surg. 1970;120(2):275–8.

59. Kazprzak F, Raithel D. Eversion carotid endarterectomy. Technique and early results. J Cardiovasc Surg. 1989;30:495.

60. Darling RC 3rd, Paty PS, Shah DM, Chang BB, Leather RP. Eversion endarterectomy of the internal carotid artery: technique and results in 449 procedures. Surgery. 1996;120(4):635–9.

61. Morris G, Lechter A, DeBakey M. Surgical treatment of fibromuscular disease of the carotid arteries. Arch Surg. 1968;96:636–43.

62. Mathias K. A new catheter system for percutaneous transluminal angioplasty (PTA) of carotid artery stenoses. Fortschr Med. 1977;95:1007–11.

63. Roffi M, Mathias K. History of carotid artery stenting. J Cardiovasc Surg. 2013;54(1):1–10.

64. Mathias K, Jager H, Hennigs S, Gissler HM. Endoluminal treatment of internal carotid artery stenosis. World J Surg. 2001;25(3):328–34.

65. Crawley F, Clifton A, Buckenham T, Loosemore T, Taylor RS, Brown MM. Comparison of hemodynamic cerebral ischemia and microembolic signals detected during carotid endarterectomy and carotid angioplasty. Stroke. 1997;28(12):2460–4.

66. Jordan WD Jr, Voellinger DC, Doblar DD, Plyushcheva NP, Fisher WS, McDowell HA. Microemboli detected by transcranial Doppler monitoring in patients during carotid angioplasty versus carotid endarterectomy. Cardiovasc Surg. 1999;7(1):33–8.

67. Theron J, Raymond J, Casasco A, Courtheoux F. Percutaneous angioplasty of atherosclerotic and postsurgical stenosis of carotid arteries. AJNR Am J Neuroradiol. 1987;8(3):495–500.

68. Zahn R, Mark B, Niedermaier N, Zeymer U, Limbourg P, Ischinger T, et al. Embolic protection devices for carotid artery stenting: better results than stenting without protection? Eur Heart J. 2004;25(17):1550–8.

69. Parodi JC, La Mura R, Ferreira LM, Mendez MV, Cersosimo H, Schonholz C, et al. Initial evaluation of carotid angioplasty and stenting with three different cerebral protection devices. J Vasc Surg. 2000;32(6):1127–36.

70. Mahoney EM, Greenberg D, Lavelle TA, Natarajan A, Berezin R, Ishak KJ, et al. Costs and cost-effectiveness of carotid stenting versus endarterectomy for patients at increased surgical risk: results from the SAPPHIRE trial. Catheter Cardiovasc Interv. 2011;77(4):463–72.

71. Howard VJ, Meschia JF, Lal BK, Turan TN, Roubin GS, Brown RD Jr, et al. Carotid revascularization and medical management for asymptomatic carotid stenosis: protocol of the CREST-2 clinical trials. Int J Stroke. 2017;12(7):770–8.

72. Premarket Approval: United States Food & Drug Administration. Available from: https://www.accessdata.fda.gov/scrIpts/cdrh/cfdocs/cfpma/pma.cfm?id=P040012.

73. Decision Memo for Carotid Artery Stenting (CAG-00085R) 2005. Available from: https://www.cms.gov/medicare-coverage-databas.

74. Bergeron P. Direct percutaneous carotid access for carotid angioplasty and stenting. J Endovasc Ther. 2015;22(1):135–8.

75. Malas MB, Leal J, Kashyap V, Cambria RP, Kwolek CJ, Criado E. Technical aspects of transcarotid artery revascularization using the ENROUTE transcarotid neuroprotection and stent system. J Vasc Surg. 2017;65(3):916–20.

76. Alpaslan A, Wintermark M, Pinter L, Macdonald S, Ruedy R, Kolvenbach R. Transcarotid artery revascularization with flow reversal. J Endovasc Ther. 2017;24(2):265–70.

77. Blaisdell WF, Clauss RH, Galbraith JG, Imparato AM, Wylie EJ. Joint study of extracranial arterial occlusion. IV. A review of surgical considerations. JAMA. 1969;209(12):1889–95.

78. Fields WS, Maslenikov V, Meyer JS, Hass WK, Remington RD, Macdonald M. Joint study of extracranial arterial occlusion. V. Progress report of prognosis following surgery or nonsurgical treatment for transient cerebral ischemic attacks and cervical carotid artery lesions. JAMA. 1970;211(12):1993–2003.

79. Walker MD, Marler JR, Goldstein M, et al. Endarterectomy for asymptomatic carotid artery stenosis. JAMA. 1995;273(18):1421–8.

80. Halliday A, Harrison M, Hayter E, Kong X, Mansfield A, Marro J, et al. 10-year stroke prevention after successful carotid endarterectomy for asymptomatic stenosis (ACST-1): a multicentre randomised trial. Lancet. 2010;376(9746):1074–84.

81. European Carotid Surgery Trialists' Collaborative Group. Randomised trial of endarterectomy for recently symptomatic carotid stenosis: final results of the MRC European carotid surgery trial (ECST). Lancet. 1998;351(9113):1379–87.

82. North American Symptomatic Carotid Endarterectomy Trial. North American symptomatic carotid endarterectomy trial. Methods, patient characteristics, and progress. Stroke. 1991;22(6):711–20.

83. North American Symptomatic Carotid Endarterectomy Trial Collaborators. Beneficial effect of carotid endarterectomy in symptomatic patients with high-grade carotid stenosis. N Engl J Med. 1991;325(7):445–53.

84. Wholey MH, Jarmolowski CR, Wholey M, Eles GR. Carotid artery stent placement–ready for prime time? J Vasc Interv Radiol. 2003;14(1):1–10.

85. Coward LJ, Featherstone RL, Brown MM. Safety and efficacy of endovascular treatment of carotid artery stenosis compared with carotid endarterectomy: a Cochrane systematic review of the randomized evidence. Stroke. 2005;36(4):905–11.

86. Alberts MJ. Results of a multicenter prospective randomized trial of carotid artery stenting vs. carotid endarterectomy. Stroke. 2001;32(Suppl 1):325.

87. Ederle J, Featherstone RL, Brown MM. Randomized controlled trials comparing endarterectomy and endovascular treatment for carotid artery stenosis: a Cochrane systematic review. Stroke. 2009;40(4):1373–80.

88. Brott TG, Hobson RW 2nd, Howard G, Roubin GS, Clark WM, Brooks W, et al. Stenting versus endarterectomy for treatment of carotid-artery stenosis. N Engl J Med. 2010;363(1):11–23.

History of Vertebral Artery Surgery

5

Sachinder Singh Hans

The vertebral artery as an anatomical entity was first reported by the studies of Willis (1664) and Quain from anatomical dissection [1]. Like other major developments in the field of vascular reconstruction, vascular trauma played a major role in initiating vertebral artery reconstruction for managing the symptoms of hindbrain ischemia. Dietrich in 1831 first proposed the ligation of the distal vertebral artery in the occipito-atloid region and in the atlantoaxial region [2]. Maisonneuve (1857) successfully ligated the vertebral artery at the level of the sixth cervical vertebrae for control of bleeding following a stab wound. The patient died 1 month later from septic cerebral embolism [3]. Andrew Smyth performed the first elective ligation of the vertebral artery in 1864 in order to control bleeding from erosion of the vertebral artery caused by tuberculosis abscess [3]. Moniz performed the first vertebral arteriography in 1932. Matas performed successful excision of the vertebral artery aneurysm between the occiput and the atlas from a posterior approach. Schumacher and Carter reported 4 vertebral aneurysms in 1946 out of 364 cases of arterial trauma. Rich et al. reported 8 (1.4%) cases of vertebral artery pseudoaneurysms or arteriovenous fistulas out of series of 558 vascular injuries [3]. Elkin and Harris reported ten cases of arteriovenous aneurysms of the vertebral artery with proximal and distal ligation of the vertebral artery [3]. Crawford et al. described the technique of trans-subclavian endarterectomy for treatment of basilar insufficiency [4]. In 1963, Powers et al. described the presenting symptoms of vertebral artery insufficiency in greater detail along with results of surgical treatment [5]. In 1970, Wylie and Ehrenfeld described the anastomosis of the proximal vertebral artery to the common carotid artery [6]. In 1973, Carney performed side to side subclavian-vertebral anastomosis as well as segmental resection of the vertebral artery followed by primary anastomosis at the level of C2.

Berguer, Andaya, and Bauer described the vein bypass from subclavian to proximal vertebral artery in 1977. In the same year, Cormier and Laurian presented an extensive experience in vertebral reconstructions [7]. Carney and associates performed the first vein bypass from the common carotid artery to the distal vertebral artery.

George and Laurian reported their experience in 1980 with special reference to operations on the third portion of the vertebral artery [8]. Giangola et al. in 1991 reported 136 vertebral artery reconstructions performed since 1964 [9]. These authors performed vertebral artery angioplasty with vein patch, carotid to vertebral artery bypass,

S. S. Hans
Medical Director of Vascular and Endovascular Services, Henry Ford Macomb Hospital, Clinton Township, MI, USA

Chief of Vascular Surgery, St. John Macomb Hospital, Warren, MI, USA

Department of Surgery, Wayne State University School of Medicine, Detroit, MI, USA

© The Editor(s) (if applicable) and The Author(s) 2018
S. S. Hans (ed.), *Extracranial Carotid and Vertebral Artery Disease*,
https://doi.org/10.1007/978-3-319-91533-3_5

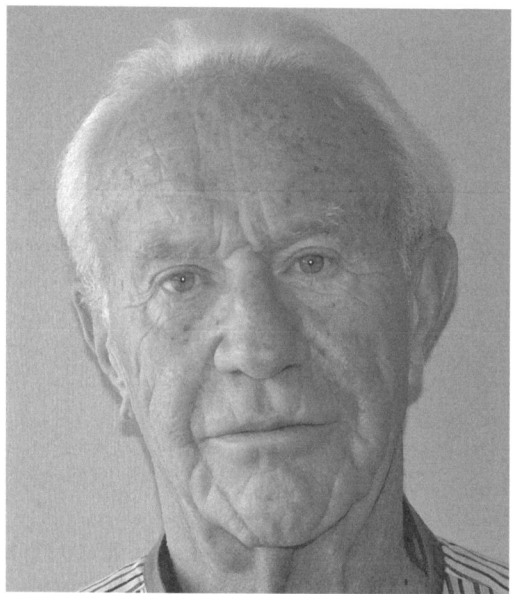

Fig. 5.1 Dr. Ramon Berguer (1941–)

and reimplantation of the vertebral artery into the common carotid artery. Berguer emphasized that nearly all proximal vertebral artery reconstructions can be performed by transposing its first segment to the common carotid artery with excellent patency of 99% at 5 years [10]. The same author described the reconstruction of distal vertebral artery by using vein bypass from the common carotid artery [11]. The other options include transposition of the external carotid artery to vertebral artery, transposition of the occipital artery to vertebral artery, and transposition of the vertebral artery to high cervical ICA. For all of these options, exposure of the third portion of the vertebral artery at the level of C1–C2 is necessary as more length of the vertebral artery is accessible between the two transverse processes and is distal to the site where the vertebral artery may be compressed by osteophytes secondary to degenerative cervical osteoarthritis. In addition, vertebral artery usually reconstitutes at this level in patients when vertebral artery (V2) has occluded in its intracervical course [11]. Dr. Ramon Berguer (Fig. 5.1) had made the greatest contributions in the field of vertebral artery reconstruction during the past 50 years. He has seminal publications

pertaining to vertebral artery reconstruction and has also published two books in the management of carotid and vertebral artery disease as an editor and sole author [10–12].

Extracranial vertebral artery disease can also be managed by endovascular techniques such as angioplasty and stenting as sophisticated new endovascular techniques are being introduced. Surgical treatment for vertebral artery atherosclerotic lesions may become less common as the endovascular management evolves.

Review Questions
1. The first successful excision of vertebral artery aneurysm was performed by:
   A. Moniz
   B. Matas
   C. Schumacher and Carter
   D. Rich

   Answer: B

2. Subclavian to vertebral artery bypass was first performed by:
   A. Wylie
   B. Berguer
   C. Carney
   D. Crawford

   Answer: B

3. Elective ligation of vertebral artery to control bleeding was first performed by:
   A. Moniz
   B. Maisonneuve
   C. Andrew Smyth
   D. Powers

   Answer: C

References

1. Quain R. The anatomy of the arteries of the human body, with its applications to pathology and operative surgery. In: lithographic drawings with practical commentaries. London: Taylor and Walton; 1844.
2. Dietrich. Transactions of the first Pan-American Medical Congress. Medicine. Washington: Government Printing Office; 1895.

3. Carney AL. Vertebral artery surgery: historical development, basic concepts of brain hemodynamics, and clinical experience of 102 cases. Adv Neurol. 1981;30:249–82.
4. Crawford ES, De Bakey ME, Fields WS. Roentgenographic diagnosis and surgical treatment of basilar artery insufficiency. JAMA. 1958;168(5):509–14.
5. Powers SR Jr, Drislane TM, Iandoli EW. The surgical treatment of vertebral artery insufficiency successes and failures. Arch Surg. 1963;86(1):60–4.
6. Wylie EJ, Ehrenfeld WK. Extracranial occlusive cerebrovascular disease: diagnosis and management. Philadelphia: W. B. Saunders; 1970.
7. Cormier JM, Laurian C. Surgical management of vertebral-basilar insufficiency. J Cardiovasc Surg. 1976;17(3):205–23.
8. George B, Laurian C. The vertebral artery. Pathology and surgery. New York: Springer; 1987.
9. Giangola G, Imparato AM, Riles TS, Lamparello PJ. Vertebral artery angioplasty in patients younger than 55 years: long-term follow-up. Ann Vasc Surg. 1991;5(2):121–4.
10. Buerger R. Vertebral artery reconstructions. Ann Surg. 1981;193:441–7.
11. Buerger R, Morasch MD, Kline RA. A review of 100 consecutive reconstructions of the distal vertebral artery for embolic and hemodynamic disease. J Vasc Surg. 1998;27(5):852–9.
12. Berguer R, Andaya LV, Bauer RB. Vertebral artery bypass. Arch Surg. 1976;111:976–9.

Noninvasive Vascular Lab Testing for Carotids, Vertebrals, and Transcranial Doppler

6

Hosam Farouk El Sayed, Nicolas J. Mouawad, and Bhagwan Satiani

Overview

Cerebrovascular angiography remains the gold standard for evaluation of extracranial cerebrovascular disease. However, this procedure is invasive and carries definite risks including access site complications, contrast-related complications, and even embolic-related neurologic deficits that can reach 1% of angiography diagnostic procedures [1]. Over the past several decades, there have been significant advances in the development of noninvasive diagnostic modalities for extracranial cerebrovascular disease including computed tomographic angiography (CTA), magnetic resonance angiography (MRA), and ultrasound.

Ultrasound was first applied to study the carotid circulation as early as 1954, but it was not until 1967 that its clinical application in velocity detection was reported. In 1971, Hokanson, working in Eugene Strandness' laboratory at the University of Washington in Seattle, provided the first noninvasive visualization of an arterial segment using pulsed Doppler methods [2, 3].

The goals of noninvasive testing of cerebrovascular disease include:

1. To distinguish normal from diseased vessels
2. To classify the degree of stenosis of the carotid artery
3. To determine the surface and internal features of the atherosclerotic plaque
4. To assess the cerebral collateral circulation
5. To be safe and cost-effective

From the clinical point of view, the primary goal is to identify patients who are at risk for stroke and who may benefit from specific treatment options. A secondary goal is to document progressive or recurrent disease in patients already known to be at risk.

Carotid Artery and Vertebral Artery Duplex

Noninvasive carotid testing can be considered as either indirect or direct. The indirect tests, such as supraorbital Doppler and oculoplethysmography, are of limited value and no longer widely used. Duplex scanning has become the standard noninvasive method for extracranial carotid evaluation. This combination of B-mode imaging, pulsed Doppler spectral analysis, and color flow imaging provides both anatomic and physiologic information on the vessels of inter-

H. F. El Sayed · B. Satiani (✉)
Department of Surgery, Division of Vascular Surgery and Diseases, The Ohio State University College of Medicine, Columbus, OH, USA
e-mail: bhagwan.satiani@osumc.edu

N. J. Mouawad
McLaren Bay Region Hospital, Bay City, MI, USA

© The Editor(s) (if applicable) and The Author(s) 2018
S. S. Hans (ed.), *Extracranial Carotid and Vertebral Artery Disease*,
https://doi.org/10.1007/978-3-319-91533-3_6

est [4, 5]. B-mode imaging, which is essentially gray-scale imaging, has been used to evaluate the carotid plaque morphology at the level of the carotid bifurcation and to assess the histologic features of the plaques; however, the clinical relevance of this information is somewhat controversial [6, 7] (Fig. 6.1). The B-mode can classify plaques according to their echogenicity into hypoechoic-like soft plaques, hyperechoic-like calcific plaques, or isoechoic (Fig. 6.2). It can also detect if the plaque is of homogeneous or heterogeneous echogenicity that may be attributed to the presence of intra-plaque hemorrhage. This feature has been noted more frequently in patients with neurologic events than in asymptomatic carotid stenosis [2]. However, B-mode imaging cannot be used to determine the size of the arterial lumen or the degree of stenosis because the interface between the arterial wall and the flow in blood is not always clearly seen. Also, acoustic shadowing from calcified plaques may prevent thorough visualization of the arterial wall and lumen [8] (Fig. 6.3). These limitations are overcome by adding pulsed Doppler flow sampling, i.e., duplex technology. Using B-mode imaging as a guide for the precise placement of the pulsed Doppler gate, velocity measurements and spectral sound analysis of the Doppler signals can be used to determine the degree of stenosis in the carotid (Fig. 6.4). The color duplex scanner utilizes many sampling sites to determine the

backscattered frequency and visually depicts this information as a real-time flow image. The color depiction of the frequencies facilitates the examination and identification of focal areas of abnormal flow patterns. In other words, the color flow imaging presents simultaneous flow information on the entire image [2] (Fig. 6.3). The accuracy of carotid duplex in evaluating carotid disease has been reported by multiple investigators to be in the 90% or more range [9–12]. It should be noted that some degree of variability is unavoidable in physiologic measurements such as duplex scanning. In the carotid duplex scan, the greatest variability or mismatch compared to a gold standard such as arteriography is in the moderately stenotic internal carotid arteries. The agreement is much better or >95% for normal arteries or those with greater than 70% stenosis. Studies have shown that the agreement between duplex scanning and arteriography is equivalent to the agreement between two radiologists interpreting the same arteriograms [5, 13].

The extracranial vertebral-basilar duplex examination includes longitudinal B-mode scan of the vertebral artery in the mid-cervical portion followed by the origin and the most distal portion accessible in the neck. Duplex ultrasound allows evaluation of the vertebral artery flow between the transverse processes in 96–100% of cases and visualization of the vertebral artery origins in 65–90% of the patients [14]. The spectrum of

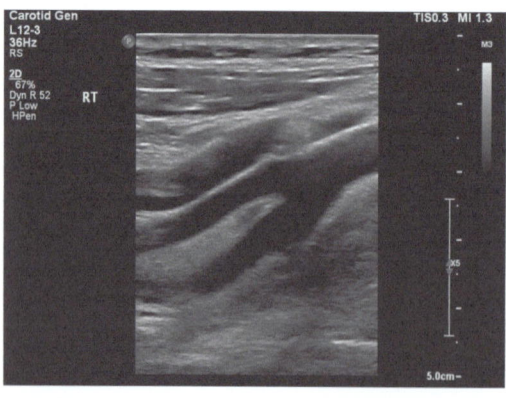

Fig. 6.1 Sagittal view of the carotid bifurcation in B-mode showing a normal carotid bifurcation

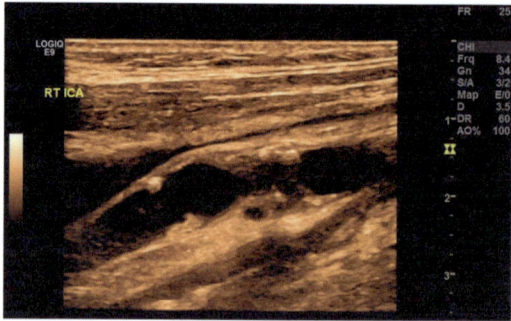

Fig. 6.2 Sagittal B-mode view of the internal carotid artery showing a mixed plaque with both hyperechoic (white) and hypoechoic (dark or black) areas within the plaque

Fig. 6.3 Internal carotid color flow image showing calcified plaque (in white) with shadowing under it (red arrow). Abnormal spectral Doppler signals are obtained in an area of less calcification showing probable 50–69% stenosis based upon our criteria

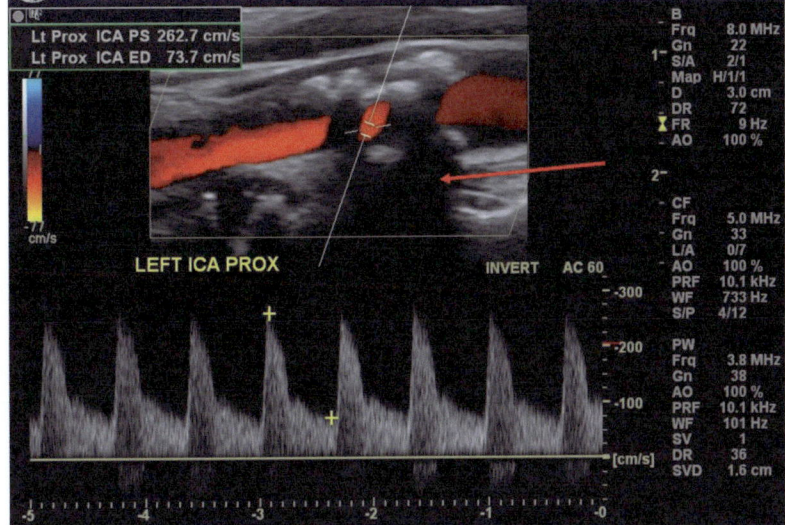

Fig. 6.4 Color flow and spectral Doppler image of the left internal carotid artery showing peak systolic velocities of 636 cm/s and end-diastolic velocities of 182 cm/s consistent with a 70–99% stenosis. The color image also shows color "aliasing" indicating a high-grade lesion

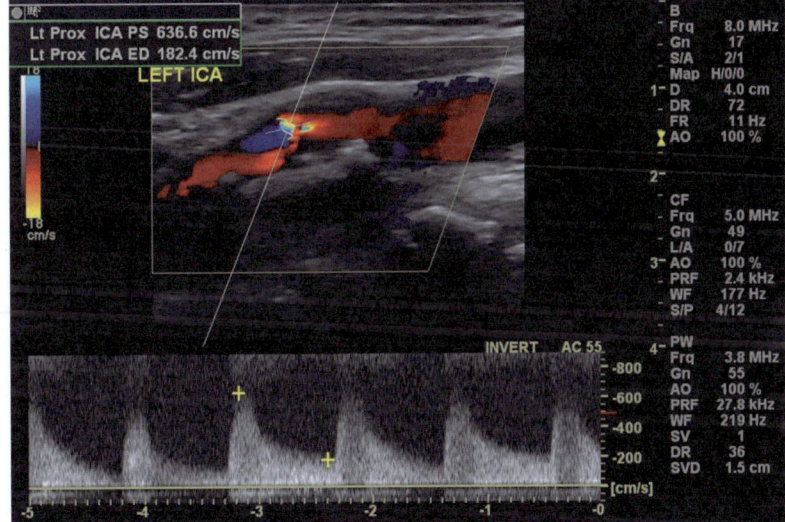

vertebral pathology detectable by duplex scanning includes:

1. Vertebral artery occlusion or absence of flow
2. Hypoplastic vertebral artery
3. Subclavian steal

Unfortunately, there are no established criteria for grading various degrees of extracranial vertebral artery stenosis [14]. The normal flow of the vertebral is antegrade with a peak systolic velocity in the vertebral artery of 40–50 cm/s (Fig. 6.5). The velocity may be low in subdominant or hypoplastic vertebral artery. Subclavian artery steal is a hemodynamic phenomenon indicating stenosis or occlusion of the proximal subclavian artery where flow in the vertebral artery is reversed (Fig. 6.6). The "hyperemia" test can provoke flow reversal in patients with latent steal. A blood pressure cuff is inflated in the ipsilateral arm to supra-systolic values, and the patient is asked to perform physical exercise

Fig. 6.5 Color flow image of the vertebral artery showing antegrade flow. Red arrow indicated acoustic shadowing from the vertebral process through which the vertebral artery travels

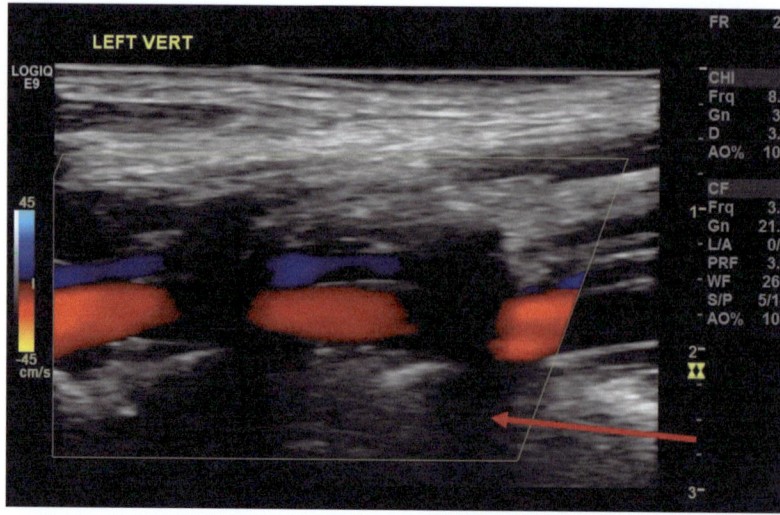

Fig. 6.6 Spectral Doppler showing reverse or retrograde flow in the vertebral artery. Color part of the image also confirms retrograde flow with the blue color indicating flow going away from the Doppler probe

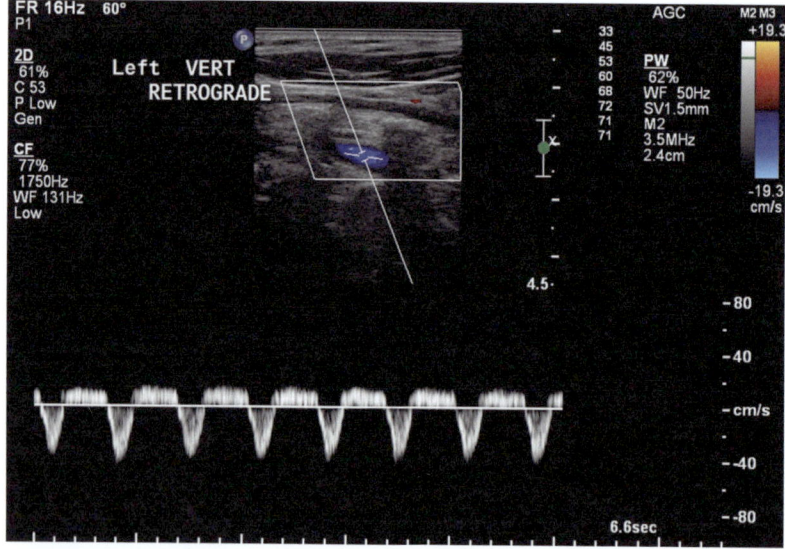

with that arm to increase the metabolic demand and vasodilatation. Upon sudden cuff release, a systolic flow reversal with low diastolic antegrade flow is seen indicating latent steal [14] (Fig. 6.7). The so-called alternating flow signal ("bunny rabbit") or total reversal of flow at rest represents different stages of subclavian steal phenomenon (Fig. 6.7). It is called a syndrome if clinical symptoms of posterior circulation ischemia develop [14, 15].

Indications of Carotid and Vertebral Scanning

Vascular laboratories are currently charged with assessing appropriateness of testing by both third-party reimbursement agencies and accrediting bodies. There are established guidelines for appropriateness of testing but may vary by country, state to state, and by insurer carrier [16, 17]. Laboratory personnel must stay current with

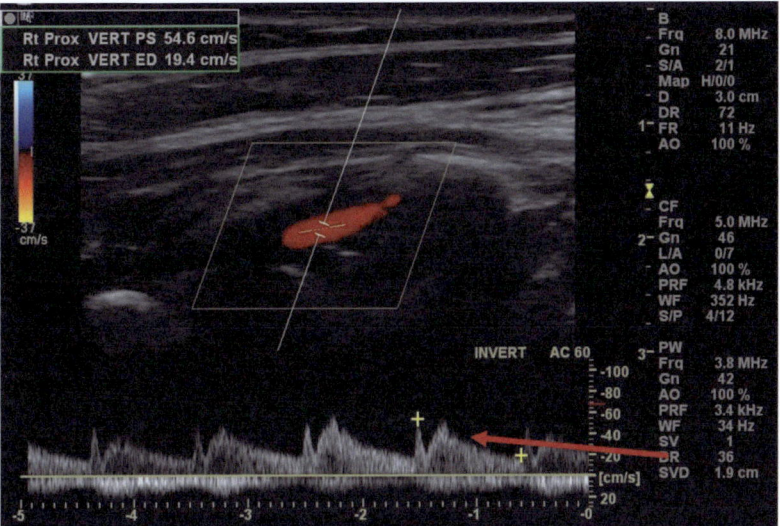

Fig. 6.7 Spectral Doppler showing a "bunny rabbit" waveform indicating latent or occult subclavian stenosis

what are determined to be appropriate indicators in their region. Generally accepted indications include but are not limited to:

- Stroke
- Transient ischemic attacks including weakness of one side of the face, slurred speech, weakness of a limb, or hemispheric field defects
- Amaurosis fugax/other visual disturbances
- Non-hemispheric neurologic symptoms and syncope
- Carotid bruit
- Pulsatile neck mass
- Follow-up of carotid endarterectomy
- Anatomic delineation of carotid system for head and neck surgery
- Follow-up of asymptomatic carotid stenosis
- Preoperative evaluation—heart and other major surgeries
- Injury or trauma to the neck
- Suspicion of subclavian steal

If indications are not documented, or if there is a question regarding the appropriateness of the indications, the referring physician should be contacted for clarification. It is also important to check with the specific state Medicare carrier or other

third-party carriers if the laboratory is not sure of the appropriateness of the indication for the study.

Contraindications and Limitations of Scanning

The presence of open neck wounds at the site of scanning, central venous lines, dressings of surgery, and staples are all limitations to scanning as scanning may not be possible in those situations.

Patients with previous radical neck dissections or other procedures with or without radiation may be easier examined using extra gel. Patients who cannot lie flat can be scanned sitting in a wheelchair or bed. Patients with deep muscular necks may require alternate transducers from those usually chosen to one that allows deeper penetration. Markedly calcific vessels will make assessment by both B-mode and Doppler difficult. Multiple views may allow the examiner to visualize differing segments in each view for adequate assessment.

Equipment and Supplies

A high-resolution duplex ultrasound system equipped with Doppler spectral analysis is standard. Transducers commonly used are a 5–10 MHZ frequency linear transducer, although transducers in the range of 5–7.5 MHZ imaging frequencies or less, which allow adequate B-mode as well as velocity assessment, might also be used in most patients. Higher frequencies may be needed in thin necks and lower frequencies in deep or muscular necks. Hardcopy documentation can be done using videotape, color printers, optical disk, or other permanent storage. Blood pressure cuffs of varying sizes are used to measure systemic blood pressure and perform subclavian steal studies. Ultrasound gel should also be available, preferably warm.

Protocol of Examination

Each vascular lab must have a standardized and documented protocol for carotid insonation. Any variations in technique from the standard protocol should be documented for reference in follow-up studies. The criteria of diagnosis are based on velocity data, so consistency is very important when comparing studies. An angle of 60° between the vessel axis and the sample volume should be maintained when performing velocity measurements. If not obtainable due to severe angulation or other technical factors, an angle of less than 60° should be used. This information should be considered at the time of interpretation. Angles above 60° should never be used as small errors in angle measurement will cause large errors in velocity calculation. The sample volume should be placed in the center stream (or center of the jet in stenosis) in the vessel and should be as small as possible. Both transverse and longitudinal scan planes should be used. Any measurement of vessel diameter or diam-

eter reduction should be performed in transverse, and any Doppler velocity waveform should be obtained in the longitudinal view.

Interpretation and Diagnostic Criteria

A carotid duplex ultrasound report should include estimation of the degree of stenosis, plaque characterization, vertebral artery flow, and the presence of any incidental findings such as dissections, tumors, intimal flaps, and aneurysms that need to be mentioned to the treating physicians. Each vascular lab has its own diagnostic criteria and standard report for carotid and vertebral duplex ultrasound ideally based upon internal validation by correlating with other diagnostic modalities including CTA, MRA, and carotid angiograms. Our institutional internally validated criteria for carotid duplex interpretation are shown in Fig. 6.8.

The overall accuracy of the test is the statistical analysis that allows the comparison between the relationship of sensitivity and specificity. In practice, the accuracy of carotid duplex ultrasound can vary widely among vascular laboratories, and this variation has been identified to be clinically significant [18].

The most common utilized criteria for carotid duplex ultrasonography are listed in the consensus document from the Society of Radiologists in Ultrasound (SRU) that was convened in October 2002 (Table 6.1). Importantly, these recommended criteria were based on an analysis of several published studies and anecdotal experiences of the panelists [14, 15].

Our Duplex Ultrasound Criteria for Internal Carotid Artery Stenosis

Stenosis Category, %	PSV (cm/sec)	EDV (cm/sec)	IC/CC ratio
< 50	< 135	<40	
50-69%	135-284	>40	2-4
70-99%	>285	>85	>4
Preocclusive	Minimal flow		
Occlusion	No detectable flow		

Fig. 6.8 Carotid duplex interpretation criteria used in the Ross Heart and Vascular Center, Ohio State University Vascular Laboratory

Table 6.1 Consensus conference panel duplex ultrasound criteria for diagnosis of internal carotid stenosis

Degree of stenosis	Internal carotid artery peak systolic velocity	Internal carotid artery end-diastolic velocity	Internal carotid artery-to-common carotid artery peak systolic velocity ratio	Presence of plaque
Normal	<125 cm/s	<40 cm/s	<2.0	No plaque or intimal thickening is visible
<50% stenosis	<125 cm/s	<40 cm/s	<2.0	Plaque or intimal thickening is visible
50–69% stenosis	125–230 cm/s	40–100 cm/s	2–4	Plaque is visible
≥70% stenosis to near occlusion	>230 cm/s	>100 cm/s	>4	Visible plaque and lumen narrowing are seen
Near occlusion	High, low, or undetectable	Variable	Variable	Markedly narrowed lumen at color Doppler
Total occlusion	Undetectable	Not applicable	Not applicable	No detectable patent lumen at gray-scale

Data from Grant EG, et al. Carotid artery stenosis: grayscale and Doppler ultrasound diagnosis—Society of Radiologists in Ultrasound consensus conference. Ultrasound Q. 2003;19(4):190–8

AbuRahma and colleagues critically appraised the SRU criteria to evaluate its accuracy and recommended amending the moderate category criteria of 50–69% to increase accuracy [18]. This evaluation reports the validation of the consensus criteria for normal internal carotid arteries as well as varying degrees of stenosis. The sensitivity, specificity, and overall accuracy are reasonably good for normal carotids as well as <50% stenosis; however, improvement was possible in the 50–69% range [19]. It is important to note that the consensus criteria themselves were not validated and, in fact, served as a baseline for vascular laboratories that have not validated their own criteria. Therefore, it is imperative that institutions internally validate their own criteria.

Institutions have applied the consensus criteria to their center's data to determine the true accuracy by correlating it with angiographic data. Furthermore, the IAC issued a "white paper" and recommended that vascular laboratories use SRU Consensus Conference Criteria for interpretation of internal carotid stenosis (Table 6.1). However, given the large variability among institutions, the IAC also noted that "facilities which have rigorously internally validated their own criteria may continue to use these criteria at the present time" [20, 21]. As such, we maintain a rigorous quality control of our carotid duplex ultrasound testing and continue to use our own criteria with an accuracy of over 90% [16].

Carotid duplex ultrasound has been correlated with angiographic findings in native unstented carotid arteries. Duplex criteria and accuracy assessment are not well established following carotid angioplasty and stenting. In fact, studies have demonstrated that velocity criteria for the native carotid arteries classify angiographically normal stented carotid arteries as being stenotic—these elevated velocities are likely secondary to altered compliance within the stent-artery complex. As such, a different set of criteria are used to evaluate flow velocities in stented carotid arteries—these again should be internally validated [22]. The accuracy of velocity criteria following carotid artery stenting is not standardized, and follow-up carotid ultrasounds are mandatory to be compared to earlier velocity evaluations after stenting.

Plaque Characterization

Studies have shown that the plaque structure at the carotid artery bifurcation is related to the risk of causing neurologic symptoms of TIA or stroke. This has led to the concept of "unstable" plaques, which have been determined to lead to plaque rupture and neurologic symptoms [23, 24]. Conventional angiography, although considered to be the gold standard in determining the degree of stenosis of the carotid artery, lacks the ability to provide information about the plaque structure and hence the risk of becoming symptomatic [25].

Studies have shown that vulnerable or unstable plaques are the ones that have large extracellular lipid-rich core, thin fibrous caps, reduced smooth muscle density, and increased numbers of activated macrophages and are more likely to be associated with plaque rupture and neurologic symptoms [26, 27]. High-resolution ultrasound using B-mode scanning can identify the characteristics of unstable (vulnerable) plaques in carotid artery disease based on echogenicity (brightness), homogeneity, and surface characteristics. Echogenicity reflects the overall brightness of the plaque with the term hyperechoic referring to echogenic (white) and the term hypoechoic referring to echolucent (black or dark) plaques [28]. The reference structure to which plaque echo density should be compared to is the blood for hypoechoic, the sternomastoid muscle for isoechoic, and the bone for hyperechoic plaques [29]. Hypoechoic plaques have been found to have significantly higher risk of being symptomatic than hyperechoic plaques. Homogeneity on the other hand implies the uniformity of the echogenicity of the plaque. Homogeneous plaques are the ones that have a uniform consistency irrespective of whether they are predominantly hypoechoic or hyperechoic. The term heterogeneous should be used for plaques of non-uniform consistency, i.e., having both hypoechoic and hyperechoic components. Studies have shown that heterogeneous plaques are more associated with symptoms and if found in asymptomatic patients, they are more prone to develop symptoms subsequently [30, 31]. As far as surface

characteristics of plaques, they are classified into smooth surface plaques when the surface has a smooth continuous boundary, irregular when there is uneven or pitted boundary and ulcerated when pocked or there is a crater like defect with sharp margins. Studies have also shown that irregular or ulcerated plaques are more commonly associated with symptoms compared with smooth-surfaced plaques [32, 33].

In general, complicated carotid plaques that are more associated with ipsilateral neurological symptoms have the ultrasound characteristics of being echolucent, heterogeneous with irregular or ulcerated surface that contrasts with uncomplicated plaques that are usually in asymptomatic patients that are usually hyperechoic, homogeneous with smooth surface without ulceration [34, 35].

Vertebral Artery Flow

Bilateral vertebral artery flow direction and flow characteristics should be identified during the ultrasound examination. Normally, the flow in the vertebral arteries is antegrade toward the head. No flow in one or both vertebral arteries indicates total occlusion of that vessel. Sometimes, in cases of distal vertebral artery occlusion, a "thumping" sound may be encountered at the lower part of the neck which indicates that the blood flow is striking against the occlusion then briefly reversing. In cases of asymmetric flow in both vertebral arteries or suspicion of vertebral steal, blood pressure discrepancy between both arms must be identified, and hyperemia test as mentioned above can be used as a provocative test to unmask subclinical vertebral artery steal [14, 15].

Incidental Findings

Any coincidental findings during the carotid and vertebral duplex examination should be identified and recorded in the final ultrasound report, e.g., enlarged lymph node, an incidental thyroid nodule, suspicion of carotid body tumor, and so forth.

Unusual Findings on Noninvasive Carotid Exam

Sometimes, noninvasive carotid studies can identify unusual exam findings other than the evaluation of carotid bifurcation atherosclerotic disease. Some of these findings are:

- Dissection or intimal flaps caused by tearing of the intimal wall: in dissections, flow enters under the intima creating a separate flow channel. Intimal flaps will cause localized flow disturbances related to the size and extent of the intimal flap(s). Dissections are found in head and neck injury as well as extensions of aortic dissections. They can be spontaneous or related to blunt trauma.
- Fibromuscular dysplasia (FMD): affects mid-/distal ICA. It is characterized by homogeneous fibrous material in the wall associated with multiple areas of stenosis in the mid- and distal ICA indicated by superimposed high- and low-velocity signals.
- Carotid body tumor: usually located in between the ICA and ECA. It is highly vascularized and usually perfused by the ECA. On noninvasive carotid studies, it appears as a vascularized mass splaying the ICA and ECA widely apart.
- Carotid aneurysm: this is an extremely rare diagnosis. The majority is atherosclerotic in nature, but other causes include previous trauma, prior surgery, and more rarely postpartum. However, most patients that are sent to the vascular laboratory with a suspected carotid aneurysm due to a pulsatile mass in the neck have a tortuous or redundant CCA or prominent innominate artery or subclavian and not really aneurysm cases.

Limitations of Carotid Duplex Scanning

Certain clinical situations pose challenges to the examination and interpretation of carotid duplex examination and should be kept in mind while interpreting the results of the examination. In those situations, it is usually not enough to rely solely on carotid duplex examination results and other noninvasive studies including CTA and MRA, or carotid angiograms are needed to supplement the results of the noninvasive testing. Some of these situations are:

- The presence of contralateral carotid occlusion: cases of contralateral carotid occlusion can be associated with increased compensatory flow in the ipsilateral ICA which can overestimate the degree of ipsilateral stenosis, something that should be interpreted with caution.
- Excessive tortuosity or looping of the carotids: it can be difficult to insonate the vessels at the needed 60-degree angle to the vessel, which again can overestimate the degree of stenosis due to overestimation of the flow velocities.
- Excessive carotid plaque calcification: in these cases, some areas of the vessel can be hidden by the shadowing cast by the excessive calcification. Velocities of flow cannot be evaluated in those hidden areas, which may be the most stenotic area of the vessel. As such, having a lower velocity may be due to the inability to see the area of the high velocity causing underestimation of the degree of stenosis in these vessels. Care must be taken to insonate the vessel at different angles to evaluate the area of concern hidden behind the calcification, but sometimes that cannot be accomplished. Reports in these studies should mention the limitations cast by the calcification and warn the treating physicians of the possible underestimation of the degree of stenosis.
- Presence of tandem carotid lesions: disease proximal or distal to the carotid bifurcation may cause a decrease in the velocity in a bifurcation stenosis because of decreased inflow in case of proximal lesions or increased resistance in more distal lesions. In cases of ipsilateral proximal CCA or brachiocephalic artery disease, the waveforms in the distal CCA and ICA can be dampened and have delayed systolic rise time or low slope to peak systole as compared to the contralateral side leading to

underestimation of the stenosis. In cases of significant distal disease in the ICA, the waveforms can become more of a high resistance signal where there is a sharp systolic rise time and significant reduction in diastolic flow that can go down to zero in cases of total distal ICA occlusion.

- Cardiovascular status: may affect the velocity waveforms. The presence of hypertension or tachycardia may result in increased pulsatility in the absence of carotid stenosis. Diffuse cerebrovascular disease may result in bilateral high resistant waveforms in the absence of cervical disease. Decrease cardiac output may cause waveform damping and possibility flow to zero in diastole. These changes could be erroneously attributed to proximal or distal disease. In these cases, symmetrical findings may clue the examiner that these are systemic changes and avoid a false-positive diagnosis.

Carotid Endarterectomy Based on Duplex Scanning Alone

Continued improvements in the accuracy and reliability of carotid duplex scanning, along with mounting demands to minimize both costs and risks of medical care, have prompted most surgeons to consider performing carotid endarterectomy based on the clinical evaluation and duplex scan findings alone [36, 37]. Carotid bifurcation lesions which are suitable for endarterectomy in both asymptomatic patients and patients with hemispheric neurologic symptoms can be accurately detected by duplex scanning. While duplex scanning does not provide any direct information on arterial lesions involving the proximal aortic arch branches or the intracranial circulation, significant occlusive lesions proximal or distal to the carotid bifurcation are uncommon and rarely have an adverse effect on the outcome of carotid endarterectomy. Furthermore, most stenoses in the proximal brachiocephalic vessels can be suspected based on common carotid flow abnormalities or unequal arm blood pressures that can provoke then the evaluation using other modalities of imaging.

Experience with duplex scanning in patients undergoing carotid endarterectomy indicate that the results of arteriography rarely alter the clinical treatment plan when a technically adequate duplex scan shows an 80–99% stenosis in asymptomatic patients or an ipsilateral 50–99% stenosis in patients with hemispheric neurologic symptoms [38]. Arteriography is most likely to influence clinical decisions when the carotid duplex scan is nondiagnostic, when the lesion appears to extend beyond the carotid bifurcation, when there is one of the limitations described previously, or when the internal carotid stenosis is less than 50% in a patient with focal neurologic deficit that corresponds to the mildly diseased vessel [4].

Newer Advances

Debate continues about screening asymptomatic patients with duplex scanning. The US Preventive Services Task Force has advised against ultrasound screening of the asymptomatic general population. The value of densitometric analysis and echogenicity of carotid plaques by duplex scanning has shown that predominantly echolucent plaques are associated with about a 2.6-fold increased risk of ipsilateral stroke in patients with 50% or greater stenosis [39]. Carotid intima-media thickness (CIMT) continues to be used in research studies to assess cardiovascular risk but lacks data for widespread use at this point. Microbubble contrast agents have been introduced to detect carotid ulceration. Contrast-enhanced ultrasound has demonstrated superior sensitivity and diagnostic accuracy in detecting ulceration compared to standard duplex scanning [40]. Similarly, 3D sonography is being utilized to detect and improve image quality and quantify plaque morphology and echomorphology [41].

Transcranial Doppler

Transcranial Doppler (TCD) is a noninvasive method of evaluating blood flow in the circle of Willis in the brain through the intact skull. It was

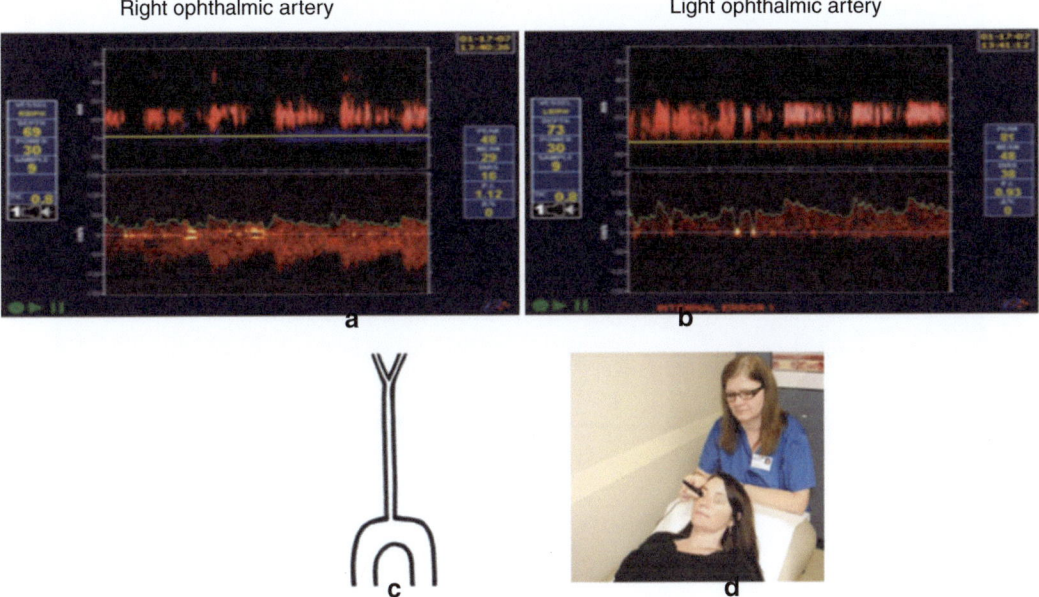

Fig. 6.9 Normal transorbital exam. Both ophthalmic blood flows are antegrade and are shown in images (**a**) and (**b**) (red). A vertebral artery map is depicted in image (**c**) and (**d**) sonographer position for transorbital scanning. Courtesy of Dr. Zsolt Garami, The Houston Methodist Hospital

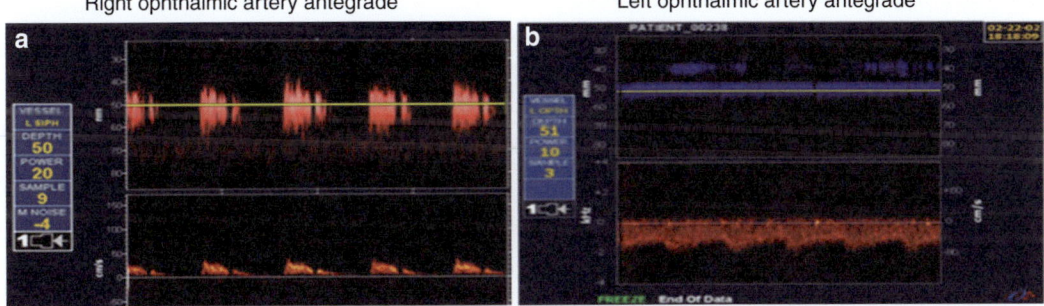

Fig. 6.10 Transcranial Doppler study in a patient with an occluded left internal carotid artery. Right ophthalmic artery flow is antegrade (**a**) (red), while the left ophthal-mic artery flow is retrograde (**b**) (blue). Courtesy of Dr. Zsolt Garami, The Houston Methodist Hospital

first introduced by Rune Aaslid et al. in 1982 [42]. A low-frequency 2-MHz pulsed Doppler is used to evaluate the intracranial middle cerebral artery, anterior cerebral artery, the posterior cerebral artery, and the distal internal carotid, ophthalmic, vertebral, and basilar artery through transtemporal, transorbital, submandibular, and transforaminal windows in the skull [43] (Figs. 6.9, 6.10, 6.11, and 6.12). Using the Doppler probe, the depth of insonation can be specified by selecting a specific pulse repetition frequency that is based on the average speed of sound in soft tissue, thus locating the signals originating from a specific depth. The machine emits the sound pulse and waits for the time needed to make a round trip to and from a specific depth and then senses the returning signals. The machine then can determine the flow patterns including direction of flow in the vessel, pulsatility index, and velocity based on Doppler shift principle [38]. Each intracranial vessel can be insonated through a specific bone window and at a specific depth.

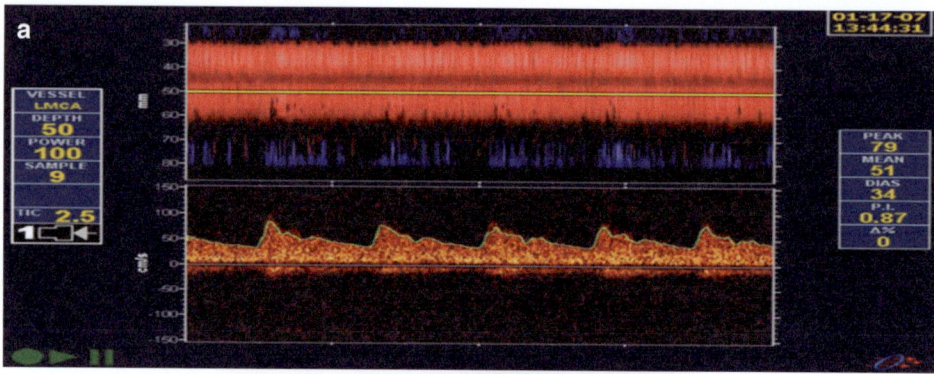

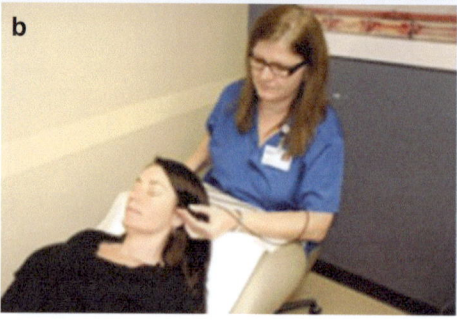

Fig. 6.11 Sonographer demonstrating technique with a transtemporal window (**b**). Normal middle cerebral artery (MCA) flow. MCA M-mode fills screen from 65 to 30 mm depth (pulsatility index normal 0.6–1.1) (**a**). Courtesy of Dr. Zsolt Garami, The Houston Methodist Hospital

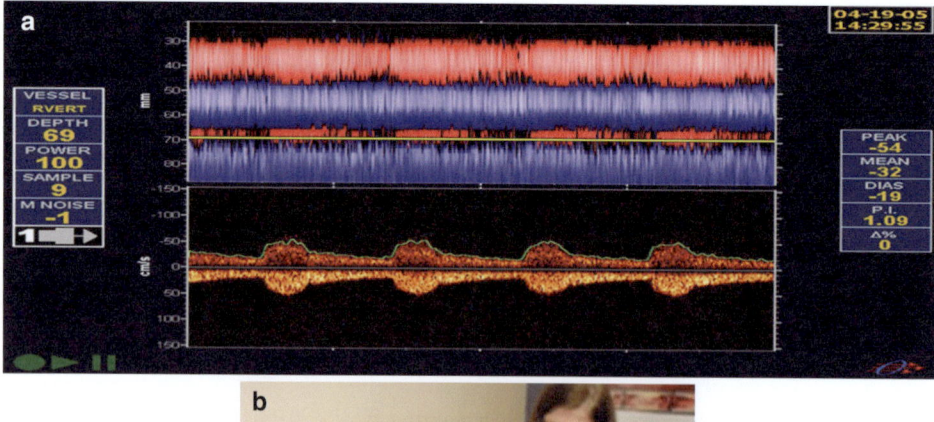

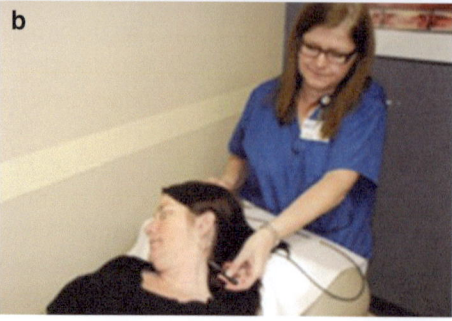

Fig. 6.12 Sonographer demonstrating technique of a transforaminal window (**b**). Right vertebral artery and posterior inferior cerebellar artery (PICA) normal flow. At 69 mm depth, the vertebral artery flow is below the baseline (blue), and the PICA flow is above the baseline (red) (**a**). Courtesy of Dr. Zsolt Garami, The Houston Methodist Hospital

Table 6.2 Guidelines for normal transcranial Doppler study interpretation

Artery	Window	Depth (mm)	Flow direction	Mean velocity
MCA	Temporal	30–60	Toward	55 ± 12
ACA	Temporal	60–85	Away	50 ± 11
PCA	Temporal	60–70	Bidirectional	40 ± 10
TICA	Temporal	55–65	Toward	39 ± 9
ICA (siphon)	Orbital	60–80	Bidirectional	45 ± 15
OA	Orbital	40–60	Toward	20 ± 10
VA	Occipital	60–80	Away	38 ± 10
BA	Occipital	80–110	Away	41 ± 10

ACA anterior cerebral artery, *BA* basilar artery, *ICA* internal carotid artery, *MCA* middle cerebral artery, *OA* ophthalmic artery, *PCA* posterior cerebral artery, *TICA* terminal internal carotid artery, *VA* vertebral artery
Data from Stone PA and Hass SM. Vascular laboratory: arterial duplex scanning. In: Cronenwett JL and Johnston KW, editors. Rutherford's vascular surgery, chap. 16, 8th ed. Philadelphia: Elsevier Saunders; 2014. p. 230–57

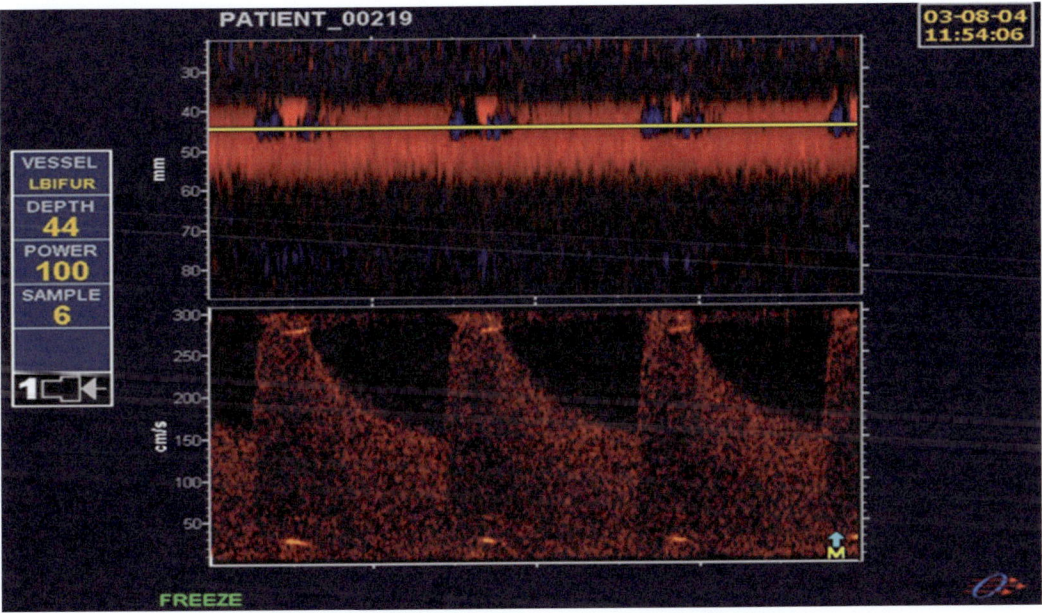

Fig. 6.13 Left middle cerebral artery (MCA) stenosis showing elevated velocity in the left MCA as well as post-stenotic turbulence. Courtesy of Dr. Zsolt Garami, The Houston Methodist Hospital

Listed in Table 6.2 are the normal depth, direction, window, and velocity measurements in each of the intracranial vessels [43, 44]. Recently, power motion mode (PMD) was invented by Moehring and Spencer to facilitate and streamline TCD [45]. This technique uses overlapping Doppler samples to simultaneously display flow signal intensity and direction over 6 cm of intracranial space. PMD provides a color-coded display of all flow signals over the specified range of depths. The brighter colors reflect stronger

intensities and the direction is also determined. The PMD provides a road map that can serve as a guide for more complete spectral analysis [43, 45] (Figs. 6.9, 6.10, 6.11, 6.12, and 6.13). The TCD has multiple capabilities including:

- Diagnosis of intracranial stenosis and occlusion based on focal velocity increase, post-stenotic turbulence, and discrepancy between the two sides as well as reversed direction in specified vessels (Fig. 6.13)

- Detection and monitoring of vasospasm following subarachnoid hemorrhage and following aneurysm clipping [46]
- Evaluation of intracranial effects of extracranial obstructions including assessment of collateral flow pathways [47]
- Detection of cerebral emboli [45]
- Evaluation and monitoring of intracranial blood flow during surgical procedures including carotid procedures and aortic arch and cardiac procedures [48, 49]
- Detection and evaluation of patent foramen ovale before, during, and after closure [47]
- Evaluation of cerebral autoregulation [50, 51]
- Support of the diagnosis of brain death [52]
- Prognosis and effects on treatment in acute stroke patients [53]
- Detects feeder arteries in AVMs

Transcranial Doppler is a portable and inexpensive tool for evaluating cerebrovascular circulation in relation to multiple disease states and intervention. However, TCD requires intense in-depth training as well as experience in both performing and interpreting the test results [41]. Also, temporal windows needed for most of the evaluations are absent in 5–15% of patients due to inability of the ultrasound beam to penetrate the skull, in which case, the test cannot be performed [42].

Conclusions

While advances continue in equipment, technology, and data related to improving accuracy of duplex scanning of the cerebrovascular system, the test has become a reliable and accurate diagnostic tool in the management of diseases related to the cerebrovascular system. This chapter explains the basic physiology, protocols, criteria, limitations, and common usage of duplex scanning of the carotid, vertebral, and transcranial arteries.

Review Questions

1. In carotid duplex ultrasonography, the greatest variability or mismatch compared to a gold standard catheter-based arteriography is in:
   A. Minimal degree of stenosis (<50%)
   B. Moderate degree of stenosis (50–69%)
   C. Severe degree of stenosis (>70%)
   D. Carotid occlusion (100%)

   Answer: B

2. The ideal angle of insonation when interrogating the carotid artery is:
   A. 30°
   B. 45°
   C. 60°
   D. 90°

   Answer: C

3. Echogenicity on B-mode imaging is based on a comparison to a reference structure. Please select the appropriate combination:
   A. Blood for hyperechoic
   B. The omohyoid muscle for hypoechoic
   C. The sternocleidomastoid muscle for isoechoic
   D. Bone for hypoechoic

   Answer: C

4. The following flow pattern is identified in subclavian steal phenomenon:
   A. Reversal of flow in the internal carotid artery
   B. Reversal of flow in the vertebral artery
   C. Reversal of flow in internal mammary artery
   D. Reversal of flow in the subclavian artery

   Answer: B

References

1. Study design for randomized prospective trial of carotid endarterectomy for asymptomatic atherosclerosis. The Asymptomatic Carotid Atherosclerosis Study Group. Stroke. 1989;20(7):844–9.
2. AbuRahma AF. Overview of various noninvasive cerebrovascular techniques. In: AbuRahma AF, Bergan JJ, editors. Noninvasive vascular diagnosis: a practical guide to therapy. 2nd ed. London: Springer; 2007. p. 50–9.
3. Mozersky DJ, Hokanson DE, Sumner DS, Strandness DE Jr. Ultrasonic visualization of the arterial lumen. Surgery. 1972;72(2):253–9.
4. Zierler RE, Kohler TR, Strandness DE Jr. Duplex scanning of normal or minimally diseased carotid arteries: correlation with arteriography and clinical outcome. J Vasc Surg. 1990;12(4):447–54; discussion 54-5.
5. Dawson DL, Zierler RE, Strandness DE Jr, Clowes AW, Kohler TR. The role of duplex scanning and arteriography before carotid endarterectomy: a prospective study. J Vasc Surg. 1993;18(4):673–80; discussion 80-3.
6. Aburahma AF, Thiele SP, Wulu JT Jr. Prospective controlled study of the natural history of asymptomatic 60% to 69% carotid stenosis according to ultrasonic plaque morphology. J Vasc Surg. 2002;36(3):437–42.
7. Gronholdt ML, Nordestgaard BG, Schroeder TV, Vorstrup S, Sillesen H. Ultrasonic echolucent carotid plaques predict future strokes. Circulation. 2001;104(1):68–73.
8. AbuRahma AF, Jarrett KS. Duplex scanning of the carotid arteries. In: AbuRahma AF, Bergan JJ, editors. Noninvasive vascular diagnosis: a practical guide to therapy. 2nd ed. London: Springer; 2007. p. 60–88.
9. Polak JF, Dobkin GR, O'Leary DH, Wang AM, Cutler SS. Internal carotid artery stenosis: accuracy and reproducibility of color-Doppler-assisted duplex imaging. Radiology. 1989;173(3):793–8.
10. Spadone DP, Barkmeier LD, Hodgson KJ, Ramsey DE, Sumner DS. Contralateral internal carotid artery stenosis or occlusion: pitfall of correct ipsilateral classification—a study performed with color-flow imaging. J Vasc Surg. 1990;11(5):642–9.
11. Mattos MA, Hodgson KJ, Ramsey DE, Barkmeier LD, Sumner DS. Identifying total carotid occlusion with colour flow duplex scanning. Eur J Vasc Surg. 1992;6(2):204–10.
12. Londrey GL, Spadone DP, Hodgson KJ, Ramsey DE, Barkmeier LD, Sumner DS. Does color-flow imaging improve the accuracy of duplex carotid evaluation? J Vasc Surg. 1991;13(5):659–63.
13. Moneta GL, Edwards JM, Chitwood RW, Taylor LM Jr, Lee RW, Cummings CA, et al. Correlation of North American Symptomatic Carotid Endarterectomy Trial (NASCET) angiographic definition of 70% to 99% internal carotid artery stenosis with duplex scanning. J Vasc Surg. 1993;17(1):152–7; discussion 7-9.
14. Ribo M, Alexandrov AV. Vertebral artery ultrasonography. In: AbuRahma AF, Bergan JJ, editors. Noninvasive vascular diagnosis: a practical guide to therapy. 2nd ed. London: Springer; 2007. p. 97–102.
15. Bornstein NM, Norris JW. Subclavian steal: a harmless haemodynamic phenomenon? Lancet. 1986;2(8502):303–5.
16. American College of Cardiology Foundation (ACCF), American College of Radiology (ACR), American Institute of Ultrasound in Medicine (AIUM), American Society of Echocardiography (ASE), American Society of Nephrology (ASN), Intersocietal Commission for the Accreditation of Vascular Laboratories (ICAVL), Society for Cardiovascular Angiography and Interventions (SCAI), Society of Cardiovascular Computed Tomography (SCCT), Society for Interventional Radiology (SIR), Society for Vascular Medicine (SVM), Society for Vascular Surgery (SVS), American Academy of Neurology, American Podiatric Medical Association, Society for Clinical Vascular Surgery, Society for Cardiovascular Magnetic Resonance, Society for Vascular Ultrasound, Peripheral Vascular Ultrasound, Mohler ER, Gornik HL, Gerhard-Herman M, et al. ACCF/ACR/AIUM/ASE/ASN/ICAVL/SCAI/SCCT/SIR/SVM/SVS 2012 appropriate use criteria for peripheral vascular ultrasound and physiological testing part I: arterial ultrasound and physiological testing: a report of the American College of Cardiology Foundation Appropriate Use Criteria Task Force, American College of Radiology, American Institute of Ultrasound in Medicine, American Society of Echocardiography, American Society of Nephrology, Intersocietal Commission for the Accreditation of Vascular Laboratories, Society for Cardiovascular Angiography and Interventions, Society of Cardiovascular Computed Tomography, Society for Interventional Radiology, Society for Vascular Medicine, and Society for Vascular Surgery. J Vasc Surg. 2012;56:e17–51.
17. Satiani B, Masterson L, Kudlaty E, Starr JE, Go MR. Significant cost savings can result from accurate coding of carotid duplex indications and elimination of inappropriate tests. J Angiol Vasc Surg. 2016;1:002.
18. Shakhnovich I, Kiser D, Satiani B. Importance of validation of accuracy of duplex ultrasonography in identifying moderate and severe carotid artery stenosis. Vasc Endovasc Surg. 2010;44(6):483–8.

19. AbuRahma AF, Srivastava M, Stone PA, Mousa AY, Jain A, Dean LS, et al. Critical appraisal of the Carotid Duplex Consensus criteria in the diagnosis of carotid artery stenosis. J Vasc Surg. 2011;53(1):53–9; discussion 9-60.

20. Braun RM, Bertino RE, Milbrandt J, Bray M, Society of Radiologists in Ultrasound Consensus Criteria to a Single Institution Clinical Practice. Ultrasound imaging of carotid artery stenosis: application of the Society of Radiologists in Ultrasound Consensus Criteria to a Single Institution Clinical Practice. Ultrasound Q. 2008;24(3):161–6.

21. Shaalan WE, Wahlgren CM, Desai T, Piano G, Skelly C, Bassiouny HS. Reappraisal of velocity criteria for carotid bulb/internal carotid artery stenosis utilizing high-resolution B-mode ultrasound validated with computed tomography angiography. J Vasc Surg. 2008;48(1):104–12; discussion 12-3.

22. Lal BK, Hobson RW 2nd, Goldstein J, Chakhtoura EY, Duran WN. Carotid artery stenting: is there a need to revise ultrasound velocity criteria? J Vasc Surg. 2004;39(1):58–66.

23. Sabetai MM, Tegos TJ, Nicolaides AN, El-Atrozy TS, Dhanjil S, Griffin M, et al. Hemispheric symptoms and carotid plaque echomorphology. J Vasc Surg. 2000;31(1 Pt 1):39–49.

24. Tegos TJ, Sabetai MM, Nicolaides AN, Elatrozy TS, Dhanjil S, Stevens JM. Patterns of brain computed tomography infarction and carotid plaque echo-genicity. J Vasc Surg. 2001;33(2):334–9.

25. Nicolaides AN, Griffin M, Kakkos SK, Geroulakos G, Kyriacou E, Georgiou N. Ultrasonic characterization of carotid plaques. In: AbuRahma AF, Bergan JJ, editors. Noninvasive vascular diagnosis: a practical guide to therapy. 2nd ed. London: Springer; 2007. p. 127–48.

26. Davies MJ, Richardson PD, Woolf N, Katz DR, Mann J. Risk of thrombosis in human atherosclerotic plaques: role of extracellular lipid, macrophage, and smooth muscle cell content. Br Heart J. 1993;69(5):377–81.

27. Falk E. Why do plaques rupture? Circulation. 1992;86(6 Suppl):III30–42.

28. de Bray JM, Baud JM, Delanoy P, Camuzat JP, Dehans V, Descamp-Le Chevoir J, et al. Reproducibility in ultrasonic characterization of carotid plaques. Cerebrovasc Dis. 1998;8(5):273–7.

29. Polak JF, Shemanski L, O'Leary DH, Lefkowitz D, Price TR, Savage PJ, et al. Hypoechoic plaque at US of the carotid artery: an independent risk factor for incident stroke in adults aged 65 years or older. Cardiovascular Health Study. Radiology. 1998;208(3):649–54.

30. Liapis CD, Kakisis JD, Kostakis AG. Carotid stenosis: factors affecting symptomatology. Stroke. 2001;32(12):2782–6.

31. Carra G, Visona A, Bonanome A, Lusiani L, Pesavento R, Bortolon M, et al. Carotid plaque morphology and cerebrovascular events. Int Angiol. 2003;22(3):284–9.

32. Iannuzzi A, Wilcosky T, Mercuri M, Rubba P, Bryan FA, Bond MG. Ultrasonographic correlates of carotid atherosclerosis in transient ischemic attack and stroke. Stroke. 1995;26(4):614–9.

33. Golledge J, Cuming R, Ellis M, Davies AH, Greenhalgh RM. Carotid plaque characteristics and presenting symptom. Br J Surg. 1997;84(12):1697–701.

34. Geroulakos G, Ramaswami G, Nicolaides A, James K, Labropoulos N, Belcaro G, et al. Characterization of symptomatic and asymptomatic carotid plaques using high-resolution real-time ultrasonography. Br J Surg. 1993;80(10):1274–7.

35. O'Donnell TF Jr, Erdoes L, Mackey WC, McCullough J, Shepard A, Heggerick P, et al. Correlation of B-mode ultrasound imaging and arteriography with pathologic findings at carotid endarterectomy. Arch Surg. 1985;120(4):443–9.

36. Moore WS, Ziomek S, Quinones-Baldrich WJ, Machleder HI, Busuttil RW, Baker JD. Can clinical evaluation and noninvasive testing substitute for arteriography in the evaluation of carotid artery disease? Ann Surg. 1988;208(1):91–4.

37. Norris JW, Halliday A. Is ultrasound sufficient for vascular imaging prior to carotid endarterectomy? Stroke. 2004;35(2):370–1.

38. Moore WS. For severe carotid stenosis found on ultrasound, further arterial evaluation is unnecessary. Stroke. 2003;34(7):1816–7; discussion 9.

39. Gupta A, Kesavabhotla K, Baradaran H, et al. Plaque echolucency and stroke risk in asymptomatic carotid stenosis: a systematic review and meta-analysis. Stroke. 2015;46:91–7.

40. Kate GL, van Dijk AC, van den Oord SC, et al. Usefulness of contrast-enhanced ultrasound for detection of carotid plaque ulceration in patients with symptomatic carotid atherosclerosis. Am J Cardiol. 2013;112:292–8.

41. Yao J, van Sambeek MR, Dall'Agata A, et al. Three-dimensional ultrasound study of carotid arteries before and after endarterectomy: analysis of stenotic lesions and surgical impact on the vessel. Stroke. 1998;29:2026–31.

42. Aaslid R, Markwalder TM, Nornes H. Noninvasive transcranial Doppler ultrasound recording of flow velocity in basal cerebral arteries. J Neurosurg. 1982;57(6):769–74.

43. Ribo M, Alexandrov AV. Transcranial Doppler sonography. In: AbuRahma AF, Bergan JJ, editors. Noninvasive vascular diagnosis: a practical guide to therapy. 2nd ed. London: Springer; 2007. p. 103–26.

44. Adams R, McKie V, Nichols F, Carl E, Zhang DL, McKie K, et al. The use of transcranial ultrasonography to predict stroke in sickle cell disease. N Engl J Med. 1992;326(9):605–10.

45. Moehring MA, Spencer MP. Power M-mode Doppler (PMD) for observing cerebral blood flow and tracking emboli. Ultrasound Med Biol. 2002;28(1):49–57.

46. Newell DW, Grady MS, Eskridge JM, Winn HR. Distribution of angiographic vasospasm after sub-

arachnoid hemorrhage: implications for diagnosis by transcranial Doppler ultrasonography. Neurosurgery. 1990;27(4):574–7.

47. Kelley RE, Namon RA, Juang SH, Lee SC, Chang JY. Transcranial Doppler ultrasonography of the middle cerebral artery in the hemodynamic assessment of internal carotid artery stenosis. Arch Neurol. 1990;47(9):960–4.

48. Gaunt ME, Martin PJ, Smith JL, Rimmer T, Cherryman G, Ratliff DA, et al. Clinical relevance of intraoperative embolization detected by transcranial Doppler ultrasonography during carotid endarterectomy: a prospective study of 100 patients. Br J Surg. 1994;81(10):1435–9.

49. Cao P, Giordano G, Zannetti S, De Rango P, Maghini M, Parente B, et al. Transcranial Doppler monitoring during carotid endarterectomy: is it appropriate for selecting patients in need of a shunt? J Vasc Surg. 1997;26(6):973–9; discussion 9-80.

50. Mancini M, De Chiara S, Postiglione A, Ferrara LA. Transcranial Doppler evaluation of cerebrovascular reactivity to acetazolamide in normal subjects. Artery. 1993;20(4):231–41.

51. Sugimori H, Ibayashi S, Irie K, Ooboshi H, Nagao T, Fujii K, et al. Cerebral hemodynamics in hypertensive patients compared with normotensive volunteers. A transcranial Doppler study. Stroke. 1994;25(7):1384–9.

52. Ducrocq X, Braun M, Debouverie M, Junges C, Hummer M, Vespignani H. Brain death and transcranial Doppler: experience in 130 cases of brain dead patients. J Neurol Sci. 1998;160(1):41–6.

53. Demchuk AM, Burgin WS, Christou I, Felberg RA, Barber PA, Hill MD, et al. Thrombolysis in brain ischemia (TIBI) transcranial Doppler flow grades predict clinical severity, early recovery, and mortality in patients treated with intravenous tissue plasminogen activator. Stroke. 2001;32(1):89–93.

Cerebrovascular Imaging (CT, MRI, CTA, MRA)

7

Brent Griffith, Brendan P. Kelley, Suresh C. Patel, and Horia Marin

Introduction

There are a number of imaging modalities available for evaluating the vasculature of the head and neck, including duplex ultrasound (DUS), computed tomography angiography (CTA), magnetic resonance angiography (MRA), and conventional digital subtraction angiography (DSA). Each modality has its own advantages and disadvantages, and each offers different degrees of sensitivity and specificity for various disease processes. Thus, the clinical scenario and clinical question must be considered in choosing the most appropriate imaging modality.

In addition to modality-specific considerations, patient factors must also be taken into account. For example, the presence of certain cardiac devices or metal within the patient, morbid obesity, or extreme claustrophobia may preclude patients from undergoing assessment with MRI. Similarly, poor renal function or contrast allergies may prevent a contrast-enhanced examination, making non-contrast MRA techniques the better choice. As such, an understanding of the strengths and weaknesses of each modality within various clinical contexts is necessary in order to optimize the clinical workup of cerebrovascular disease.

This chapter will focus on MR and CT techniques for cerebrovascular imaging. Duplex ultrasound and digital subtraction angiography are covered in detail in other chapters.

Magnetic Resonance Imaging (MRI) and Magnetic Resonance Angiography (MRA)

MRI

Vascular imaging with MRI is accomplished with a specific technique, MR angiography. However, it is important to remember even nonvascular MR sequences offer valuable information regarding the vasculature, primarily by the way of "flow voids," and should be closely assessed whenever routine MR imaging is performed.

Flow Voids

In general, images from standard MR sequences are created by signals arising from within *stationary tissues*. Thus, fast-moving blood, such as within the carotid and vertebral arteries, actually results in a *normal absence of signal* or a "flow void," within the vessel lumen [1]. Assessment of these "flow voids" should be a routine part of any MRI interpretation, especially in the head and neck as their presence or absence can provide valuable information with regard to flow dynamics and integrity of the vascular structures [1].

B. Griffith (✉) · B. P. Kelley · S. C. Patel · H. Marin
Radiology, Henry Ford Health System,
Detroit, MI, USA
e-mail: brentg@rad.hfh.edu

© The Editor(s) (if applicable) and The Author(s) 2018
S. S. Hans (ed.), *Extracranial Carotid and Vertebral Artery Disease*,
https://doi.org/10.1007/978-3-319-91533-3_7

85

The most obvious example leading to an absent flow void, and the situation with clinical implications, is slow or absent flow within a vessel, such as in the case of occlusion or distal to a high-grade stenosis. In this situation, the intraluminal blood behaves like stationary tissue, resulting in an absent flow void within the affected vessel. This is an important finding as it can indicate the need for dedicated vascular imaging.

It is important to remember, however, that factors other than flow velocity can also affect an intraluminal flow void, particularly when coupled with slow intraluminal flow. An example is in the setting of parallel orientation of a vessel within the imaging plane, such as in the third segment of the vertebral artery. In this situation, the flowing blood undergoes relaxation prior to leaving the imaging plane, which creates signal within the vessel lumen and leads to absence, or reduction, of the normal flow void.

MRA

Vascular imaging with MRI is known as MR angiography (MRA). MRA is the only available vascular imaging technique that can be performed without the injection of contrast medium—a technique referred to as time-of-flight (TOF) MRA. This feature is especially useful in patients with chronic kidney disease, in whom renal function must be taken into consideration, as well as in patients with allergies to contrast material. An additional benefit of MRA, in contrast to CT angiography and catheter angiography, is its ability to be performed without the use of ionizing radiation.

Time-of-Flight MR Angiography (TOF MRA)

In contrast to routine MRI, which creates images from stationary tissues, TOF MRA *suppresses signal from stationary tissues*, instead using the movement of blood within the vessel lumen to create signal [1]. This creation of signal within the vessel from flowing blood is termed "flow-related enhancement." In order to isolate flow within the arteries, venous "flow-related enhance-

ment" is excluded by the use of saturation bands above the imaging volume, which saturates flow occurring in the cranial to caudal direction.

TOF MRA can be performed using both 2D and 3D acquisition modes. 2D TOF MRA uses multiple thin slices stacked in a plane perpendicular to the course of traversing blood vessels. An advantage of the 2D acquisition mode is a shorter imaging time and better sensitivity to slow flow. It can also be used to image longer vessel segments by increasing the number of image slices. The disadvantages of 2D TOF MRA include a decreased sensitivity to in-plane flow and decreased spatial resolution due to relatively thick imaging slices. In addition, "stair-step" artifact may be seen, which is significantly worsened with patient motion (Fig. 7.1a).

3D TOF MRA is more commonly used to evaluate the head and circle of Willis given the smaller coverage area needed. The greatest advantage of the 3D acquisition mode is its superior spatial resolution. In addition, because it is obtained using isotropic voxels, it can be reformatted in any direction. Disadvantages of the 3D acquisition are its insensitivity to slow flow and longer acquisition length. In addition, because it is not obtained with individual slices, patient motion affects the entire imaged volume rather than a single slice.

Challenges of TOF MRA

There are a number of challenges that can be encountered with TOF MRA. A few of these include:

- *T1 shortening*—Flowing blood creates hyperintense signal within the vessel lumen (i.e., flow-related enhancement). However, because TOF MRA is obtained using a T1-weighted sequence, any other cause of T1 shortening (e.g., subacute blood products, fat, and melanin) also appears as hyperintense signal. This can both mimic and obscure vascular pathology. This can be especially problematic in the setting of arterial dissection, as the intramural hematoma can demonstrate T1 hyperintense signal, mimicking normal flow-related enhancement and obscuring the arterial dissection (Fig. 7.1b, c).

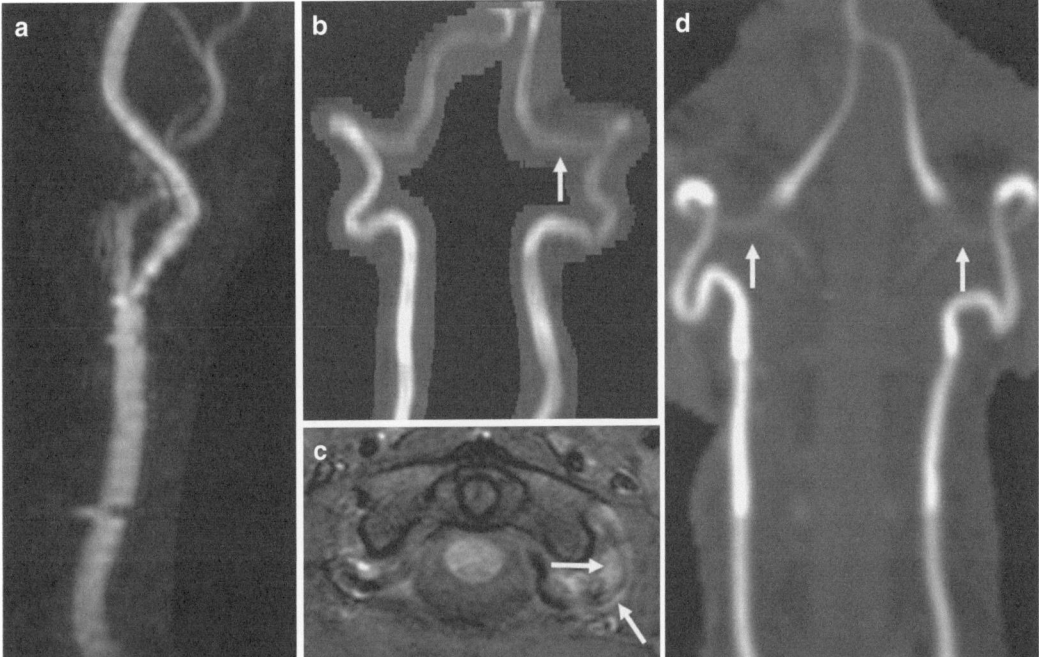

Fig. 7.1 Potential pitfalls in MRA. (**a**) Stair-step artifact is visible within the common carotid artery and carotid bulb on this 2D TOF MRA due to patient motion. (**b**, **c**) TOF MRA (**b**) in a patient with left vertebral artery dissection demonstrates only mild asymmetric signal loss within the V3 segment with apparently preserved luminal caliber. However, an axial T1-weighted fat-saturated sequence (**c**) clearly demonstrates T1 hyperintense hemorrhage within the vessel wall, which mimicked flow-related enhancement on the TOF MRA. (**d**) TOF MRA demonstrating symmetric diminished flow-related enhancement within the V3 segments of the bilateral vertebral arteries due to in-plane saturation artifact

- *Signal saturation due to slow, reversed, or in-plane flow*—TOF MRA relies on the movement of blood in and out of the imaging plane to create signal. Blood flow within a vessel parallel to the scan plane, or blood that is flowing too slowly within a vessel, can become desaturated (Fig. 7.1d). This desaturation leads to loss of flow-related enhancement and can mimic a vessel stenosis or occlusion. Similarly, blood flowing in the cranial to caudal direction (e.g., reversed vertebral artery flow in the setting of subclavian steal) will also demonstrate absent flow-related enhancement. This phenomenon, along with motion, is also responsible for a lower diagnostic value of TOF MRA in the analysis of the origin of the great vessels from the aortic arch due to signal saturation caused by in-plane flow in the aortic arch.

- *Flow-related artifact*—Complex blood flow (e.g., turbulence, non-laminar, flow separation) results in phase dispersion with associated loss of signal on TOF MRA [2]. This is commonly seen at areas of stenosis and can lead to an overestimation of the degree of stenosis. In addition, artifactual loss of signal intensity is commonly seen at the carotid bulb due to flow separations, flow reversal, and secondary flows [3]. Unfortunately, because atherosclerotic plaques also tend to occur at this location, this artifact can sometimes be mistaken for a true stenotic defect (Fig. 7.2) [3].

- *Lack of surrounding anatomic detail*—Because TOF MRA suppresses signal from stationary tissues, anatomy surrounding the vessels is difficult to evaluate on the source images.

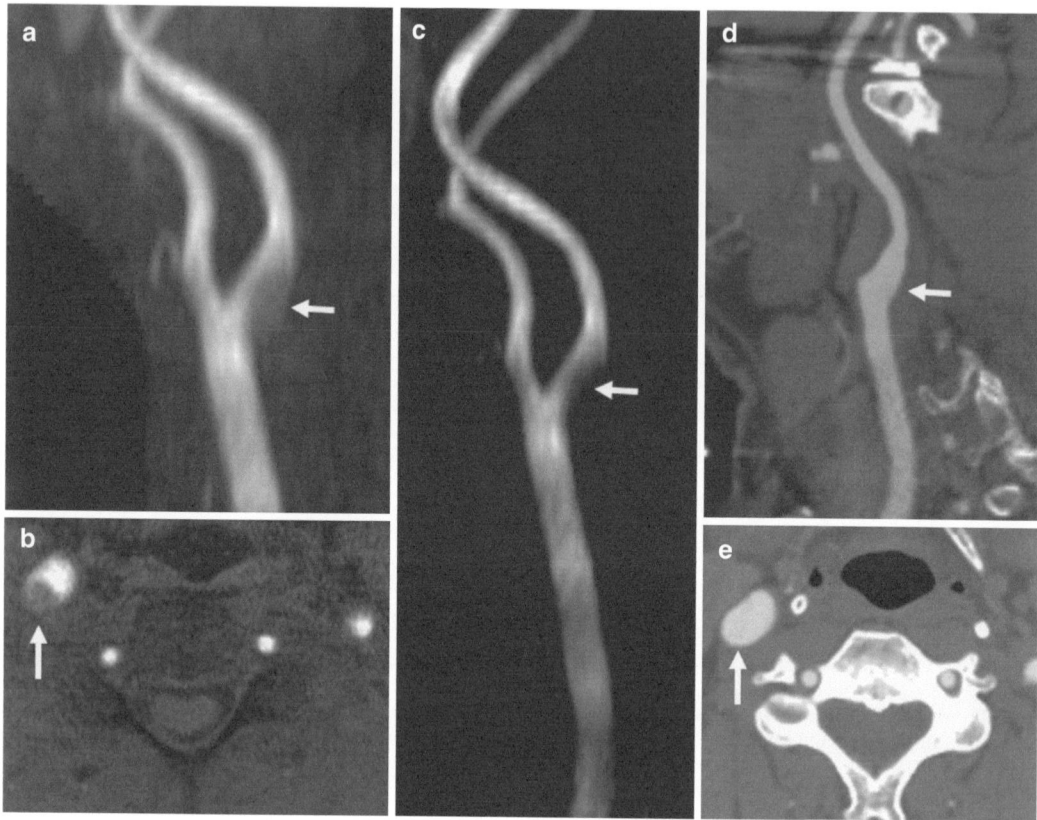

Fig. 7.2 Flow artifact at the carotid bulb. (**a–c**) TOF MRA demonstrates vague signal loss within the posterior aspect of the right carotid bulb (**a** and **b**). With improper windowing, this signal loss can be mistaken for an athero-sclerotic plaque with stenosis. (**d, e**) Curved planar reformat (**d**) and axial (**e**) CT angiographic images demonstrate a widely patent right carotid bulb confirming flow-related artifact responsible for the defect seen on MRA

Contrast-Enhanced MR Angiography (CE-MRA)

As opposed to TOF MRA, which produces signal from the flowing blood itself, CE-MRA relies on an intravascular contrast agent to directly generate signal within the vessel lumen. One benefit of CE-MRA relative to TOF MRA is its ability to acquire the same imaging volume in a shorter period of time using a single breath hold, even while imaging a larger field of view. CE-MRA is also typically acquired in the coronal plane, which allows analysis of the origins of the great vessels from the aortic arch. In addition, CE-MRA is more accurate than TOF MRA in the setting of slow-flow or high-grade stenosis, which can be overestimated with TOF

MRA. The main limitation of CE-MRA is a lower spatial resolution, which is traded off for a shorter acquisition time.

Phase-Contrast MR Imaging (PC-MRI)

PC-MRI is an additional non-contrast imaging technique that can be used in MR angiography, although in assessing head and neck vasculature is most often used for MR venography. A potential advantage of PC-MRI is its ability to provide information about the direction and velocity of flowing blood. Disadvantages of PC-MRI are its sensitive imaging parameters and small field of view often required to avoid significant artifacts.

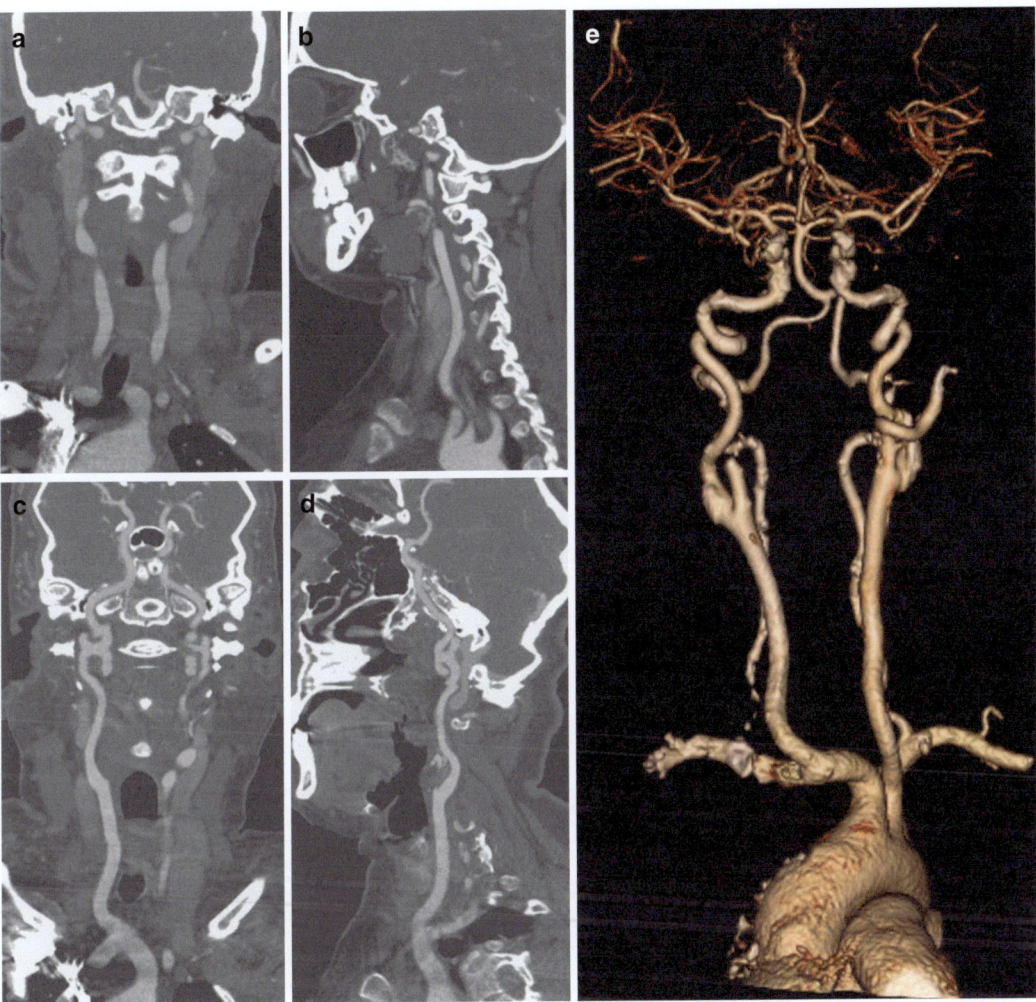

Fig. 7.3 CT angiography post-processing. Coronal (**a**) and sagittal (**b**) multiplanar reconstructions can be acquired directly from the CT scanner at the time of image acquisition. Curved planar reformats (**c**, **d**) and 3D volume-rendered images (**e**) can then be created with the use of post-processing software. Notice how the curved planar reformats allow for the entire vessel to be visualized in a single image—in this case in the coronal (**c**) and sagittal (**d**) planes

Computed Tomography Angiography (CTA)

While selective catheter angiography using digital subtraction angiography (DSA) remains the gold standard in cerebrovascular imaging, multidetector CTA represents a less invasive alternative that is both fast, reliable, and adequate for most indications of vascular imaging in routine clinical practice [4]. CTA is performed following the rapid intravenous infusion of iodinated contrast and requires proper bolus timing for the most accurate assessment.

CTA is performed in the axial plane following the rapid intravenous infusion of iodinated contrast. Axial images can then be reformatted in any imaging plane, although typically in the coronal and sagittal plane. In addition to the reformatted images produced by the scanner at the time of imaging, advanced post-processing techniques allow for a wide variety of additional evaluation tools, including 3D volume and surface-rendered images, curved planar reformats, as well as various segmentation techniques designed to isolate anatomy of interest (i.e., vessels) from surrounding structures (e.g., bone) (Fig. 7.3).

In comparison with MRA, CTA is faster, easier to acquire, and less expensive and offers higher spatial resolution without the same susceptibility to motion- or flow-related artifacts. Also, in contrast to DSA, CTA allows for simultaneous evaluation of the vessel wall and vessel lumen, as well as visualization of surrounding anatomy.

Disadvantages of CTA include patient exposure to ionizing radiation, iodinated contrast allergies, and the potential risk of contrast-induced nephropathy. An additional disadvantage of CTA, or any contrast-enhanced imaging technique, is the reliance on appropriate timing of imaging in relationship to the contrast bolus administration. This timing can be influenced by multiple patient factors, including cardiac output and intravascular blood volume, as well as equipment-specific technical factors (e.g., CT scanner speed). Failure to take these factors into account can result in lower-quality examinations.

Anatomy

Extracranial Vasculature

Blood supply to the head and neck comes from branches of the aortic arch, the great vessels, including the brachiocephalic trunk (innominate artery), left common carotid artery, and left subclavian artery. The brachiocephalic trunk then divides into the right subclavian artery and right common carotid artery.

Carotid Arteries

Both common carotid arteries bifurcate in the midcervical region, giving rise to the external and internal carotid arteries.

The external carotid arteries supply blood to the cervical and facial soft tissues, sinonasal cavity, oral cavity and pharynx, external ear, and soft tissues of the scalp. In addition, the middle meningeal branch of the external carotid artery enters the intracranial cavity through the foramen spinosum, supplying blood to the meninges.

The extracranial ICA (cervical segment) has no visible branches and enters the skull base via the carotid canal, located in the petrous portion of the temporal bone. It then traverses the petrous

bone before emerging within the cavernous sinus. The intracranial ICA is subdivided into the cavernous, clinoid, ophthalmic, and communicating segments.

Vertebral Arteries

The vertebral arteries arise as the first and largest branches of their respective subclavian arteries. The vertebral arteries are divided into four segments.

The first segment (V1; prevertebral segment) begins at the vessel origin from the subclavian artery and ends as the vessel enters the transverse foramen, which usually occurs at the C6 level [5].

After entering the transverse foramen, the second segment (V2; foraminal segment) ascends within the cervical transverse foramina from the sixth to the third cervical vertebra. The left transverse foramen is generally larger than the right, and the right vertebral artery is more commonly the hypoplastic vessel [6, 7].

The V3, or extraspinal segment of the vertebral artery, extends from the C2 transverse process to the artery's entry through the dura mater [8]. The course and anatomy of the V3 segment are complex with redundancy resulting in loops and bends that allow for mobility of the vessel with head rotation [8].

The two vertebral arteries then penetrate the dura and the arachnoid membrane at the level of the foramen magnum to enter the intracranial cavity (V4; intradural segment). The V4 segments eventually join to form the basilar artery.

Circle of Willis and Collateral Pathways

Arterial circulation in the head and neck provides a number of collateral pathways for blood flow as a means of protecting the brain from the effects of an isolated arterial occlusion or stenosis. Knowledge of these collateral pathways is essential when evaluating head and neck vasculature.

Extracranial Pathways

The most well-known extracranial collateral pathway is an anastomosis between branches of the internal and external carotid arteries occurring through the orbit and at the level of the meninges. This circulation pathway occurs by way of end-to-end connections between the ophthalmic artery, a branch of the internal carotid artery, and facial, sinonasal, and meningeal branches of the ipsilateral external carotid artery. If blood flow within the internal carotid artery becomes insufficient, flow through the branches of the external carotid artery can reverse the direction of flow within the ophthalmic artery, thereby providing a supply of blood to the ICA and circle of Willis.

Intracranial Pathways

The circle of Willis creates an important source of intracranial collateral flow, connecting the right-to-left circulation via the anterior communicating artery and the anterior-to-posterior circulation via the posterior communicating arteries. The circle of Willis is usually able to adequately compensate for occlusion of a single artery proximal to the circle. Because of its importance, it is critical that the circle of Willis be evaluated when contemplating vascular interventions in the neck. A comprehensive vascular analysis should also include assessment of the relative contribution of each of the vertebral arteries to the posterior circulation.

Pathology

Atherosclerosis

Carotid artery disease is responsible for 10–20% of ischemic strokes [9]. As such, screening for atherosclerotic disease involving the carotid artery is an important tool in stroke prevention as it can identify patients at greatest risk for stroke and triage them to the appropriate treatment.

Evaluation of Carotid Stenosis

CTA

CTA performed for evaluation of suspected carotid or vertebral artery stenosis should include from the level of the aortic arch to the circle of Willis. This is especially important in the setting of known atherosclerotic disease or associated risk factors, in order to exclude the possibility of tandem stenotic lesions [4]. Common locations for tandem lesions of atherosclerotic carotid stenosis in the head and neck include luminal narrowing of the cervical ICA at or near its origin with a separate more distal area of stenosis within the intracranial ICA. Identification of tandem lesions prior to intervention is crucial because patients who undergo carotid endarterectomy to address cervical ICA stenosis may remain symptomatic if the downstream intracranial ICA stenosis is not also addressed [4].

One limitation of CTA in the assessment of stenosis is the presence of dense atherosclerotic calcification, which can obscure contrast within the vessel lumen and result in an overestimation of the degree of stenosis [4, 10]. This can be improved by careful adjustment of the window and level setting prior to assessing luminal caliber. In addition, regardless of atherosclerotic calcification, assessment of arterial stenosis can be inaccurate if axial images do not represent a true cross section of the vessel, such as with a tortuous vessel. In these situations, curved planar reformats can be helpful to ensure a true cross-sectional measurement [4, 11].

MRA

MRA noninvasively generates high-resolution images of the carotid arteries without the use of contrast material. However, MRA, and in particular TOF MRA, has specific pitfalls and limitations. One important example is in distinguishing high-grade stenosis (near-occlusion) from complete occlusion—in these situations CTA and/or CE-MRA is superior to TOF MRA (Figs. 7.4 and 7.5) [4]. Generally speaking, MRA is thought to overestimate the degree of stenosis, particularly on axial TOF MRA source data without MIP and MPR reformats [4, 11]. However, correlation with angiography suggests that, despite these limitations, high-quality TOF MRA in the evaluation of extracranial carotid and vertebral artery disease can have a sensitivity of 97–100% and specificity of 82–96% under optimal conditions [12]. One important note should be made that MRA is not limited in the setting of vascular calcification and should be the modality of choice when calcification limits duplex or CTA.

Fig. 7.4 Ulcerated atherosclerotic plaque and severe stenosis. (**a**) Maximal intensity projection rendering from TOF MRA of the neck demonstrates narrowing of the left carotid bulb with a flow gap in the proximal left internal carotid artery (solid arrow), as well as an ulcerated plaque as evidenced by an outpouching of flow-related enhancement projecting posteriorly from the proximal carotid bulb (dashed arrow). (**b**) Sagittal curved planar reformat from CTA demonstrates severe stenosis correlating with the flow gap on MRA (solid arrow) along with contrast filling the ulcerated plaque at the proximal carotid bulb (dashed arrow). (**c**) Axial CTA image demonstrates the small residual lumen (arrow) at the site of severe stenosis due to a mixed density atherosclerotic plaque

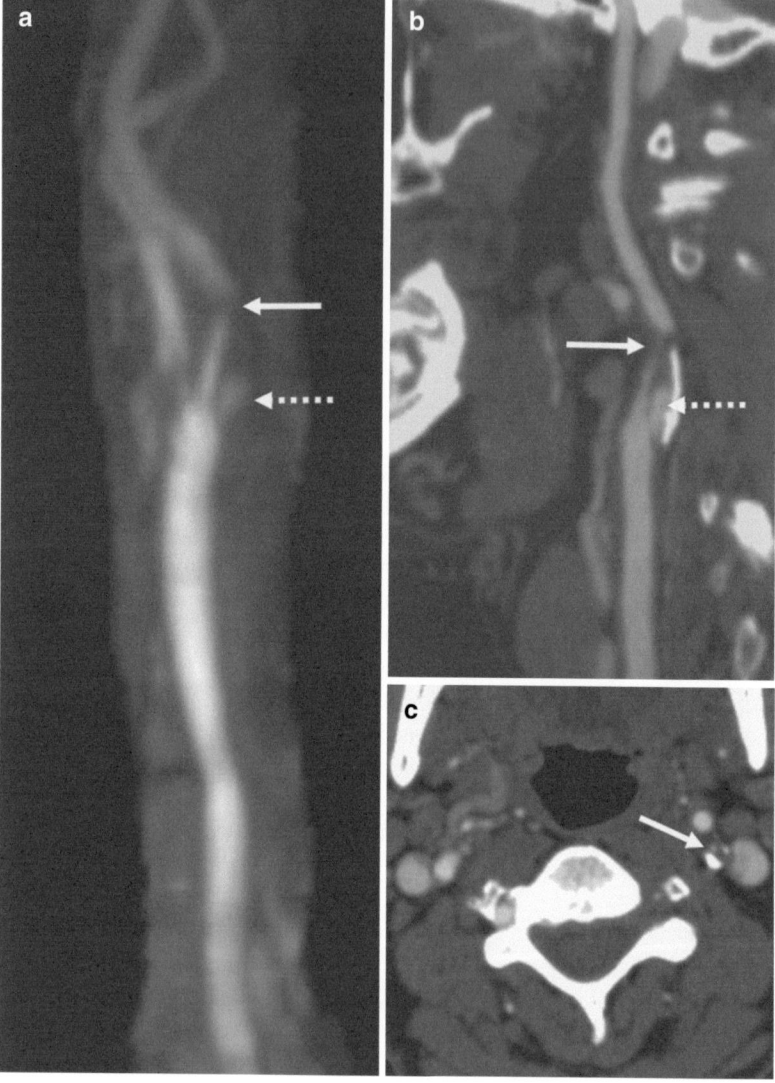

Assessing the Degree of Stenosis

Measuring the degree of carotid stenosis is typically performed using methods derived from two prior studies, the North American Symptomatic Carotid Endarterectomy Trial (NASCET) and the European Carotid Surgery Trial (ECST). Although both methods originally assessed degree of stenosis using conventional angiogram, both are routinely applied to cross-sectional imaging techniques.

The NASCET method assesses the luminal diameter at the point of greatest stenosis and at the normal part of the ICA beyond the carotid bulb. The percent stenosis is determined by cal-

culating the ratio of these two measurements: (1 − [diameter at maximal stenosis/diameter at the normal ICA]) * 100%) (Fig. 7.6) [13, 14]. In comparison, the ECST method determines the percentage diameter stenosis at the point of maximum narrowing, using as the denominator an estimate of the original width of the artery at this point of maximal narrowing [15]. One caveat to keep in mind is that assessment of the degree of stenosis is limited if the NASCET method is used in the setting of near-occlusion, as this often results in narrowing of the post-stenotic ICA secondary to reduced flow and ultimately leads to an underestimation of the degree of stenosis

Fig. 7.5 Near-occlusion of the carotid. (**a**) Maximal intensity projection rendering from TOF MRA of the neck demonstrates apparent occlusion of the left internal carotid artery beyond the carotid bulb as evidenced by abrupt loss of flow-related enhancement (solid arrow). (**b**) Sagittal maximal intensity projection reformat from CTA demonstrates a tiny residual patent lumen of the internal carotid artery compatible with a "string sign" (solid arrows). (**c**) Axial CTA image demonstrates a tiny residual lumen (arrow) within the internal carotid artery. In addition, note the importance of proper timing of the contrast bolus as this acquisition was performed too late as evidenced by venous enhancement and poor arterial opacification

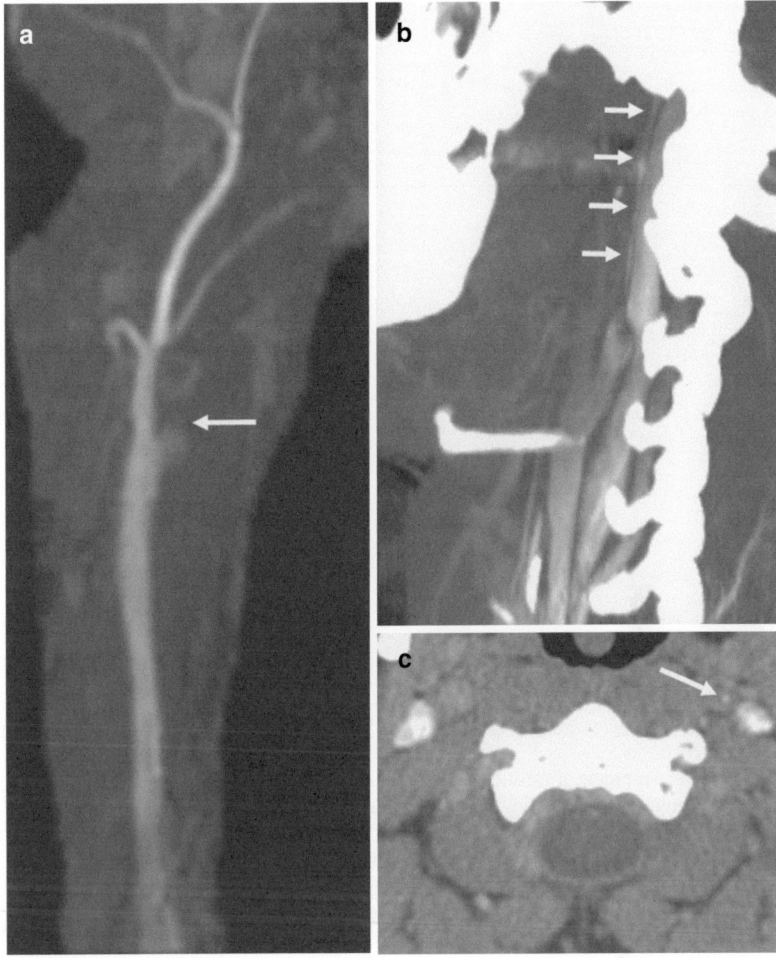

[14]. In the original NASCET reports, these near-occlusions were identified and assigned as 95% stenosis [14].

Carotid Plaque Characterization

The degree of carotid stenosis remains the standard imaging parameter used to report the extent and severity of carotid artery stenosis and is also the primary clinical criteria used for predicting the risk of stroke related to atherosclerotic disease [16, 17]. However, beyond simply the degree of stenosis, disruption of a pre-existing carotid atherosclerotic plaque with subsequent plaque rupture and thromboembolism is also thought to be an important cause of ischemic stroke (Fig. 7.7) [18]. The vulnerability of an atherosclerotic plaque to disruption is thought to be related to the plaque's intrinsic composition.

As such, characterization of plaque morphology can be helpful to identify those plaques at greatest risk of leading to subsequent cerebrovascular events and properly triaging those patients to the appropriate treatment.

Intraplaque hemorrhage has long been recognized as an important component of a complex atherosclerotic plaque. However, a number of additional plaque features have also been shown to be associated with an increased risk of stroke, including common carotid artery intima-media thickness, plaques with thin fibrous caps and large lipid cores, as well as plaque ulceration [16]. In contrast to these high-risk features, plaques with high calcium content are thought to be associated with a lower risk of stroke, particularly when the calcification is located superficially [19].

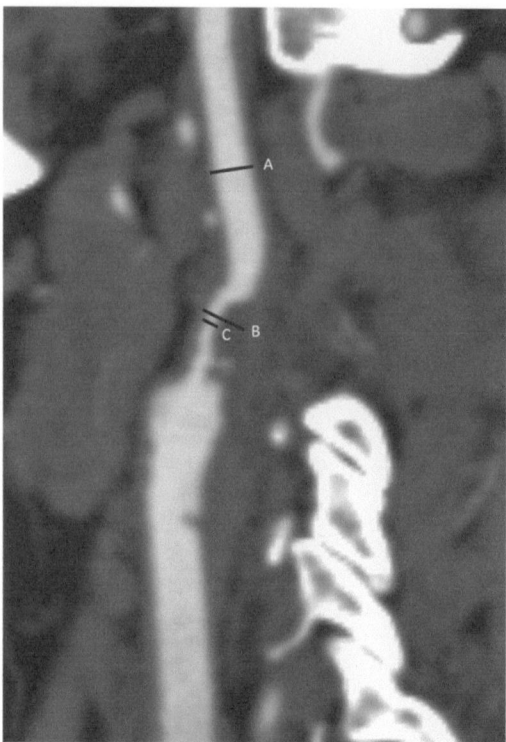

Fig. 7.6 Measurement of carotid stenosis. Sagittal curved planar-reformatted image from CTA demonstrates methods for stenosis measurements used with the North American Symptomatic Carotid Endarterectomy Trial (NASCET) and the European Carotid Surgery Trial (ECST) methods. Stenosis measured by NASCET = (1 − [C/A]) * 100%. Stenosis measured by ECST = (1 − [C/B]) * 100%

MRI can identify the lipid-rich necrotic core and the fibrous capsule with high sensitivity and specificity [20]. MRI can also distinguish between an intact thick, thin, and ruptured fibrous cap [21]. In addition, specific MRI protocols have the ability to demonstrate certain plaque components, including calcium, lipid, and fibrocellular element, as well as thrombus within the plaques [22]. Contrast agents can also be used to evaluate atherosclerotic plaque, which not only improves visualization of the degree of stenosis but also facilitates further characterization of the vessel wall, as enhancing regions on MRI have been shown to strongly correlate with regions of neovascularity and inflammation on histology [23].

CTA, while highly accurate in identifying calcification, has been less reliable in describing carotid plaque morphology. In a prior study by Wintermark et al., there was only a 72.6% agreement between CTA and histologic examination in carotid plaque characterization [16]. CTA showed perfect concordance with histologic examinations for the presence of calcifications and also performed well in detecting ulcerations and in measuring the fibrous cap thickness [16]. However, while showing good correlation with histology for large lipid cores and large hemorrhages, the reliability was otherwise limited for these components due to significant overlap between densities associated with lipid-rich necrotic cores, connective tissue, and hemorrhage [16].

Recurrent Carotid Stenosis After Carotid Revascularization

Neointimal hyperplasia is the most common pathophysiology of restenosis after carotid stenting [24]. Neointimal hyperplasia generally occurs in the first few months after carotid stenting and is uncommon to be encountered after the first 24 months [24].

Doppler ultrasonography is a reliable tool to evaluate for in-stent restenosis, keeping in mind that peak velocity for both systolic and diastolic flow is slightly higher inside the stent than in native arteries [25, 26]. Evaluation with Doppler US can be limited by anatomic factors, particularly in evaluation of the distal end of the stent, which can be overcome with CTA (Fig. 7.8), MRA, or DSA.

Cross-sectional imaging is relatively limited in accurate analysis of the luminal caliber within the carotid stent, mainly because of the metallic artifact both on CTA and MRA. Beam hardening artifact on CTA is directly related to the amount of metal in the stent. This technical limitation can be overcome with specific newer CT techniques such as spectral or dual source CTA and specialized post-processing software [26]. TOF MRA has significant limitation in the assessment of in-stent

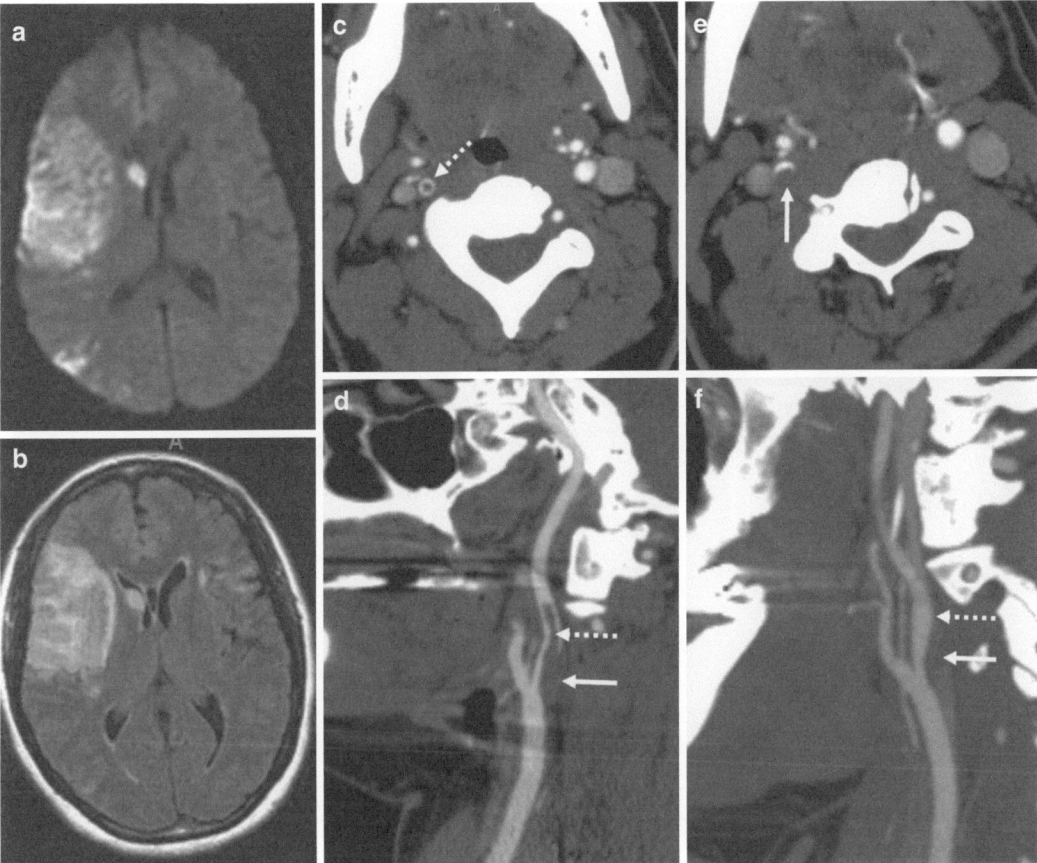

Fig. 7.7 Ruptured atherosclerotic plaque with intraluminal thrombus and acute infarct. Axial diffusion-weighted (**a**) and FLAIR (**b**) images demonstrate an acute infarct in the right middle cerebral artery territory. (**c, d**) Axial and sagittal curved planar reformatted images from CTA of the neck demonstrates a low-density, non-calcified atherosclerotic plaque at the right carotid bulb (solid arrow) with an adherent thrombus floating in the proximal internal carotid artery lumen. (**e, f**) Follow-up CTA images again demonstrate the low-density atherosclerotic plaque (solid arrow) with resolution of the intraluminal thrombus (dashed arrow)

restenosis, primarily due to limited in-stent luminal visibility with artificial luminal narrowing related to the magnetic susceptibility artifact from the metallic stent (Fig. 7.9). Slightly improved characterization is possible with CE-MRA, where the presence of an intraluminal contrast agent allows a more accurate luminal assessment [27]. Digital subtraction angiography remains the standard of imaging if restenosis is suspected by luminal narrowing on CTA or decreased flow-related enhancement on MRA.

Restenosis after carotid endarterectomy is amenable to characterization with Doppler ultrasound, CTA, or MRA, given the absence of a metallic implant. Restenosis following carotid endarterectomy usually occurs gradually with most occurring during the first 2 years after surgery [28, 29]. The primary cause of restenosis during this time period is myointimal hyperplasia, an arterial wall cellular reaction caused by surgical manipulation, with progressive atherosclerosis usually occurring later [28]. Intimal hyperplasia will present with circumferential luminal narrowing (Fig. 7.10). Recurrent atherosclerotic plaque will have similar imaging characteristics to the atherosclerotic involvement with asymmetric narrowing, calcifications, fatty content, and ulcerations.

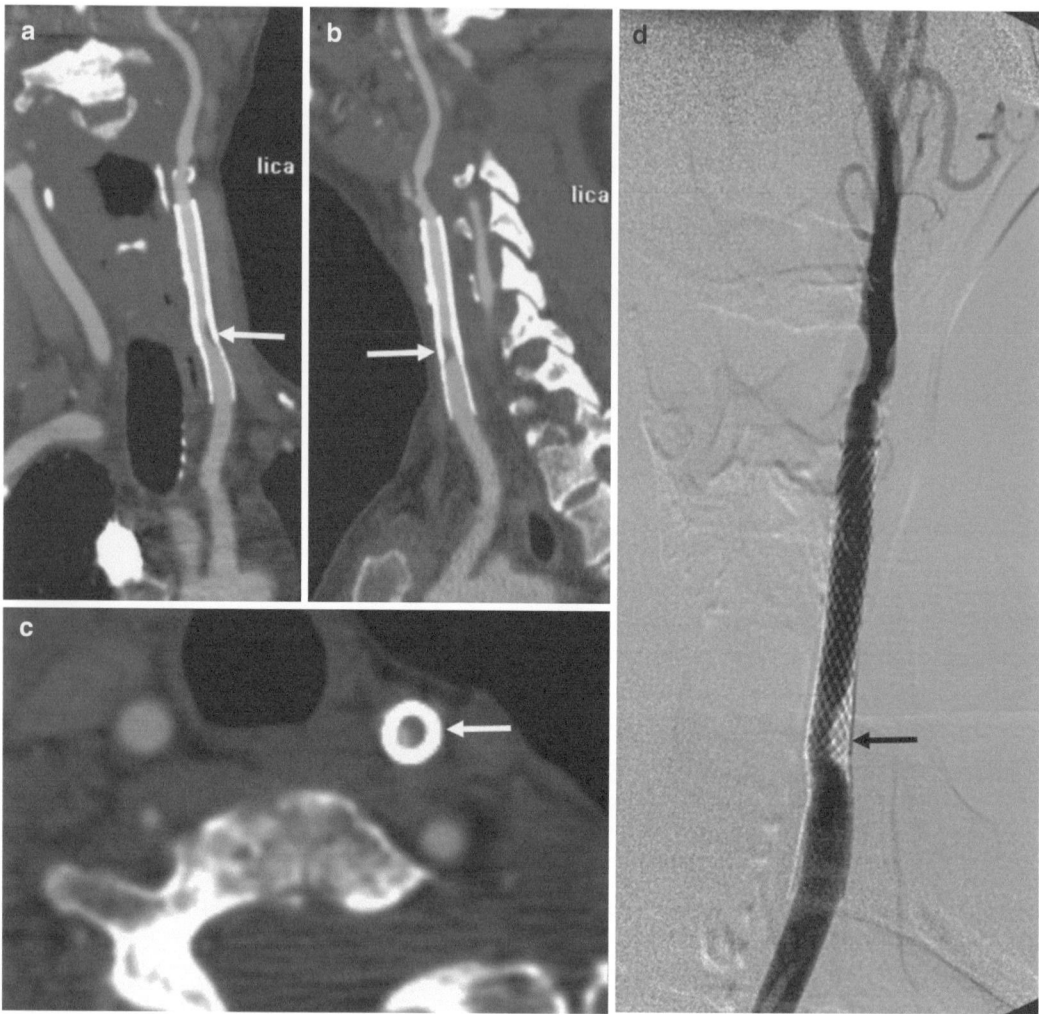

Fig. 7.8 In-stent restenosis on CT angiography. (**a–c**) Curved planar reformats (**a**, **b**), and axial (**c**) CT angiogram demonstrates the capability of CTA in assessing the stent lumen with proper windowing. In-stent restenosis is evidenced by the eccentric low density narrowing within the proximal aspect of the stent lumen. (**d**) Conventional angiogram better demonstrates the degree of luminal narrowing

Evaluation of Vertebral Artery Stenosis

Posterior circulation strokes account for 20% of all strokes. Of these strokes involving the posterior circulation, 20–25% are thought to be due to vertebral artery stenosis likely resulting in artery to artery embolization [30]. Despite this, management of vertebral artery stenosis remains somewhat uncertain due to the lack of large randomized controlled trials such as those performed for carotid stenosis.

Imaging evaluation of the vertebral arteries is more challenging relative to the carotid arteries due to their smaller size. The gold standard for evaluating vertebral artery stenosis is digital subtraction angiography. However, in terms of noninvasive imaging modalities, both CE-MRA and CTA were shown to be more sensitive than DUS for identifying vertebral artery stenosis [31].

Fig. 7.9 Technical limitation of TOF MRA in assessing in-stent restenosis. (**a**) Maximum intensity projection rendering from TOF MRA shows loss of flow-related enhancement within the cervical internal carotid artery. (**b**) Conventional angiogram demonstrates a patent lumen with narrowing distally. This case demonstrates the limitation of TOF MRA in evaluating for in-stent restenosis

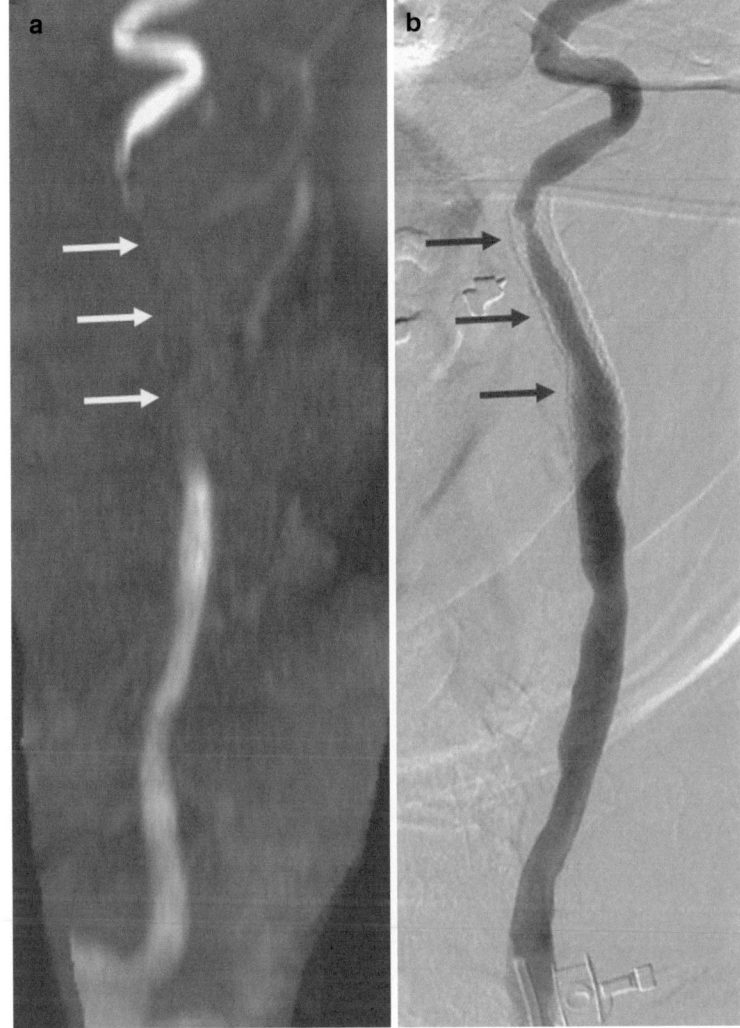

Subclavian Steal

Subclavian steal phenomenon occurs when there is high-grade stenosis or occlusion of a proximal portion of the subclavian artery with compensatory collateral flow from the contralateral side via the vertebrobasilar junction. This leads to reversal of flow within the vertebral artery ipsilateral to the diseased subclavian artery in order to maintain distal arterial supply to the affected upper extremity. This phenomenon is given the term *subclavian steal syndrome* when this reversal of vertebral artery flow results in symptoms of cerebral ischemia.

Imaging evaluation for subclavian steal must not only evaluate the vessels for patency and stenosis but also the direction of flow within the vessels. CTA and routine CE-MRA can reliably identify stenosis within the subclavian artery, but neither provides information about the direction of flow. TOF MRA is sensitive to flow direction with reversed flow leading to loss of flow-related enhancement, although it should be noted that severe stenosis and vessel occlusion would demonstrate a similar finding. However, loss of flow-related enhancement on TOF MRA images within the vertebral artery ipsilateral to a subclavian artery stenosis coupled with demonstration

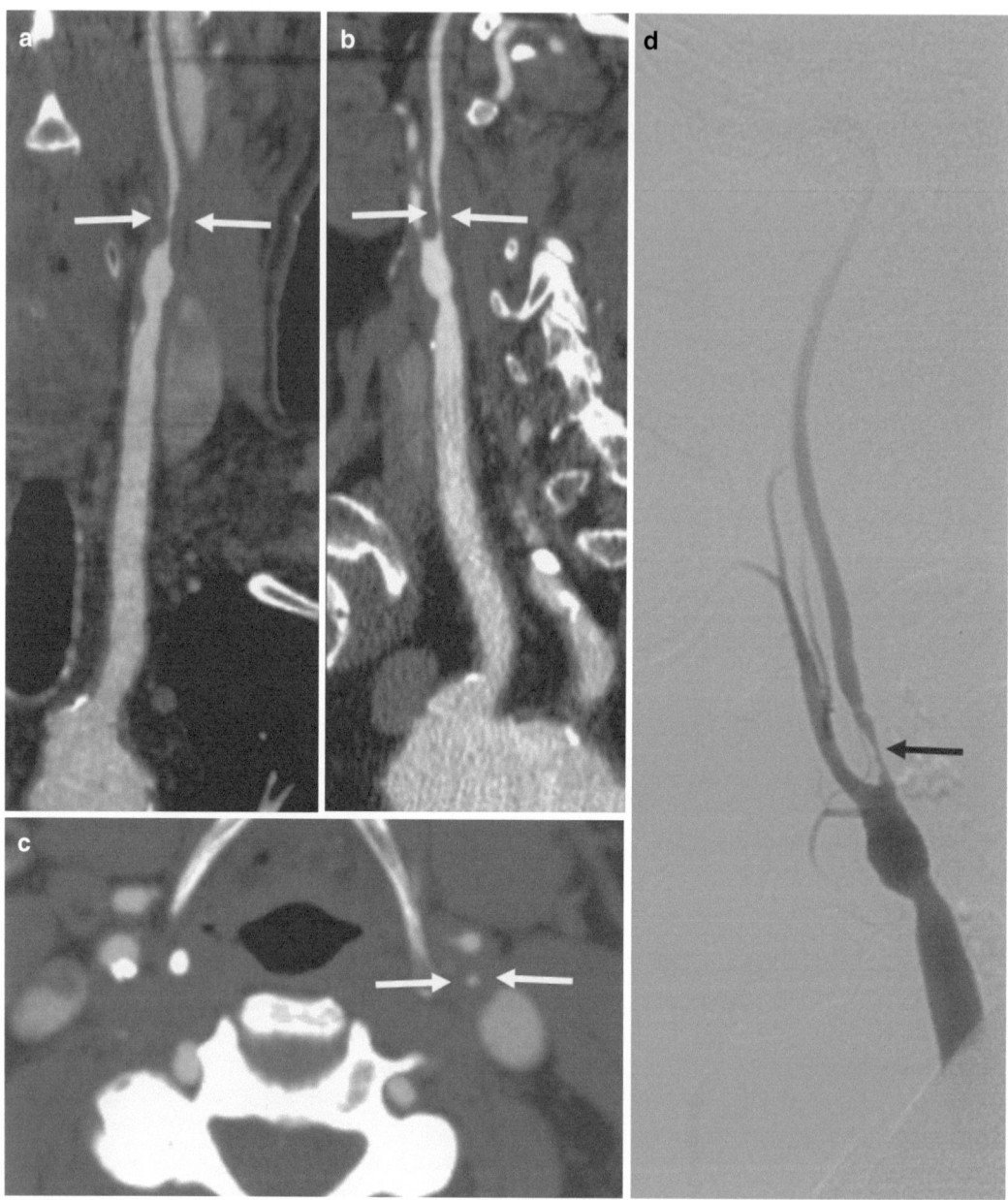

Fig. 7.10 Myointimal hyperplasia with restenosis follow-ing carotid endarterectomy. (**a**–**c**) Curved planar reformats (**a**, **b**) and axial (**c**) CT angiogram demonstrates circumfer-ential luminal narrowing within the proximal left internal carotid artery. (**d**) Conventional angiogram confirms the luminal narrowing compatible with restenosis

of vessel patency on either CTA or CE-MRA can be inferred to represent subclavian steal phenom-enon. Time-resolved CE-MRA can also be used to demonstrate delayed and retrograde filling of the affected vertebral artery (Fig. 7.11).

Radiation-Induced Carotid Stenosis

External beam radiotherapy is often necessary to treat cancers of the oral cavity, pharynx, lar-ynx, or salivary gland or lymphomas involving

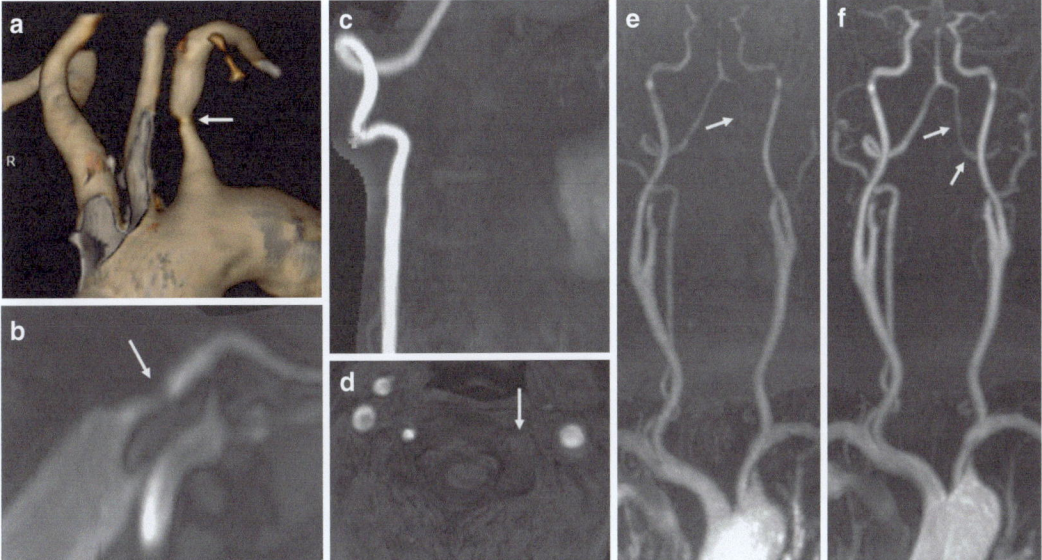

Fig. 7.11 Subclavian steal phenomenon. (**a, b**) Volume-rendered 3D image and curved planar reformat from MRA of the chest demonstrate stenosis of the proximal left subclavian artery. (**c, d**) TOF MRA images demonstrate absent flow-related enhancement within the left ver-tebral artery, which is representative of either absent, slow, or reversed flow. (**e, f**) Time-resolved contrast-enhanced MRA demonstrates delayed enhancement of the left vertebral artery, which flows in the opposite direction via the vertebrobasilar junction

the cervical lymph nodes. Radiation-induced carotid artery stenosis is reported to occur in 30–50% of patients treated with external irradiation for head and neck cancer [32]. Three types of radiation damage to the carotid artery have been described following neck irradiation. These include (1) carotid rupture, which usually occurs when radiotherapy is combined with radical neck dissection (Fig. 7.12); (2) early arterial occlusion, typically occurring within months following radiotherapy; and (3) late development of athero-sclerosis, which is the most frequent lesion and is associated with neurologic symptoms occurring several years after irradiation [33].

Causes of radiation-induced carotid stenosis include (1) damage to the vasa vasorum caus-ing ischemic necrosis with subsequent fibrosis, (2) adventitial fibrosis with narrowing, and (3) acceleration of the atherosclerotic process [34]. On imaging, radiation-induced stenoses are usu-ally long and affect arteries that are less com-monly involved with standard atherosclerosis, such as the common carotid artery (Fig. 7.13).

Correlation of the site of involvement with the initial radiation field is useful in establishing the diagnosis.

Dissection

Dissections of the carotid and vertebral arteries, although rare, are an important cause of isch-emic stroke in young- and middle-aged patients, accounting for 10–25% of such cases [35]. Dissections can be either traumatic or atraumatic in nature. Traumatic dissections are those in which a clear traumatic etiology is recognized—either from penetrating injury or blunt trauma. Atraumatic dissections can then be classified into one of two types: (1) those in which no precipi-tating factor is recognized (spontaneous) and (2) those in which there is a clearly recognized pre-ceding movement or position that is not the result of an external force (trivial trauma) [36].

Spontaneous dissections in the neck most commonly involve the ICA (68%) and less com-

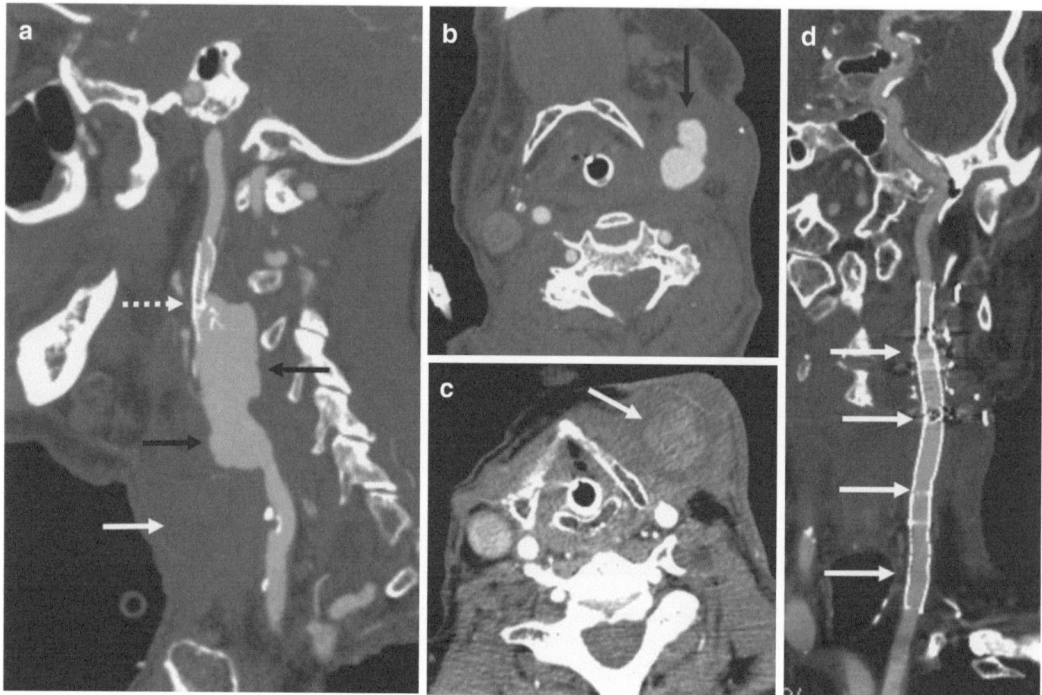

Fig. 7.12 Radiation-induced carotid artery pseudoaneurysm with rupture in patient previously treated with carotid stenting for radiation-induced stenosis. (**a–c**) CT angiogram demonstrates formation of a large pseudoaneurysm (black arrows) at the proximal aspect of the stent (dashed arrow) with a large adjacent hyperdense hematoma (white arrows). (**d**) CT angiogram following treatment with a covered stent (arrows)

monly the vertebral artery (27%), with both arteries rarely involved (5%) [37]. In addition, dissection involving multiple vessels is present in 28% of cases [37]. Risk factors that predispose patients to dissections include systemic hypertension, fibromuscular dysplasia, or other underlying connective tissue diseases. In fact, fibromuscular dysplasia can be found in up to 15% of patients with cervical artery dissection [38].

Understanding the typical locations for dissections to occur within the carotid and vertebral arteries is helpful, as it can assist in focusing one's attention to certain locations when dissection is suspected. When the carotid artery is involved, the most commonly involved segment is the high cervical segment distal to the carotid bulb, before the vessel enters the petrous segment of the carotid canal [35]. Dissections typically do not extend beyond the entry into the petrous portion of the carotid. When spontaneous dissections involve the vertebral artery, a prior study of 169 patients found that the V2 (35%) and V3 (34%) segments are more commonly involved than the V1 (20%) and V4 (11%) segments [37].

CT/CTA

Non-contrast CT of the head can sometimes provide the first evidence of a carotid dissection, demonstrating an enlarged and hyperattenuating vessel near the skull base. In the setting of traumatic dissection, CT also has the added benefit of allowing for evaluation of the surrounding soft tissues and bony structures.

On CTA, carotid dissections are typically characterized by a narrow, eccentric lumen with an increase in the overall external diameter of the vessel due to the presence of a false lumen and variable amounts of intramural blood products (Fig. 7.14). The luminal stenosis seen in the setting of a carotid dissection is typically irregular, beginning approximately 2–3 cm beyond the carotid bulb and extending for vari-

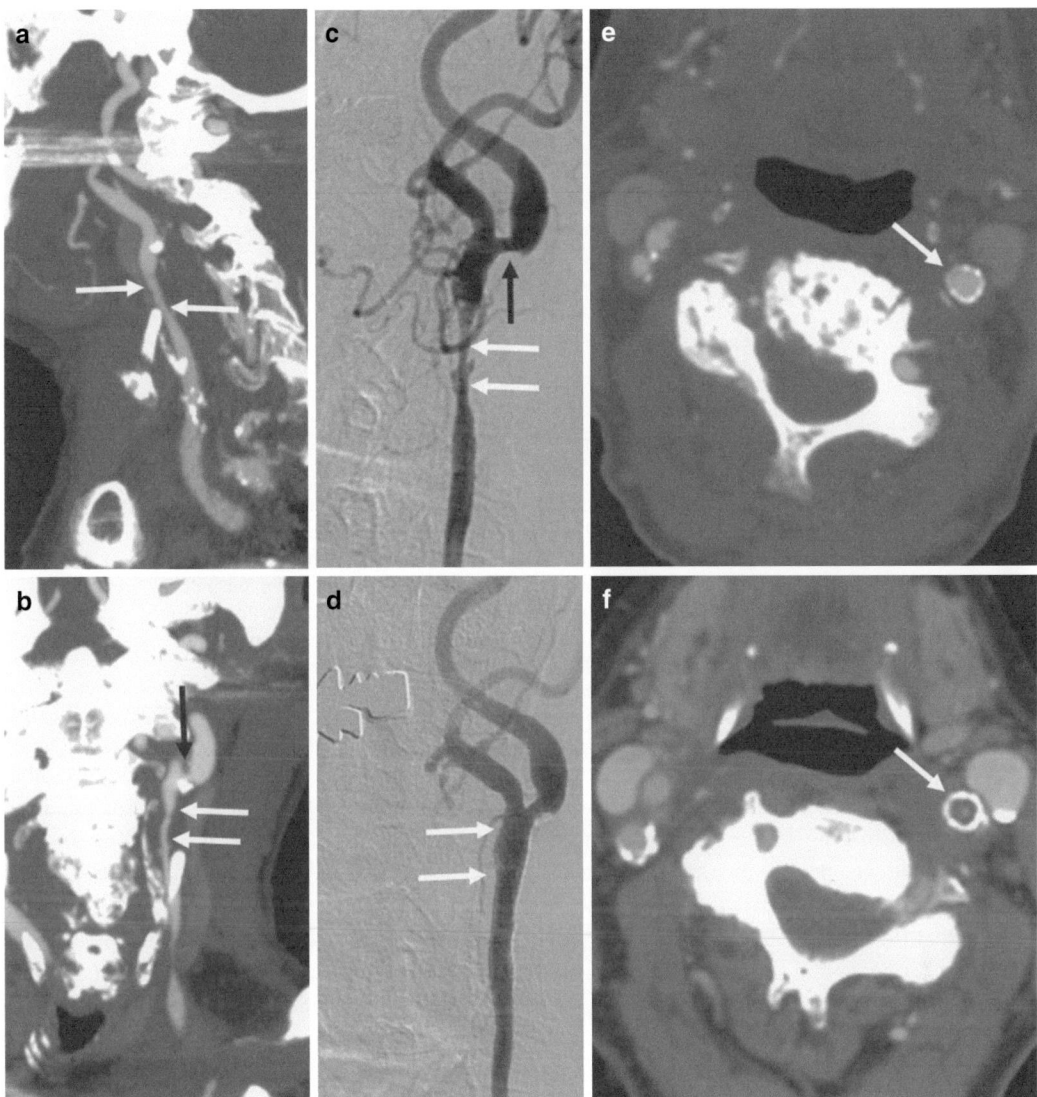

Fig. 7.13 Radiation-induced carotid stenosis followed by stenting and in-stent restenosis. (**a–c**) CT angiography (**a**, **b**) and conventional angiogram (**c**) in a patient with prior history of squamous cell carcinoma treated with radiation demonstrate a relatively long segment of stenosis (white arrows) involving the distal left common carotid artery with additional focal stenosis at the carotid bulb (black arrow). (**d**, **e**) Conventional angiogram (**d**) and axial CTA (**e**) images post-stenting demonstrate a widely patent common carotid artery lumen. (**f**) Follow-up CTA demonstrates concentric luminal narrowing within the stent compatible with in-stent restenosis

ous lengths along the artery, although generally stopping at the entry into the petrous portion of the temporal bone. It is rare for the dissection to propagate across the dura, but when this does occur, it may be associated with subarachnoid hemorrhage. When the vessel is occluded, the true lumen is completely collapsed or thrombosed, often due to significant mass effect from the false lumen and/or intramural hematoma. Pseudoaneurysms, which represent focal outpouchings of contrast at the site of a vessel wall breach, may be iatrogenic or posttraumatic and can occur either in isolation or in the setting of arterial dissection [4]. Pseudoaneurysms are typically seen in the subacute to chronic phase of the dissection.

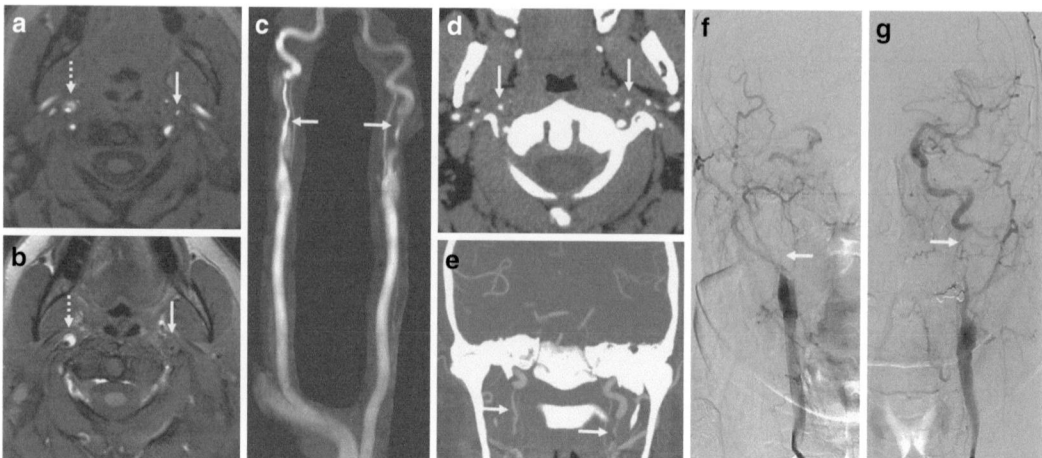

Fig. 7.14 Bilateral high cervical internal carotid artery dissection. Axial TOF MRA source images (**a**) and axial T1-weighted fat-suppressed images (**b**) demonstrate the luminal narrowing (arrow) and the mural hematoma with overall vessel expansion. On the right (dashed arrows), the T1 hyperintense crescent corresponds to subacute blood products, and on the left (solid arrows), acute mural hematoma is T1 hypointense. There is severe bilateral luminal narrowing, as seen on volume-rendered images (**c**), with flow limitation on the left demonstrated as a less robust flow-related enhancement. Corresponding axial (**d**) and coronal (**e**) CTA images demonstrate the luminal narrowing. Bilateral ICA dissection is confirmed on right (**f**) and left (**g**) digital subtraction angiography with severe luminal compromise (arrows)

MRI/MRA

Identification of an acute stroke with diffusion-weighted MR imaging of the brain, particularly in younger patients, may be the first sign of a dissection within the neck warranting further evaluation with MRA (Fig. 7.15). While intracranial dissection is rare, loss of the normal flow voids at the skull base may also warrant further evaluation with MRA.

MRA is an appealing alternative to CTA or DSA in the evaluation of arterial dissection given its ability to noninvasively demonstrate arterial flow without ionizing radiation or intravenous contrast. Axial T1-weighted MRA with fat suppression can detect high T1 signal intensity within the vessel wall or false lumen, which represents late acute/subacute blood products (methemoglobin) and is suggestive of dissection. This sign, referred to as the crescent sign, requires fat suppression for adequate visualization and may not be present during the early acute period [39, 40]. It is important to note, however, that axial T1-weighted fat-suppressed MRA images can demonstrate high signal from etiologies other than intramural hematoma as well, such as from the epidural venous plexus surrounding the vessel, slow intraluminal flow, and failure of adequate fat suppression [40]. Axial T2-weighted MR sequences may improve sensitivity for the diagnosis of dissection by providing another MR sequence to confirm hyperintense intramural blood products or demonstrate vessel wall thickening.

CTA/MRA is thought to be less sensitive in the evaluation of vertebral artery dissection given the smaller vessel size and difficulty in distinguishing a methemoglobin crescent sign from a normal venous plexus in the foramen transversarium [40]. In reality, MRI/MRA exams may not always demonstrate findings sufficient to make the diagnosis of dissection but can often identify abnormalities that raise the possibility of dissection which can then be confirmed with CTA given its ability to demonstrate additional findings indicative of dissection (e.g., intimal flaps and pseudoaneurysms) [39].

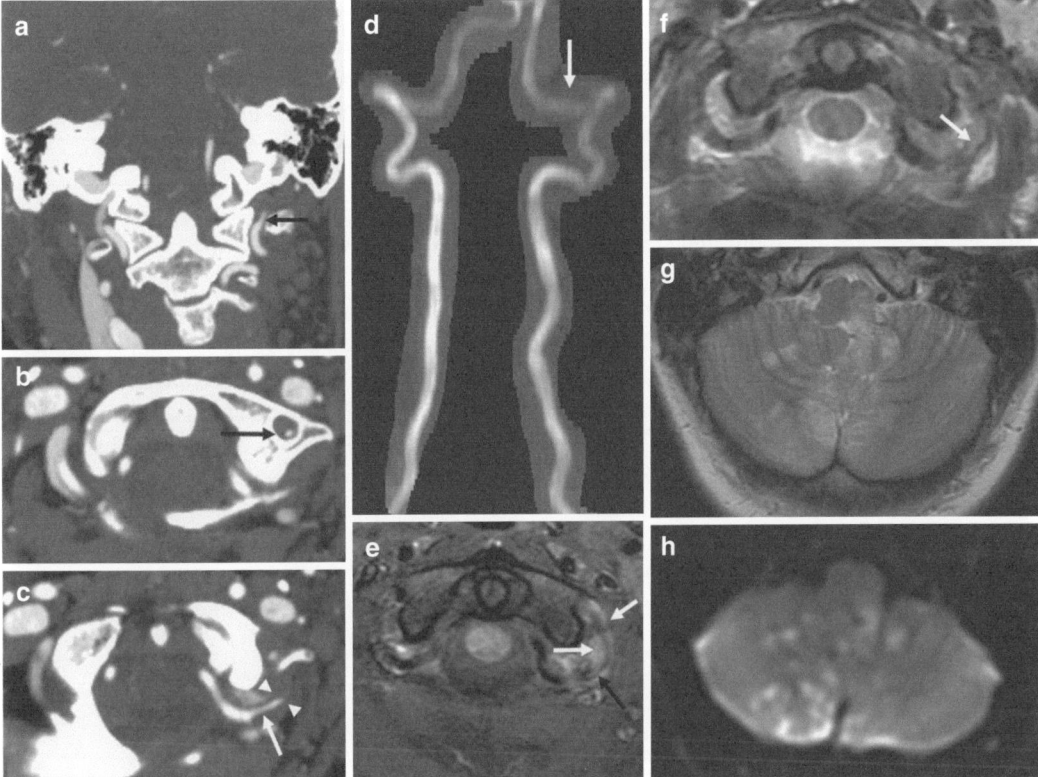

Fig. 7.15 Left vertebral artery dissection. (**a**) Coronal multiplanar reconstruction demonstrates abrupt caliber change of the left vertebral artery at the C1 transverse foramen level. (**b**) Axial CTA image demonstrates a small caliber left vertebral artery in comparison to the C1 transverse foramen, which is also eccentrically positioned within the foramen. (**c**) Axial CTA image demonstrates a small caliber left vertebral artery lumen (arrow) with an abrupt caliber change at the V3–V4 junction. The walls of the expanded left vertebral artery can be subtly identified beyond the enhancing lumen (arrowheads). (**d**) TOF MRA demonstrates subtle diminished signal intensity within the left vertebral artery. (**e**) Axial T1 fat-saturated sequence demonstrates hemorrhage within the vessel walls (white arrows) outlining the narrowed caliber flow void (black arrow). (**f**) Axial T2-weighted image demonstrates a small and irregular flow void of the left vertebral artery with surrounding hyperintense signal. (**g**, **h**) T2-weighted (**g**) and diffusion-weighted (**h**) images demonstrate acute infarcts within the left posterolateral medulla and cerebellum

Fibromuscular Dysplasia

Fibromuscular dysplasia (FMD) is an uncommon nonatherosclerotic, noninflammatory vascular disease which affects small- and medium-sized arteries [41, 42]. Although the renal vessels are classically thought to be most commonly involved, recent findings have shown that the cervical internal carotid and vertebral arteries are just as commonly affected [43]. Approximately 90% of patients with cervical FMD are women, typically in the fourth or fifth decade of life [44].

FMD has been classified into three histologic subtypes according to the portion of the arterial wall involved. These three subtypes include the intimal, medial, and adventitial forms with the medial subtype occurring in 90% of cases [44]. While oftentimes an incidental finding, FMD can result in arterial stenosis, occlusion, aneurysm, or dissection, potentially leading to clinical findings of dizziness, pulsatile tinnitus, TIA, or even stroke. As such, recognition of imaging findings suggestive of FMD is important.

The most well-recognized imaging finding of FMD is the classic "string of beads" appearance on angiography, which is characterized by alternating areas of vessel stenosis and dilatation (Fig. 7.16). This finding is seen in the most common medial variant of FMD and is suggestive of this diagnosis in the absence of another cause (vasospasm, vasculitis, etc.). The imaging appearance is due to the formation of fibromuscular ridges leading to arterial stenosis with alternating areas of arterial dilatation caused by smooth muscle loss [42]. The intimal variant of FMD is thought to be the second most common subtype and is seen on imaging as focal angiographic stenosis secondary to the nonatherosclerotic, noninflammatory accumulation of fibrous tissue in the intima [42]. The adventitial subtype of FMD occurs less than 1% of the time and is due to collagen deposition into the surrounding adventitia with extension into the periarterial tissue [42]. CTA and MRA can diagnose FMD

in demonstrating the segmental luminal caliber changes. It is important to carefully review the reformatted images in addition to the axial source images, as subtle web-like involvement is more apparent in the sagittal or coronal planes.

Vascular Malformations

Vascular malformations can occur anywhere in the head and neck but are most common in the oral cavity or nasal cavity with frequent involvement of the tongue, lips, and nasal septum [45]. Vascular malformations are classified according to their underlying vascular elements, and general categories include high flow arteriovenous malformations, venous malformations, capillary malformations, lymphatic malformations, or any combination of these groups [46]. The arterial

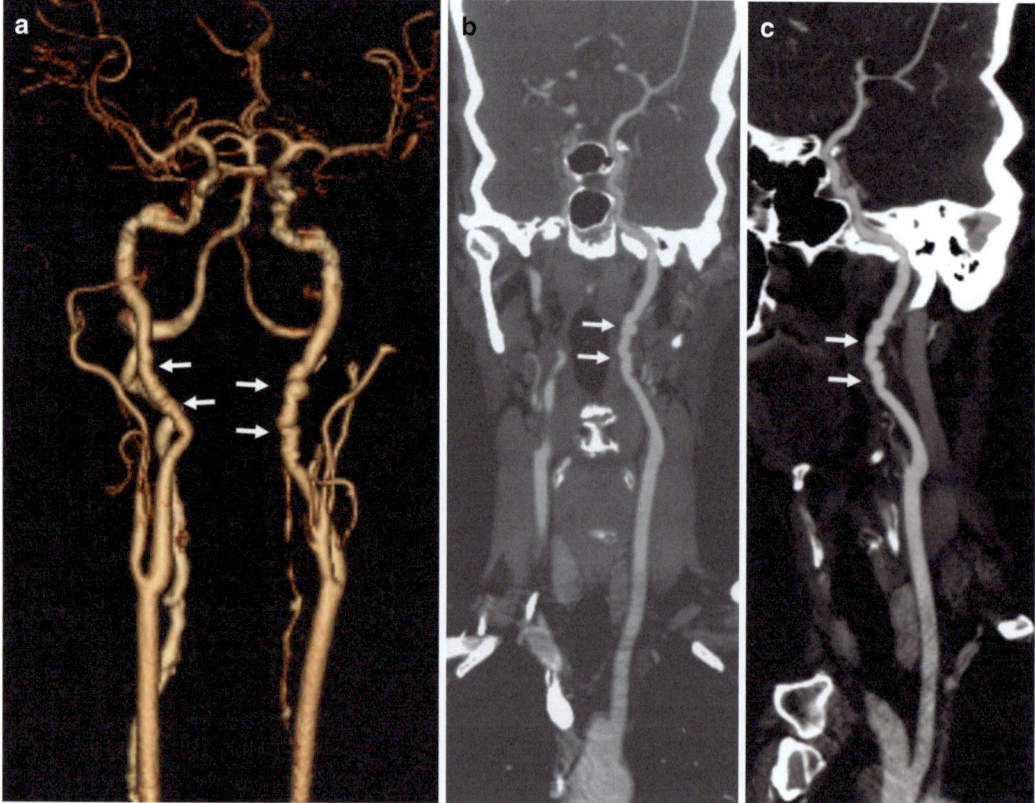

Fig. 7.16 Fibromuscular dysplasia. (**a**) Volume-rendered 3D image demonstrates a beaded appearance of both internal carotid arteries, which is also demonstrated on

coronal (**b**) and sagittal (**c**) curved planar reformatted images of the left internal carotid artery

supply to vascular malformations is dictated by their location and the adjacent native vasculature, but in the neck, these vascular lesions are often supplied by branches of the external carotid artery with additional recruitment of branches from the internal carotid artery or vertebral artery based on location and overall size [45].

High flow vascular malformations are congenital anomalies which are subdivided into arteriovenous malformations (AVMs) and arteriovenous fistulas (AVFs). AVMs typically have a nidus of abnormal vessels interposed between the arterial and venous side (Fig. 7.17), whereas AVFs consist of direct connection of a feeding artery to the draining vein. AVFs are most commonly acquired in the setting of trauma. Both AVFs and AVMs are well visualized with MR angiography, which will demonstrate the characteristic aberrant vascular connection between one or more dilated feeding arteries and enlarged draining veins without an intervening capillary network. Dynamic angiographic techniques will typically display early venous enhancement, and gradient echo sequences will demonstrate the arterial flow voids associated with these high flow lesions.

Venous malformations are the most common vascular malformation in the neck and often present in childhood [46]. Common locations include subcutaneous tissues of the face with variable involvement of the periorbital region,

muscles of mastication, and deep neck spaces [46]. Phleboliths are commonly seen in venous malformations and are highly suggestive of this diagnosis. MRI is the preferred imaging modality for assessing venous malformations of the head and neck, with these lobulated lesions most often demonstrating T1 hypo-to-isointensity to muscle with variable T1 hyperintense hemorrhage or heterogeneous signal in the setting of internal thrombosis [46]. Venous malformations typically do not demonstrate flow voids on spin echo sequences, as these are more characteristic of high flow vascular malformations but may show signal voids on gradient echo sequences [46]. Heterogeneous post-contrast enhancement is typical and highly variable based on the underlying vascular architecture and overall size of the lesion (Fig. 7.18). CT can facilitate characterization of underlying osseous remodeling and will clearly visualize any calcified phleboliths that may be present in the lesion.

Lymphatic malformations are relatively common congenital vascular anomalies in the neck caused by abnormal lymphangiogenesis. Like arterial or venous malformations, lymphatic malformations are characterized by a structurally abnormal morphology of vessels rather than abnormal proliferation or neoplasia [46]. Seventy-five percent of lymphatic malformations are found in the neck, demonstrate cystic MRI

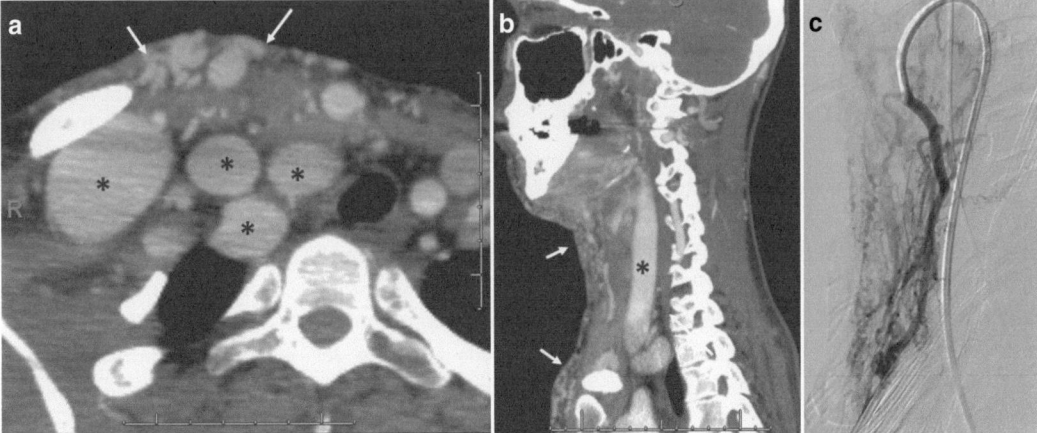

Fig. 7.17 Arteriovenous malformation. Axial (**a**) and sagittal (**b**) CT angiography and lateral view DSA (**c**) demonstrates diffuse arteriovenous malformation throughout the right anterolateral neck (arrow). There are markedly enlarged arteries and veins (*)

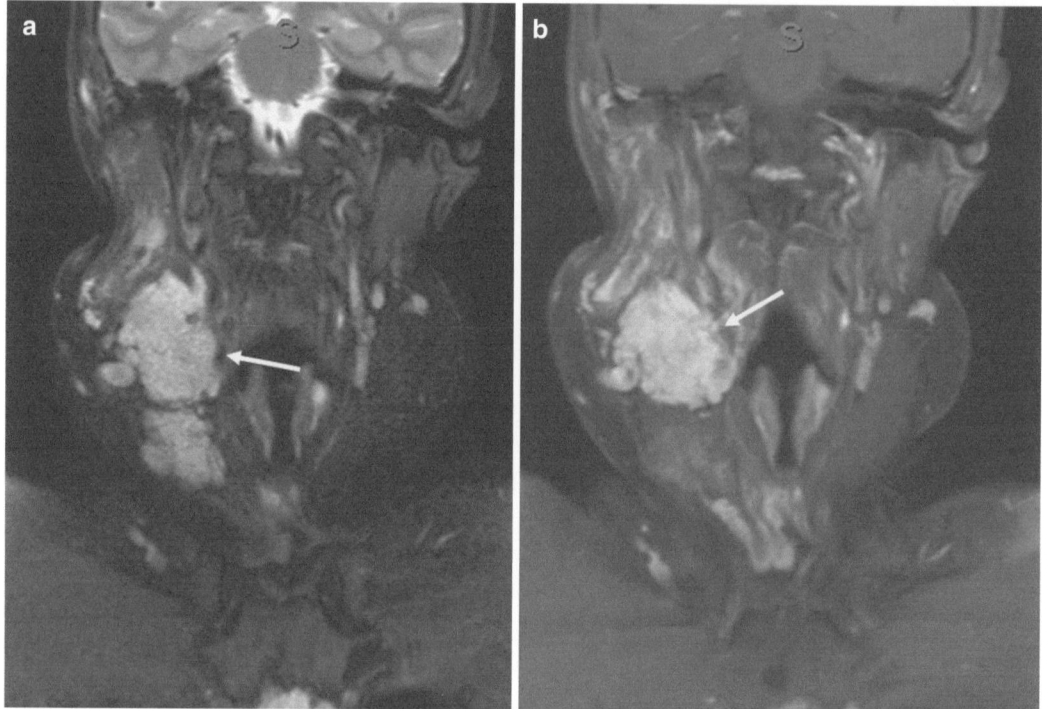

Fig. 7.18 Venous vascular malformation. Coronal fat-suppressed T2-weighted (**a**) and post-contrast T1-weighted (**b**) MR images demonstrate a lobulated hyperintense lesion in the right deep neck spaces corresponding to a vas-cular malformation (arrow). Relatively homogeneous enhancement and T2 hyperintensity is highly suggestive of a venous vascular malformation

features consisting of T2 hyperintensity with T1 hypointensity, and are classified as macrocystic or microcystic based on the size of their cystic components. The internal walls of these cystic structures are often not visible by imaging but may show subtle enhancement on post-contrast MRI (Fig. 7.19). Microcystic lymphatic mal-formations have more crowded septa because of their smaller cystic spaces and therefore may show more overall post-contrast enhancement. Internal hemorrhage can occur and will display layering blood with MR signal characteristics based on the age of blood products. If a lymphatic malformation is a mixed vascular lesion such as a venolymphatic malformation, the venous compo-nent is best identified on contrast-enhanced MRI.

Vascular Neoplasms in the Neck

Vascular neck lesions are grouped into the fol-lowing general categories: hemangiomas, glomus tumors (paragangliomas), and other (juvenile angiofibroma, angiosarcoma, Kaposi's sarcoma). All of these lesions are typically evaluated with a multimodality approach, which may include ultrasound, contrast-enhanced CT, contrast-enhanced MRI, non-contrast MRA, or catheter angiography. While discussing the imaging find-ings of each of these lesions is beyond the scope of this chapter, a few points are worth mention-ing when discussing vascular imaging of the head and neck.

Hemangiomas

Most hemangiomas can be diagnosed clinically, but imaging can be useful in atypical presenta-tions or deep lesions. Doppler ultrasound is particularly well suited for the evaluation of superficial hemangiomas of the head and neck given its ability to assess overall tumor extent and identify rich arterial and venous vascular compo-nents, but MRI has added value in cases of com-plex or deep tissue lesions. The presence of a soft

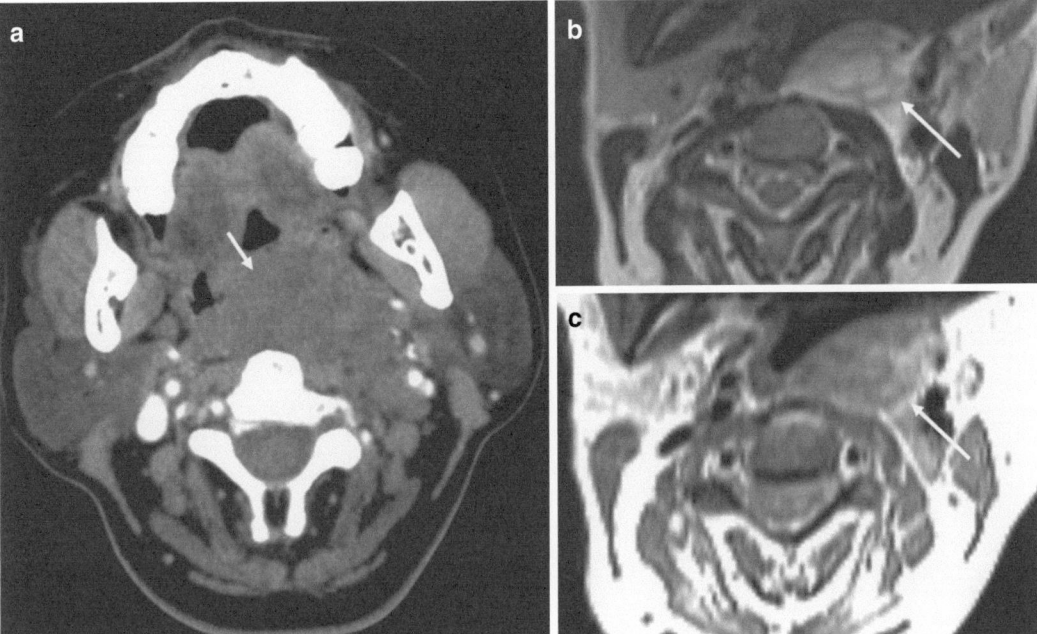

Fig. 7.19 Lymphatic vascular malformation. Axial contrast-enhanced CT images (**a**), T2-weighted (**b**), and post-gadolinium T1-weighted (**c**) MR images demonstrate a retropharyngeal mass corresponding to a vascular malformation (arrow). The lack of homogeneous enhancement and T2 hyperintensity with multiple intrinsic septa is highly suggestive of a lymphatic vascular malformation

tissue component is an important differentiating characteristic of hemangiomas compared to vascular malformations, which are purely vascular lesions [46]. Most hemangiomas are benign, such as superficial capillary, cavernous hemangiomas, or the rarer epithelioid hemangioendothelioma, but hemangiomas such as hemangiopericytoma can occur in the head and neck with variable malignant potential.

Paragangliomas

Glomus tumors, also known as paragangliomas or chemodectomas, are benign hypervascular lesions arising from neural crest cells of the autonomic nervous system and are typically seen in adults aged 40–60 years of age with a 5:1 female predominance [46]. Less than 5% of paragangliomas will undergo malignant transformation, but these tumors can often be locally aggressive [46]. By convention, these tumors are named based on their location of origin. The most common location for a paraganglioma is at

the carotid bifurcation, where they are given the name carotid body tumor, and paragangliomas in this location will characteristically splay the internal and external carotid arteries, classically with anterior displacement of the ECA and posterior displacement of the ICA (Fig. 7.20). Other locations for paragangliomas include, from superior to inferior in the head and neck, intracranially arising from parasympathetic components of Jacobsen's nerves in the middle ear near the cochlear promontory (glomus tympanicum), intracranially arising from parasympathetic components of Arnold's nerve in the jugular fossa (glomus jugulare), and extracranially at the skull base arising from the inferior vagal ganglion (glomus vagale) typically 1–2 cm below the jugular fossa or rarely from the neuroendocrine cells within the larynx. These lesions are typically evaluated with both contrast-enhanced CT and MRI. CT is extremely valuable in identifying "moth-eaten" osseous erosions of the lesions in contact with the base of the skull and

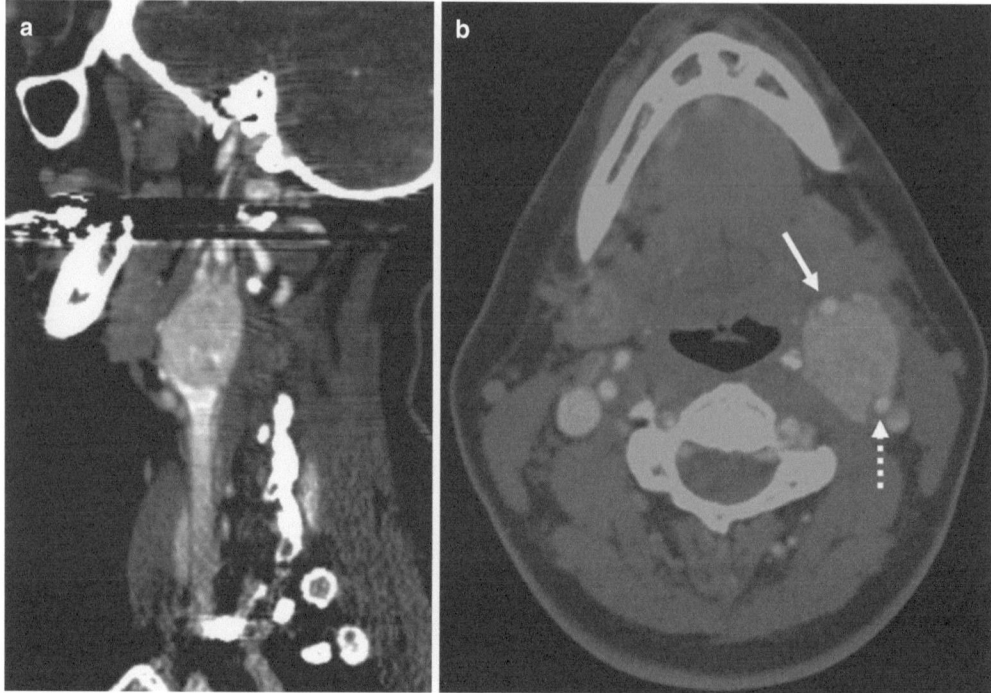

Fig. 7.20 Carotid body tumor (paraganglioma). Sagittal (**a**) and axial (**b**) CTA images demonstrate an avidly enhancing mass centered at the left carotid bifurcation splaying the internal and external carotid arteries with anterior displacement of the ECA (solid arrow) and posterior displacement of the ICA (dashed arrow). These are characteristic features of a carotid body tumor

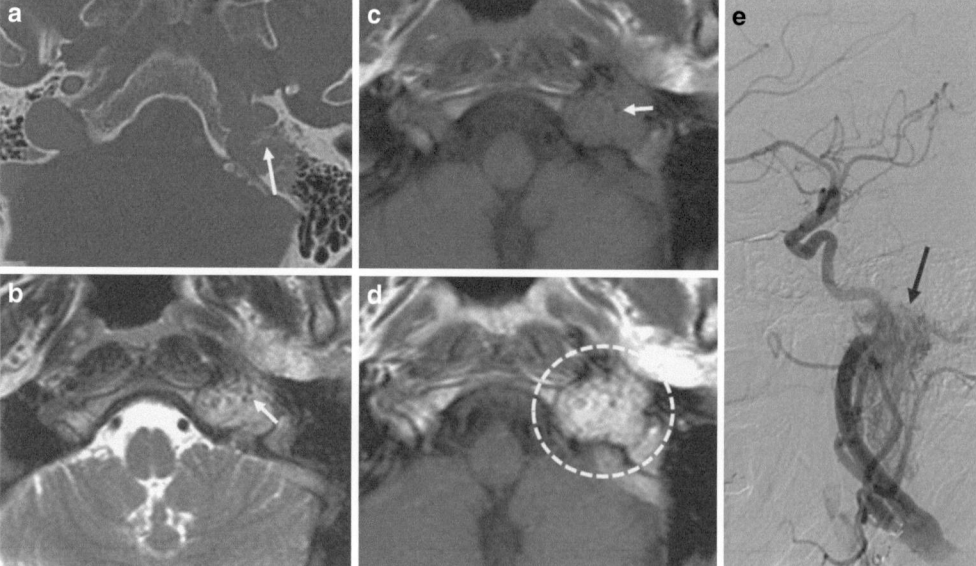

Fig. 7.21 Glomus jugulare (paraganglioma). Axial CT image (**a**) demonstrates permeative bone changes along the superolateral margin of the jugular foramen with erosive changes of the jugular spine (arrow). Axial T2-weighted (**b**), T1-weighted (**c**), and post-contrast (**d**) images demonstrate an avidly enhancing mass centered at the left jugular foramen. Hypointense foci within the mass (arrows) are due to vascular flow voids. (**e**) Preoperative angiogram shows the characteristic appearance of a hypervascular mass in the expected location of the jugular foramen with enlarged feeding arteries, intense tumor blush (arrow), and early draining veins

will classically demonstrate avid post-contrast enhancement (Fig. 7.21). Contrast-enhanced MRI will allow improved lesion characterization due to the better contrast resolution. The lesions typically display a "salt and pepper" appearance on both T1- and T2-weighted images related to the tumor stroma very rich in vessels that present as hypointense flow voids with hyperintense foci representing slow flow within vessels or blood products. MRA/CTA will demonstrate both the relationship of the lesions with the carotid artery and jugular vein, as well as the arterial supply of those lesions, which is typically via the neuromeningeal trunk of the ascending pharyngeal artery. An asymmetrically enlarged ascending pharyngeal artery is often an important diagnostic clue for paragangliomas.

Juvenile Nasopharyngeal Angiofibroma (JNA)

Juvenile nasopharyngeal angiofibromas (JNAs) are benign fibrovascular tumors which can be locally aggressive and are almost exclusively seen in adolescent males presenting with epistaxis. These lesions are thought to arise from the posterior nasal cavity in the region of the sphenopalatine foramen and typically first grow into the pterygopalatine fossa and nasal cavity with osseous destruction based on the specific pattern of local extension. These lesions can get quite large prior to clinical presentation and can even spread through the pterygomaxillary fissure into the masticator space or spread intracranially through the anterior skull base or middle cranial fossa. Characteristic patient demographic, clinical presentation, and classic imaging features are often sufficient to make this diagnosis, and biopsy of this hypervascular tumor is contraindicated given increased risk of bleeding. CT is often beneficial in assessing the degree of osseous destruction, and MRI is often necessary to fully characterize local extension in or around the skull base. Catheter angiography is performed for preoperative embolization prior to surgical resection and will characteristically demonstrate a prominent tumor blush with variable arterial supply from the ICA and ECA.

Review Questions

1. Decreased flow-related enhancement can be seen within the transverse (V3) segments of otherwise normal vertebral arteries on time-of-flight (TOF) MRA. This is due to:
   A. Slow intraluminal flow
   B. In-plane flow saturation
   C. Venous saturation pulse
   D. Turbulent flow

   Answer: B

2. Stair-step artifact is a commonly seen artifact in which of the following vascular imaging techniques:
   A. 2D time-of-flight (TOF) MRA
   B. 3D time-of-flight (TOF) MRA
   C. Contrast-enhanced (CE) MRA
   D. Phase-contrast (PC) MRA

   Answer: A

3. Which of the following atherosclerotic plaque characteristics is *not* associated with an increased risk of stroke:
   A. Intraplaque hemorrhage
   B. Large lipid core
   C. High calcium content
   D. Plaque ulceration

   Answer: C

4. Which MRI sequence can be helpful in identifying an intramural hematoma in the setting of a carotid or vertebral artery dissection?
   A. T2-weighted
   B. T1-weighted
   C. T2-weighted with fat saturation
   D. T1-weighted with fat saturation

   Answer: D

5. Which of the following imaging findings is suggestive of the diagnosis of the medial variant of fibromuscular dysplasia?
   A. Focal stenosis
   B. String sign
   C. String of beads
   D. Long segmental narrowing

   Answer: C

References

1. Pandey S, Hakky M, Kwak E, Jara H, Geyer CA, Erbay SH. Application of basic principles of physics to head and neck MR angiography: troubleshooting for artifacts. Radiographics. 2013;33(3):E113–23.
2. Sayah A, Mamourian A. Flow-related artifacts in MR imaging and MR angiography of the central nervous system. Neurographics. 2012;2:154–62.
3. Ahn KJ, You WJ, Lee JH, Kang BJ, Kim YJ, Kim BS, et al. Re-circulation artefact at the carotid bulb can be differentiated from true stenosis. Br J Radiol. 2004;77(919):551–6.
4. O'Brien WT Sr, Vagal AS, Cornelius RS. Applications of computed tomography angiography (CTA) in neuroimaging. Semin Roentgenol. 2010;45(2):107–15.
5. Schroeder GD, Hsu WK. Vertebral artery injuries in cervical spine surgery. Surg Neurol Int. 2013;4(Suppl 5):S362–7.
6. Taitz C, Nathan H, Arensburg B. Anatomical observations of the foramina transversaria. J Neurol Neurosurg Psychiatry. 1978;41(2):170–6.
7. Thierfelder KM, Baumann AB, Sommer WH, Armbruster M, Opherk C, Janssen H, et al. Vertebral artery hypoplasia: frequency and effect on cerebellar blood flow characteristics. Stroke. 2014;45(5):1363–8.
8. Ulm AJ, Quiroga M, Russo A, Russo VM, Graziano F, Velasquez A, et al. Normal anatomical variations of the V(3) segment of the vertebral artery: surgical implications. J Neurosurg Spine. 2010;13(4):451–60.
9. Expert Panel on Neurologic Imaging, Salmela MB, Mortazavi S, Jagadeesan BD, Broderick DF, Burns J, et al. ACR appropriateness criteria(R) cerebrovascular disease. J Am Coll Radiol. 2017;14(5S):S34–61. Epub 2017/05/06.
10. Lell MM, Anders K, Uder M, Klotz E, Ditt H, Vega-Higuera F, et al. New techniques in CT angiography. Radiographics. 2006;26(Suppl 1):S45–62.
11. Lell M, Fellner C, Baum U, Hothorn T, Steiner R, Lang W, et al. Evaluation of carotid artery stenosis with multisection CT and MR imaging: influence of imaging modality and postprocessing. AJNR Am J Neuroradiol. 2007;28(1):104–10.
12. Brott TG, Halperin JL, Abbara S, Bacharach JM, Barr JD, Bush RL, et al. ASA/ACCF/AHA/AANN/AANS/ACR/ASNR/CNS/SAIP/SCAI/SIR/SNIS/SVM/SVS guideline on the management of patients with extracranial carotid and vertebral artery disease: a report of the American College of Cardiology Foundation/American Heart Association Task Force on Practice Guidelines, and the American Stroke Association, American Association of Neuroscience Nurses, American Association of Neurological Surgeons, American College of Radiology, American Society of Neuroradiology, Congress of Neurological Surgeons, Society of Atherosclerosis Imaging and Prevention, Society for Cardiovascular Angiography and Interventions, Society of Interventional Radiology, Society of NeuroInterventional Surgery, Society for Vascular Medicine, and Society for Vascular Surgery. J Am Coll Cardiol. 2011;57(8):e16–94.
13. Barnett HJ, Taylor DW, Eliasziw M, Fox AJ, Ferguson GG, Haynes RB, et al. Benefit of carotid endarterectomy in patients with symptomatic moderate or severe stenosis. North American Symptomatic Carotid Endarterectomy Trial Collaborators. N Engl J Med. 1998;339(20):1415–25.
14. North American Symptomatic Carotid Endarterectomy Trial. Methods, patient characteristics, and progress. Stroke. 1991;22(6):711–20.
15. Randomised trial of endarterectomy for recently symptomatic carotid stenosis: final results of the MRC European Carotid Surgery Trial (ECST). Lancet. 1998;351(9113):1379–87.
16. Wintermark M, Jawadi SS, Rapp JH, Tihan T, Tong E, Glidden DV, et al. High-resolution CT imaging of carotid artery atherosclerotic plaques. AJNR Am J Neuroradiol. 2008;29(5):875–82.
17. Sigovan M, Bidet C, Bros S, Boussel L, Mechtouff L, Robson PM, et al. 3D black blood MR angiography of the carotid arteries. A simple sequence for plaque hemorrhage and stenosis evaluation. Magn Reson Imaging. 2017;42:95–100. Epub 2017/06/21
18. Zhao H, Zhao X, Liu X, Cao Y, Hippe DS, Sun J, et al. Association of carotid atherosclerotic plaque features with acute ischemic stroke: a magnetic resonance imaging study. Eur J Radiol. 2013;82(9):e465–70. Epub 2013/05/18
19. Wintermark M, Arora S, Tong E, Vittinghoff E, Lau BC, Chien JD, et al. Carotid plaque computed tomography imaging in stroke and nonstroke patients. Ann Neurol. 2008;64(2):149–57.
20. Yuan C, Mitsumori LM, Ferguson MS, Polissar NL, Echelard D, Ortiz G, et al. In vivo accuracy of multispectral magnetic resonance imaging for identifying lipid-rich necrotic cores and intraplaque hemorrhage in advanced human carotid plaques. Circulation. 2001;104(17):2051–6.
21. Hatsukami TS, Ross R, Polissar NL, Yuan C. Visualization of fibrous cap thickness and rupture in human atherosclerotic carotid plaque in vivo with high-resolution magnetic resonance imaging. Circulation. 2000;102(9):959–64.
22. Ricotta JJ, Aburahma A, Ascher E, Eskandari M, Faries P, Lal BK, et al. Updated Society for Vascular Surgery guidelines for management of extracranial carotid disease. J Vasc Surg. 2011;54(3):e1–31.
23. Singh N, Moody AR, Roifman I, Bluemke DA, Zavodni AE. Advanced MRI for carotid plaque imaging. Int J Cardiovasc Imaging. 2016;32(1):83–9. Epub 2015/08/22
24. Lal BK, Kaperonis EA, Cuadra S, Kapadia I, Hobson RW 2nd. Patterns of in-stent restenosis after carotid artery stenting: classification and implications for long-term outcome. J Vasc Surg. 2007;46(5):833–40.
25. Robbin ML, Lockhart ME, Weber TM, Vitek JJ, Smith JK, Yadav J, et al. Carotid artery stents: early and intermediate follow-up with Doppler US. Radiology. 1997;205(3):749–56.

26. Ringer AJ, German JW, Guterman LR, Hopkins LN. Follow-up of stented carotid arteries by Doppler ultrasound. Neurosurgery. 2002;51(3):639–43; discussion 43.

27. Frolich AM, Pilgram-Pastor SM, Psychogios MN, Mohr A, Knauth M. Comparing different MR angiography strategies of carotid stents in a vascular flow model: toward stent-specific recommendations in MR follow-up. Neuroradiology. 2011;53(5):359–65.

28. Oszkinis G, Pukacki F, Juszkat R, Weigele JB, Gabriel M, Krasinski Z, et al. Restenosis after carotid endarterectomy: incidence and endovascular management. Interv Neuroradiol. 2007;13(4):345–52.

29. Mattos MA, van Bemmelen PS, Barkmeier LD, Hodgson KJ, Ramsey DE, Sumner DS. Routine surveillance after carotid endarterectomy: does it affect clinical management? J Vasc Surg. 1993;17(5):819–30; discussion 30-1.

30. Khan S, Cloud GC, Kerry S, Markus HS. Imaging of vertebral artery stenosis: a systematic review. J Neurol Neurosurg Psychiatry. 2007;78(11):1218–25. Epub 2007/02/09

31. Khan S, Rich P, Clifton A, Markus HS. Noninvasive detection of vertebral artery stenosis: a comparison of contrast-enhanced MR angiography, CT angiography, and ultrasound. Stroke. 2009;40(11):3499–503.

32. Seto K, Yamagata K, Uchida F, Yanagawa T, Onizawa K, Bukawa H. Radiation-induced carotid artery stenosis in a patient with carcinoma of the oral floor. Case Rep Oncol Med. 2013;2013:379039. Epub 2013/07/03

33. Houdart E, Mounayer C, Chapot R, Saint-Maurice JP, Merland JJ. Carotid stenting for radiation-induced stenoses: a report of 7 cases. Stroke. 2001;32(1):118–21. Epub 2001/01/04

34. Lam WW, Leung SF, So NM, Wong KS, Liu KH, Ku PK, et al. Incidence of carotid stenosis in nasopharyngeal carcinoma patients after radiotherapy. Cancer. 2001;92(9):2357–63. Epub 2001/12/18

35. Schievink WI. Spontaneous dissection of the carotid and vertebral arteries. N Engl J Med. 2001;344(12):898–906.

36. Provenzale JM. Dissection of the internal carotid and vertebral arteries: imaging features. AJR Am J Roentgenol. 1995;165(5):1099–104.

37. Arnold M, Bousser MG, Fahrni G, Fischer U, Georgiadis D, Gandjour J, et al. Vertebral artery dissection: presenting findings and predictors of outcome. Stroke. 2006;37(10):2499–503.

38. Rodallec MH, Marteau V, Gerber S, Desmottes L, Zins M. Craniocervical arterial dissection: spectrum of imaging findings and differential diagnosis. Radiographics. 2008;28(6):1711–28.

39. Provenzale JM, Sarikaya B. Comparison of test performance characteristics of MRI, MR angiography, and CT angiography in the diagnosis of carotid and vertebral artery dissection: a review of the medical literature. AJR Am J Roentgenol. 2009;193(4):1167–74.

40. Vertinsky AT, Schwartz NE, Fischbein NJ, Rosenberg J, Albers GW, Zaharchuk G. Comparison of multidetector CT angiography and MR imaging of cervical artery dissection. AJNR Am J Neuroradiol. 2008;29(9):1753–60.

41. Furie DM, Tien RD. Fibromuscular dysplasia of arteries of the head and neck: imaging findings. AJR Am J Roentgenol. 1994;162(5):1205–9. Epub 1994/05/01

42. Olin JW, Gornik HL, Bacharach JM, Biller J, Fine LJ, Gray BH, et al. Fibromuscular dysplasia: state of the science and critical unanswered questions: a scientific statement from the American Heart Association. Circulation. 2014;129(9):1048–78. Epub 2014/02/20

43. Olin JW, Froehlich J, Gu X, Bacharach JM, Eagle K, Gray BH, et al. The United States Registry for Fibromuscular Dysplasia: results in the first 447 patients. Circulation. 2012;125(25):3182–90. Epub 2012/05/23

44. Heiserman JE, Drayer BP, Fram EK, Keller PJ. MR angiography of cervical fibromuscular dysplasia. AJNR Am J Neuroradiol. 1992;13(5):1454–7. Epub 1992/09/01

45. Kobayashi K, Nakao K, Kishishita S, Tamaruya N, Monobe H, Saito K, et al. Vascular malformations of the head and neck. Auris Nasus Larynx. 2013;40(1):89–92.

46. Gemmete JJ, Ansari SA, McHugh J, Gandhi D. Embolization of vascular tumors of the head and neck. Neuroimaging Clin N Am. 2009;19(2):181–98, Table of Contents.

Carotid and Vertebral Arteriography

Muneer Eesa

Introduction

There has been tremendous development of advanced, noninvasive cross-sectional imaging techniques for vascular evaluation of diseases of the brain, head, and neck as well as upper cervical spine. However, there remains a very important role played by invasive catheter angiography for studying the extracranial carotid and vertebral arteries. Techniques for arteriographic evaluation not only aid in diagnosing certain conditions and hence increase the confidence of surgical treatment protocols, but they also lend themselves to exploration and minimally invasive treatment modalities by endovascular means. The following sections will provide an understanding of the fundamentals of this technique by highlighting the history and evolution of catheter angiography techniques, discuss the indications and limitations of invasive catheter angiography, describe some of the associated risks involved, and provide some case scenarios as examples.

History

The development of cerebral angiography by pioneers such as Antonio Egas Moniz [1, 2] in the early part of the twentieth century was criti-cal in evaluation of not only vascular disorders of the head, neck, and brain but also led to the assessment of all types of diseases that have been until then not amenable to critical diagnosis and treatment. The initial techniques for vascular access and angiographic diagnosis involved direct carotid puncture and were in common use among the neurosurgical community. The description of percutaneous arterial access by Seldinger [3] led to the widespread adoption of catheter angiography. This would eventually lead to the routine use of cerebral angiography for the diagnosis of vascular disorders of the central nervous system. Carotid and vertebral angiography was also in common use for evaluation of masses and space-occupying lesions of the central nervous system long before the development of the first-generation computed tomography scanners [4]. This would serve as a very useful tool for evaluation of tumors and other space-occupying lesions for localization prior to neurosurgical intervention.

The description of the use of a catheter for angiography of the head and neck vasculature comes from Radner [5] who inadvertently performed a vertebral arteriogram while attempting to catheterize the heart from a right radial artery approach. Catheter angiography for cervical and cerebral arteriography was mostly popular among Scandinavian abdominal radiographers, and the technique was subsequently popularized among the radiology community in North America. The

M. Eesa
Department of Radiology, Foothills Medical Center, University of Calgary, Calgary, AB, Canada

© The Editor(s) (if applicable) and The Author(s) 2018
S. S. Hans (ed.), *Extracranial Carotid and Vertebral Artery Disease*,
https://doi.org/10.1007/978-3-319-91533-3_8

development of catheter angiography eventually led to surgical treatments for a variety of conditions but also the inevitable development of endovascular treatments for a variety of vascular disorders.

Ligation treatment for tumors of the head and neck had been described by surgical methods as early as 1904 by James Dawbarn [6], and early adopters of an endovascular approach used various embolic agents for simulating this devascularization from within the vasculature through direct exposure of the feeding vessels and subsequently using appropriate delivery catheters. Eventually the use of endovascular treatment extended to the intracranial circulation for treatment of cerebral vascular lesions, pioneered by Lussenhop and Spence in the middle part of the twentieth century who used a surgical cut down to expose the internal carotid artery and used methacrylate spheres to treat an arteriovenous malformation of the brain [7].

Evolution of Angiography

Early device development for angiography, specifically the design and production of catheters and wires for angiography, proceeded at a pace far slower than that for operative neurosurgery and vascular surgery. Early catheters for the performance of angiography were used primarily by peripheral, abdominal, and cardiac angiographers. These groups represented a larger patient population and gave the impetus for companies to improve existing designs. The earliest designs for catheters were available in a format that required shaping the tips in vitro and were especially important in supra-aortic cervical vascular access through the aortic arch, given the variations in aortic arch types, branch anatomy patterns, as well as increasing vessel tortuosity with advanced patient age. Numerous pre-shaped designs soon began to be available pioneered by experts with special interest in neurovascular diagnoses.

Advancements in engineering technology would soon see the development of smaller microcatheters and microwires which would eventually lead to the development of advanced endovascular treatment strategies for vascular diseases of the extracranial carotid and vertebral arterial system.

Noninvasive Imaging

Doppler Ultrasound

The use of gray-scale and color Doppler ultrasound techniques serves as a useful tool in the screening of vascular disorders of the extracranial carotid and vertebral arterial tree. These techniques are primarily used for the evaluation of vascular stenosis and obstructive disease but also play a role in evaluation of low flow and high flow head and neck vascular malformations.

Computed Tomography (CT) Scanning

CT scans have undergone rapid development since the first scanners in the early 1970s to the latest generation multidetector scans that can complete scan acquisitions and generate images in a matter of mere seconds. Combining the impressive capability of modern scanners with the addition of contrast media administered through the intravenous route, exquisite images of the extracranial carotid and vertebral arterial anatomy can be obtained for careful evaluation. Modern post-processing capabilities available at the scanner level and by the using third-party software can be utilized to generate multiplanar reconstructions and three-dimensional models. These can be used by surgeons and interventionalists to plan surgical or endovascular treatments.

Magnetic Resonance Imaging (MRI)

MRI is also a useful tool in the diagnostic evaluation of the extracranial carotid and vertebral arteries. MRI has the advantage of improved tissue contrast and with administration of vascular-specific, gadolinium-based contrast agents can be used to specifically image the vessels. MRI also has the advantage to obtain temporal information with sequences such as TRICKS (time-resolved imaging of contrast kinetics) or TWIST (time-resolved angiography with stochastic trajectories) sequences by obtaining a series of image acquisitions in separate phases of arterial flow obtained at rates as fast as 1–2 frames per second. Gadolinium-based contrast agents are contraindicated in patients with renal disease. There are MRI sequences such as time of flight angiography and phase-contrast imaging that do not require the use of gadolinium-based contrast and can be used in a limited manner in evaluation of the extracranial arterial vascular tree.

The advent of noninvasive vascular angiographic techniques may be considered an impediment to the educational opportunities of trainees in neuro-endovascular techniques as the volume of catheter angiography have significantly decreased. There are however enough indications for performance of catheter angiography that would enable trainees to develop this skill set to a degree that would enable the safe performance of not only diagnostic angiography but also extend that knowledge base and experience to the therapeutic aspects of cervical and cerebral vascular diseases [8].

Indications

As mentioned previously, in the modern era of readily available noninvasive cross-sectional vascular imaging techniques, the current list of indications for invasive catheter angiography for the extracranial carotid and vertebral arteries are somewhat limited. The following table lists some of the common indications, focusing on the extracranial circulation. These will be highlighted by showing examples in the section of case scenarios.

Indications for Catheter Angiography of Extracranial Carotid and Vertebral Arteries
Clarifying degree of stenosis in occlusive disease with discordant results on Doppler, CTA, and MRA
  Evaluation of high cervical spinal vascular malformations
  Preoperative evaluation for aneurysm
  Presurgical embolization of vascular head and neck tumors
  Evaluation of vascular malformations of the head and neck
  Balloon test occlusion prior to vessel sacrifice

Contraindications

The list of contraindications for cervico-cerebral angiography has traditionally been divided into absolute and relative contraindications. A case-by-case assessment of the necessity to perform the procedure must be made depending on the acuity of the case and need for rapid diagnosis. With careful technique as well as newer access devices, etc., the procedure may be performed in clinical scenarios that have been hitherto been considered a contraindication. For instance, patients with coagulopathies may undergo catheter angiography by using a micropuncture kit and ultrasound guidance for femoral access and a closure device for hemostasis after completion of arteriography. Patients with borderline renal dysfunction may undergo angiography with a good hydration protocol and may be monitored carefully for rise in serum creatinine. Indeed, a recent meta-analysis of patients with acute stroke undergoing contrast administration showed that there is no significant association of contrast administration and acute kidney injury in stroke patients, even those with known chronic kidney disease [9]. Patients with anaphylactic reactions to iodinated contrast media may undergo selective arteriography with gadolinium-based contrast if absolutely required.

Some Contraindications to Invasive
Catheter Arteriography
Anaphylactic reaction to iodinated contrast
media
    Uncorrected coagulopathy
    Connected tissue disorders prone to ves-
sel injury, e.g., Ehlers-Danlos syndrome
(type IV)
    Severe renal dysfunction

Techniques

Pre-procedural Evaluation

A proper review of the indication for catheter angiography as well as review of noninvasive imaging modalities is a must prior to performance of angiography. A history and physical examination and review of lab work should be performed to ensure there are no contraindications or factors that may affect the technical aspects of the case. Documentation of the peripheral arterial pulses will ensure safe access. An informed consent discussion should include the benefits and risks associated with the procedure and reasonable alternatives and a discussion of why catheter angiography has been recommended.

Angiography Imaging Systems

Digital subtraction angiography has improved significantly with most modern angiography systems using flat panel detector technology with improved efficiency, greater dynamic range, and capability for cone-beam CT and rotational angiography. Modern systems are capable of imaging vessels with capability of fusing vessels with previously obtained cross-sectional images, removing metal artifact from vascular clips, stent tines, etc., and provide capability for road map guidance in 3D for vascular navigation of the peripheral vascular tree. This has indeed improved the safety of catheter angiography when compared to older generation systems [10].

Vascular Access Phase

The most common site for vascular access for the performance of diagnostic angiography of the extracranial carotid and vertebral arteries is the femoral artery. Access is usually obtained by using a percutaneous approach by using a modified Seldinger technique. A short vascular sheath is usually placed for catheter introduction and helps with exchange and usage of multiple preshaped catheters. Other access sites may be occasionally used when femoral access is difficult, such as access via the radial or brachial approach. This is especially suited for vertebral arteriography, because of the anatomical nature of access to the vertebral arterial system from the subclavian artery. Some centers perform cervical arteriography routinely through a radial approach. Special considerations for patients on antiplatelet medication and anticoagulation include the use of ultrasound for access and use of micropuncture vascular kits. If there is anticipation of aortoiliac tortuosity, consideration may be given to the use of longer vascular sheaths.

Direct carotid puncture for access is seldom used for diagnostic catheter angiography and is reserved for certain cases of treatment of intracranial conditions such as acute ischemic stroke treatment and intracranial embolization when traditional access sites have failed [11].

Choice of Catheters and Wires

There are many pre-shaped catheters available for supra-aortic vascular catheterization depending on aortic arch anatomy, patient age, and tortuosity as well as operator preference and experience (Table 8.1). Most centers will use a 5Fr system

Table 8.1 Catheters used for supra-aortic neuroangiography

Angled curve/forward curve catheters	Reverse curve catheters
Berenstein	Simmons (Sim 1, 2, 3)
Davis	Vitek (VTK)
Kumpke	Bentson (JB 2, 3)
Headhunter (H1, H3)	Mani (MAN)
Modified headhunter (H1H, HY1)	CK1
TEG-T	Newton (HN 3, 4)
Vert	
Bentson (JB 1)	
Weinberg (WNBG)	
Cerebral Burke (CBL)	

for diagnostic arteriography due to the widely available variety of catheter shapes and for the right balance of size and stiffness in a substantial proportion of the patient population that is encountered. It may be possible to perform catheter angiography in younger patients using a 4Fr system as there is a lower incidence of tortuous vascular anatomy.

Isolated angiography of the carotid and vertebral arteries is rarely performed in the pediatric population. Special consideration should be given to low profile access sheaths, smaller-sized catheters, and prudent use of fluoroscopic technique and contrast injection amounts.

Aortic arch anatomy and type is an important determinant of catheter choice. Catheters for supra-aortic neuroangiography may be broadly divided into single curve (Fig. 8.1a), double curve (Fig. 8.1b), or reverse curve (Fig. 8.1c,d) catheters. For type I and most type II arches, a variety of angled catheters may suffice to obtain access, whereas the presence of a type III arch or bovine configuration, etc. might require the use of a reverse curve catheter system.

The guidewires most commonly available for cervical arteriography are either a spring-coil guidewire with long taper such as Bentson (Cook Medical) or a hydrophilic wire with angled tip such as Glidewire (Terumo). Double flushing technique with heparinized saline to ensure no stagnant blood columns within the catheter lumen is usually sufficient. Some cases where there is anticipation of protracted catheterization times may require the use of a closed system continuous heparinized flush system. Some centers routinely use in-line air filters to reduce the risk of air embolus.

Contrast injection may be performed either by using proper hand injection of contrast, ensuring meticulous care to eliminate air bubbles or by using a power injection device at an appropriate rate and volume of contrast for the selected vessel [12].

The vascular access site may be compressed manually to achieve hemostasis with an appropriate bedrest period to follow. In patients on antiplatelet or anticoagulant medication or those patients with a coagulopathy, a closure device may be necessary to achieve hemostasis [13].

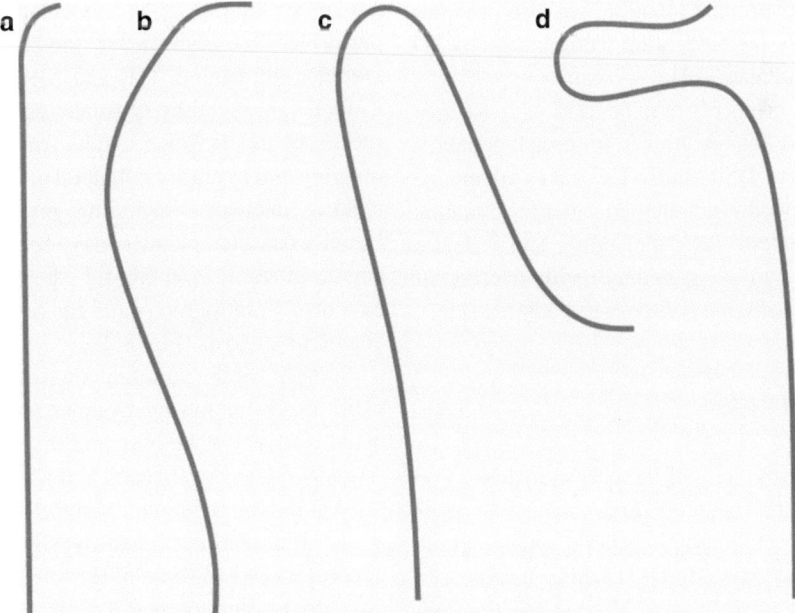

Fig. 8.1 Examples of commonly used catheters for supra-aortic neuroangiography. (**a**) Simple curve catheter: Berenstein. (**b**) Double curve catheter: Headhunter. (**c**) Reverse curve catheter: Simmons 2. (**d**) Reverse curve catheter: Vitek

Special Maneuvers and Dynamic Imaging

Invasive catheter angiography can provide additional diagnostic information as it pertains to collateral circulation by using cross-compression techniques with selective catheterization. For example, selective internal carotid angiography while compressing the contralateral internal carotid artery will provide information regarding patency of the anterior-communicating artery.

Dynamic angiography of the vertebral arteries while positioning the patient's head and neck in different positions that elicit posterior circulation symptoms may provide information on vascular lesions that may account for positional symptoms such as in patients with suspected Bowhunter's syndrome.

Advanced Angiographic Techniques

Three-dimensional rotational angiography may be incorporated into the routine angiography protocol to generate vascular models of aneurysms. This not only generates images useful for surgical and interventional planning but also provides the capability for navigation using advanced 3D road map guidance [14].

Selective protocols may be used with contrast injection and cone-beam CT rotational capabilities of modern DSA units. This takes advantage of the improved efficiency and greater dynamic range of modern flat panel units, and vascular pathologies can be generated with overlay of adjacent osseous and soft tissue structures [15].

Procedural Risks

Catheter angiography of the cervical carotid and vertebral arteries are prone to the same risks associated with angiography in general which include complications related to vascular access site bleeding and vessel injury, allergic reaction and nephrotoxicity due to iodinated contrast media,

etc. There could also be complications related to dissection of vessels from either guidewire or catheter placement and power injection devices.

However, cervico-cerebral arteriography has the added risk of neurological complications related to the vascular access of head and neck arteries. In a large study by Willinsky et al. [16], a total of 2899 consecutive cerebral DSA exams were evaluated prospectively. Permanent neurological complications were encountered in 0.5% of exams performed. The authors concluded that advancing age and pre-existing cardiovascular disease as well as increased fluoroscopy times were associated with a higher incidence of neurological complications associated with cervico-cerebral angiography.

Case Scenarios

Case #1: Extracranial Vascular Stenosis

Steno-occlusive disease of the extracranial carotid vessels and to a lesser degree the vertebral arteries is a major cause of ischemic stroke. Evaluation of the vasculature is usually performed by noninvasive modalities such as Doppler ultrasound, CT, and MR angiography. Catheter angiography is usually performed in the setting of inconclusive results from noninvasive imaging and to clarify collateral circulation when making decisions regarding revascularization. Heavily calcified plaques may obscure the actual degree of stenosis in carotid atherosclerotic disease on CT angiography and can overestimate the degree of stenosis (Fig. 8.2).

Stenoses of the vertebral arteries are less amenable to evaluation by Doppler ultrasound, and ostial disease can be obscured in the presence of artifacts related to osseous and soft tissue structures at the thoracic inlet. Vertebral ostial disease is also less well evaluated by MR angiographic techniques due to some of the same concerns but also due to limitations of coverage on most current MRI protocols.

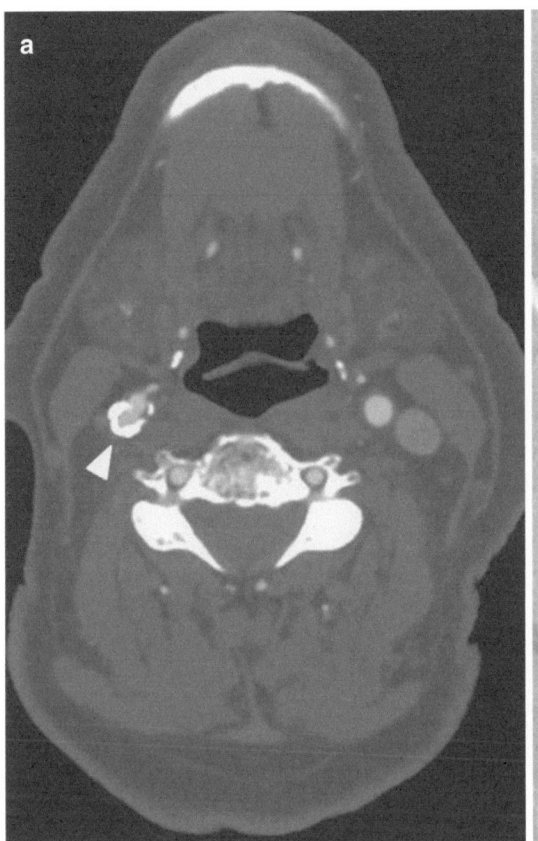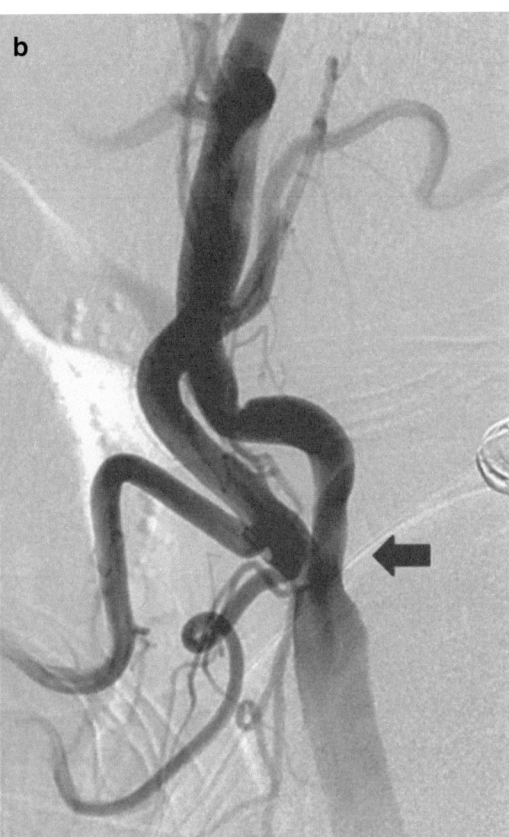

Fig. 8.2 An elderly patient presented with right hemispheric transient ischemic attack (TIA) symptoms. (**a**) CT angiography demonstrated heavily calcified plaque in relation to the right carotid bifurcation (white arrowhead).

(**b**) Catheter angiography immediately prior to planned endovascular angioplasty and stenting demonstrated non-significant stenosis, <50% (black arrow), and the patient was placed on medical management

Case #2: Aneurysms

Aneurysmal dilatation involving the cervical vasculature is less common than intracranial aneurysms. Cervical carotid aneurysms are usually contained pseudoaneurysms seen in the setting of sequelae of prior trauma and blunt vascular injury or as a sequelae of deep neck space infections. Sometimes clarification of the anatomy requires definitive catheter angiography for treatment planning. Definitive treatment of cervical aneurysms may require endovascular treatment with either coils or use of a covered stent. The specific type of treatment may dictate the need for antiplatelet therapy, and a good preoperative angiogram will help in making this determination (Fig. 8.3).

Case #3: Vascular Malformations

Vascular malformations of the head and neck region can be encountered either within the spinal column as part of the spectrum of spinal vascular malformations or in relation to the soft tissues of the head and neck such as high flow or low flow vascular malformations. There are various schemes for the classification of spinal vascular malformations and are beyond the scope of this chapter. The common spinal vascular malformations of the cervical regions that are seen in clinical practice include spina dural arteriovenous fistulae (Fig. 8.4), spinal cord vascular malformations, spinal metameric syndromes, and intracranial dural arteriovenous fistulae with spinal peri-medullary drainage.

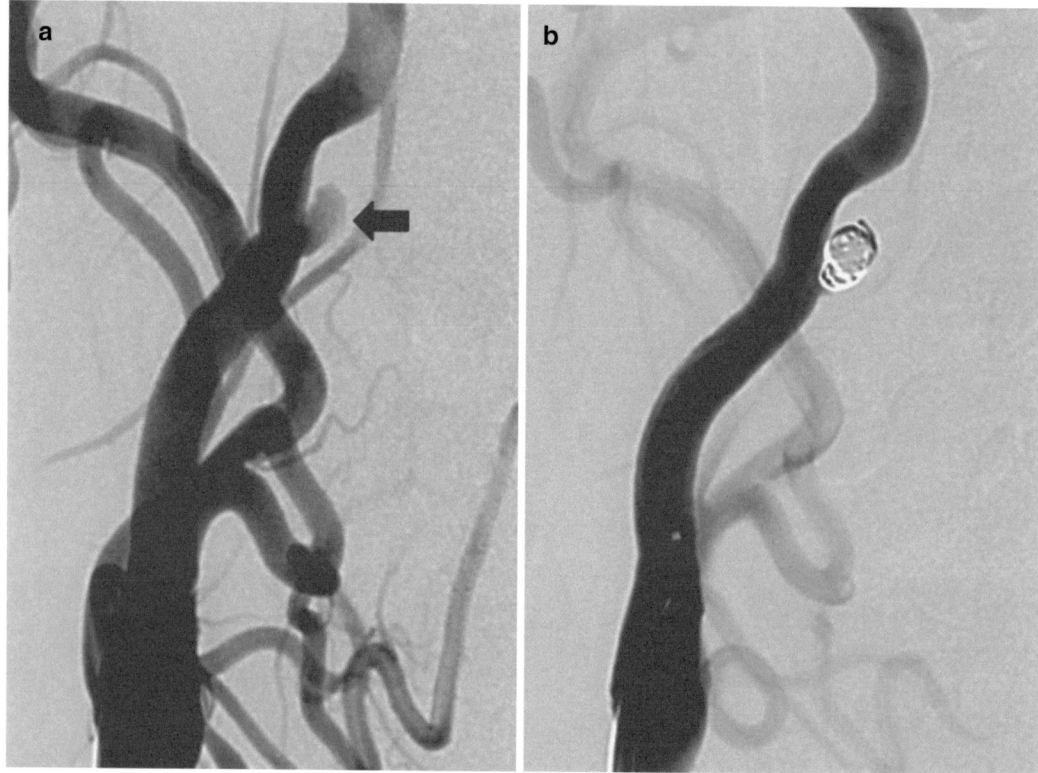

Fig. 8.3 A young patient presented with persistent right-sided neck pain following minor neck trauma 2 months prior. (**a**) Right carotid angiography demonstrates an aneurysm arising from the right internal carotid artery above the bifurcation. The aneurysm had a relatively narrow neck on angiographic evaluation. Based on the find-ings of catheter angiography, a decision was made to attempt coil obliteration of the aneurysm. (**b**) Control angiography after coil embolization demonstrates satisfactory exclusion of the aneurysm from the circulation with preserved patency of the parent vessel

Soft tissue malformations of the head and neck are a not uncommon cause of symptoms related to swelling and pain and when deep also can cause symptoms related to airway compromise and swallowing difficulties. Some indeterminate lesions will require catheter angiography to ascertain the flow characteristics as this will have implications for management (Fig. 8.5). Low flow lesions are usually amenable to percutaneous interventions, whereas high flow lesions would be best managed by a multidisciplinary approach which includes a combination of embolization and surgical resection when feasible.

Case #4: Vascular Neoplasms

Certain vascular tumors such as carotid body tumors or head and neck paragangliomas may be encountered in the head and neck region. Most of these lesions are managed by surgical resection in the appropriate context. Some surgeons may request a conventional catheter angiogram prior to surgical resection as this would determine the need and feasibility for preoperative embolization. In addition, an angiographic understanding of the regional vascular anatomy would serve as a good road map for surgical planning.

Case #5: Balloon Test Occlusion

Collateral vascular pathways play a significant role in maintaining hemodynamic balance within the head, neck, and brain circulation. These unique anatomic variations of the supra-aortic cervico-cerebral vasculature lend an opportunity for therapeutic vessel occlusions and ligation

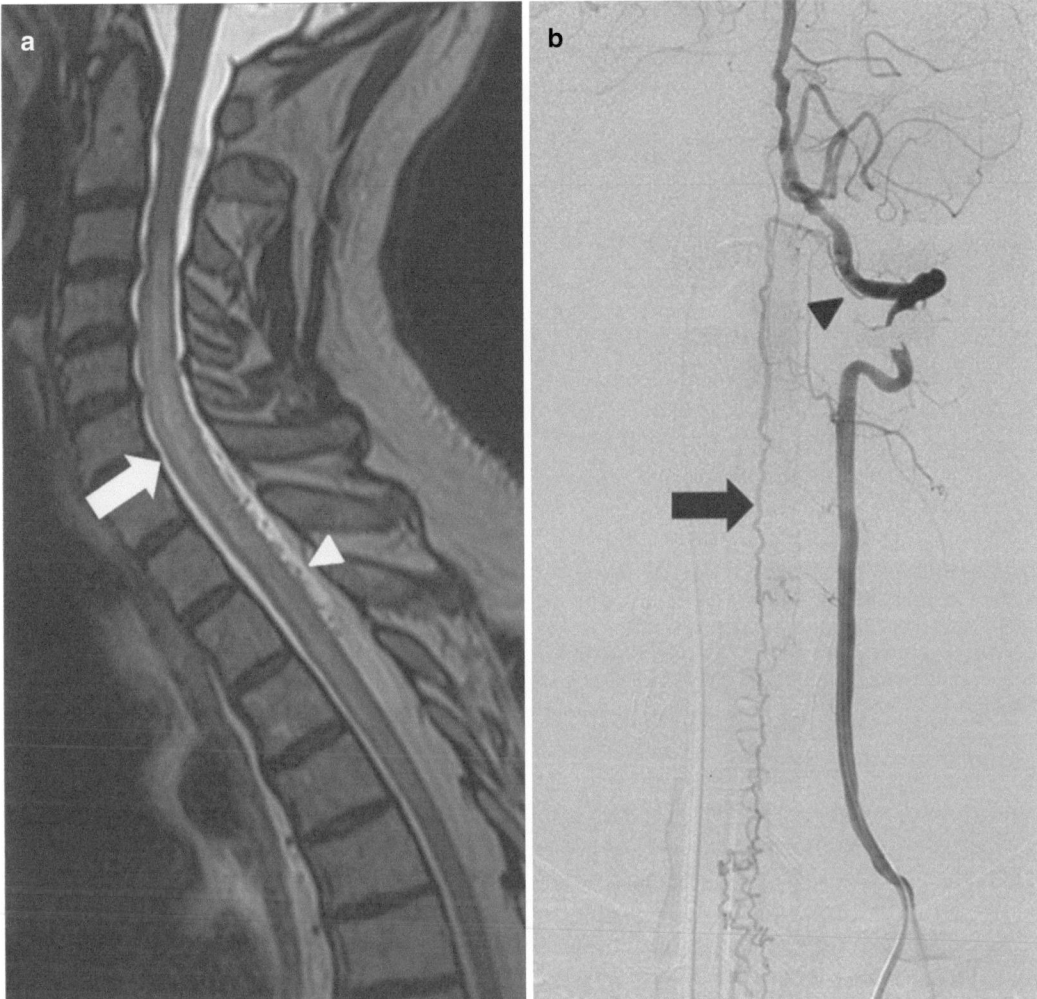

Fig. 8.4 A middle-aged male patient presented with progressive myelopathy over the past 4 months. (**a**) Sagittal T2-weighted MRI scans demonstrated abnormal cord signal change and edema centered at the mid-cervical spinal cord with extension to the upper thoracic spinal cord (white arrow) along with multiple small flow voids along the dorsal aspect of the cord (white arrowhead) highly suggestive of enlarged peri-medullary vessels. (**b**) Left vertebral angiography demonstrates a spinal dural arteriovenous fistula centered at the level of the left C1 nerve root sleeve (black arrowhead) with enlarged peri-medullary spinal veins extending caudally toward the cervicothoracic junction (black arrow)

in the setting of traumatic vascular lesions and in preparing for surgical exploration for treatment of lesions that are in close proximity to the major arteries of the head and neck as well as the skull base. Catheter angiography offers an added advantage to evaluate the collateral pathways by temporary balloon occlusion testing and in awake patients testing for neurological changes temporarily prior to definitive occlusion (Fig. 8.6). Care should be taken to adequately anticoagulate patients for the duration of testing (typically 30 min) with careful serial neurological examination during the period of occlusion. Most practitioners also institute a hypotensive challenge for the latter third of the test occlusion duration.

Case #6: Special Techniques

Modern neuroangiography imaging systems can perform advance application techniques such as rotational angiography and cone-beam CT acqui-

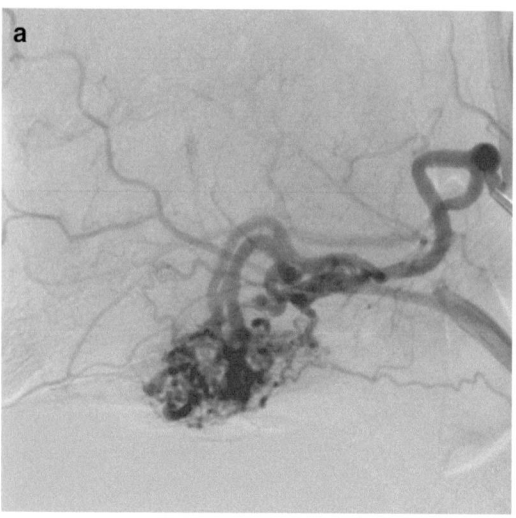 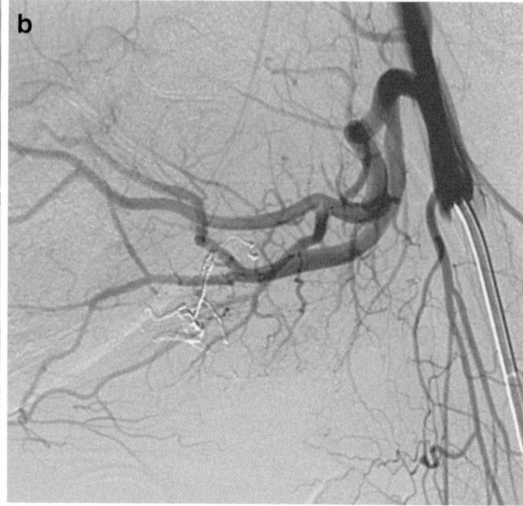

Fig. 8.5 A young patient presented with a slowly grow-ing submandibular mass for the past year. MR imaging of the neck (not shown) revealed a vascular lesion within the right submandibular space with flow voids. However, the flow of the lesion could not be determined. (**a**) Right external carotid angiography demonstrates the presence of a high flow vascular malformation supplied by branches of the right lingual artery with early draining veins drain-ing via the external jugular vein. (**b**) Due to the high flow nature of the lesion a decision was made to proceed with embolization of the lesion to be followed by surgical resection. A liquid embolic agent was used to embolize the lesion through branches of the lingual artery

sitions in the angiography suite. Modern flat panel detector units are capable of acquiring and, through software based post-processing, generat-ing images of the cervico-cerebral vasculature with exquisite details. Cone-beam CT acquisition in non-subtracted mode can demonstrate the vas-cular anatomy in relation to the regional osseous anatomy which is extremely useful in planning surgical and endovascular treatments (Fig. 8.7). Newer applications such as 3D road mapping can be useful for navigating the vasculature in complex cases for super-selective catheteriza-tion. The use of cone-beam CT angiography will also be useful in designing hybrid operating the-aters, minimizing the time between imaging and intervention. This is especially useful in trauma patients who may require surgical and endovas-cular intervention at the same time.

Limitations

The most important drawback of catheter angi-ography is the invasive nature of the procedure and the associated risks involved. As discussed above, the additional neurological risks related to catheterization of the head and neck vessels is another important limitation. However, in selected patients catheter angiography can be used as a problem-solving tool and direct man-agement. Many of these conditions have sig-nificant morbidity and mortality associated with them if left untreated, and catheter angiography may be a logical next step in the treatment para-digm. With advancements in endovascular treat-ment techniques, catheter angiography is the first step in the logical progression to treatment.

Future Directions

There are increasing reports in the literature of the use of direct carotid puncture for access to the intracranial vasculature for endovascular treatment of patients with acute ischemic stroke as well as treatment of other intracranial vascular disorders such as intracranial aneurysms and vas-cular malformations. Although its use for the sole

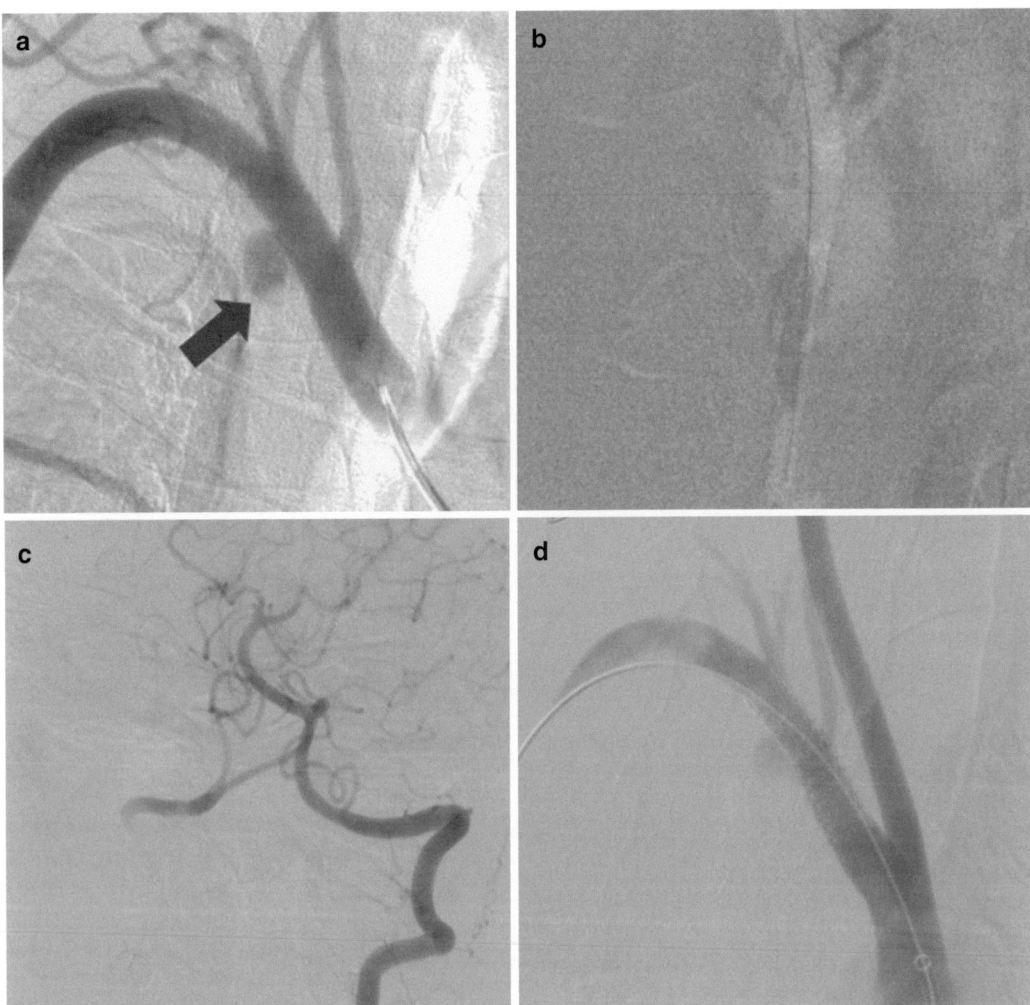

Fig. 8.6 A middle-aged patient presented with a history of trauma and CT evaluation as part of the trauma protocol demonstrated a right-sided hemothorax related to a pseudoaneurysm of the right subclavian artery. (**a**) Catheter angiography of the right subclavian artery re-demonstrated the pseudoaneurysm (black arrow) arising distal to the origin of the right vertebral artery with a relatively wide neck. Based on the morphology of the aneurysm, endovascular treatment using a stent graft was considered. (**b**) A balloon test occlusion was performed within the right vertebral artery to plan for excluding that segment of the subclavian artery. (**c**) Contralateral vertebral arteriography with balloon inflation in situ demonstrated good collateral flow and intracranial perfusion with no associated clinical neurological deficits. (**d**) A stent graft was successfully placed across the aneurysmal segment of the subclavian artery

purpose of obtaining diagnostic angiograms will be limited, this technique might find favor in the future as experience accumulates with techniques for access and closure.

Intravascular ultrasound has been used predominantly in the coronary and peripheral vasculature for evaluation of atherosclerotic plaque morphology as well as for assessing successful revascularization with stents. There are increasing reports of the use of this technology for the assessment of steno-occlusive disease in the periprocedural period for the placement of stents during endovascular revascularization [17]. This may be potentially useful in patients with severe anaphylaxis to contrast and /or renal dysfunction.

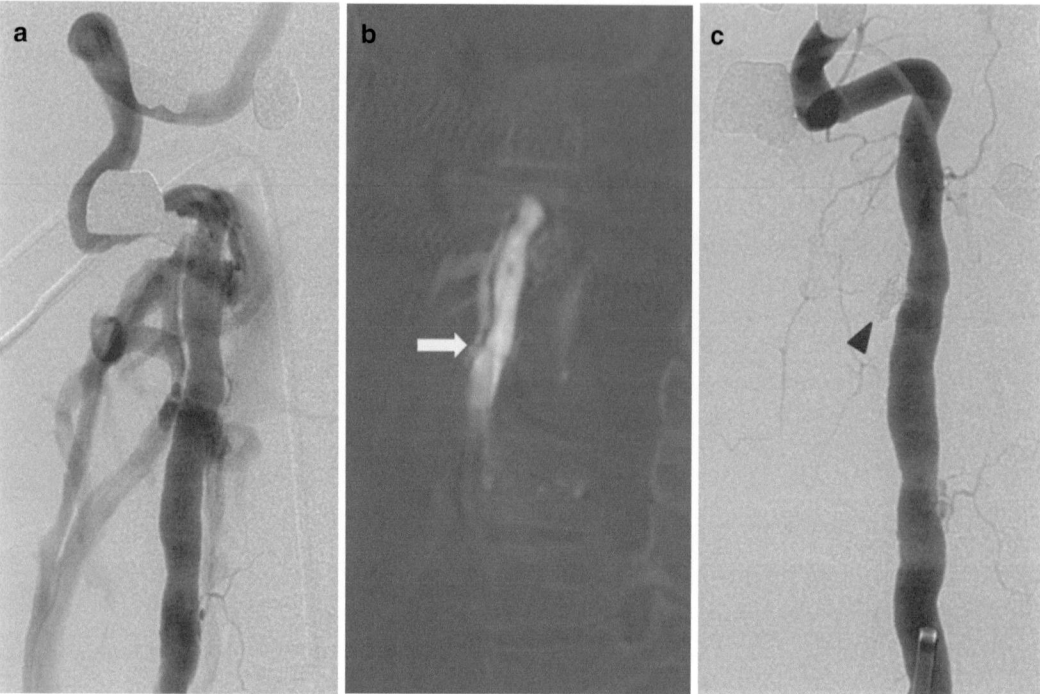

Fig. 8.7 A young patient presented with intractable tinnitus following trauma to the neck. (**a**) Right vertebral arteriography demonstrates a high flow arteriovenous shunt from the V2 segment with rapid visualization of multiple veins within the peri-vertebral venous plexus. Due to the extremely high flow nature of the shunt, an exact determination of the site of fistulation could not be determined despite high frame-rate angiography. (**b**) A dynamic cone-beam CT acquisition with dilute arteriographic contrast injection demonstrates the site of fistulation (white arrow). (**c**) The fistula was subsequently accessed using a microcatheter and embolization performed using detachable platinum coils (black arrowhead)

Conclusion

Invasive catheter angiography of the carotid and vertebral arteries has a role in the evaluation of certain pathological vascular conditions of the head and neck as outlined above. Advancements in noninvasive vascular imaging have led to a decreased need for catheter arteriography in general. However, in selected clinical settings, the technique may prove useful in the management of patients and should be utilized prudently when other means of diagnosis are inconclusive. Careful attention to technique can minimize the risks associated with this procedure. A detailed understanding of the anatomy of the extracranial carotid and vertebral arteries will aid in interpreting the angiographic images and help in planning a therapeutic intervention by surgical or endovascular means.

Review Questions
1. The technique for percutaneous vascular access for arteriography was first described by:
   A. Antonio Egas Moniz
   B. Sven Ivan Seldinger
   C. James Dawbarn
   D. Alfred Lussenhop

   Answer: B

2. Which of the following is a reverse curved catheter used in neuroangiography?
   A. Berenstein
   B. Headhunter
   C. Davis
   D. Simmons

   Answer: D

3. Which of the following is the most significant risk from carotid arteriography?
   A. Puncture site hematoma
   B. Anaphylaxis from iodinated contrast media
   C. Aortic dissection
   D. Neurological complications

Answer: D

References

1. Moniz E. L'encephalographie arterielle, son importance dans la localisation des tumeurs cerebrales. Rev Neurol (Paris). 1927;2:72–90.
2. Tondreu R. Egas Moniz 1874–1955., Father of cerebral angiography, father of psychosurgery, neurologist and psychiatrist, politician and diplomat, Nobel laureate. Radiographics. 1985;5:994–7.
3. Seldinger SI. Catheter replacement of the needle in percutaneous arteriography; a new technique. Acta Radiol. 1953;39:368–76.
4. List CF, Hodges FJ. Angiographic diagnosis of expanding intracranial lesions by vascular displacement. Radiology. 1946;47(4):319–33.
5. Radner S. Intracranial angiography via the vertebral artery. Preliminary report on a new technique. Acta Radiol. 1947;28:838–42.
6. Dawbarn R. The starvation plan for malignancy in the external carotid area. JAMA. 1904;43:792–5.
7. Luessenhop AJ, Spence WT. Artificial embolization of cerebral arteries. Report of use in a case of arteriovenous malformation. JAMA. 1960;172:1153–5.
8. Day AL, Siddiqui AH, Meyers PM, Jovin TG, Derdeyn CP, Hoh BL, et al. Training standards in neuroendo-vascular surgery: program accreditation and practitioner certification. Stroke. 2017;48(8):2318–25.
9. Brinjikji W, Demchuk AM, Murad MH, Rabinstein AA, McDonald RJ, McDonald JS, et al. Neurons over nephrons: systematic review and meta-analysis of contrast-induced nephropathy in patients with acute stroke. Stroke. 2017;48(7):1862–8.
10. Brigida R, Misciasci T, Martarelli F, Gangitano G, Ottaviani P, Rollo M, et al. Rays. 2003;28(1):21–8.
11. Mokin M, Snyder KV, Levy EI, Hopkins LN, Siddiqui AH. Direct carotid artery puncture access for endovascular treatment of acute ischemic stroke: technical aspects, advantages, and limitations. J Neurointerv Surg. 2015;7(2):108–13.
12. Yousem DM, Trinh BC. Injection rates for neuroangiography: results of a survey. AJNR Am J Neuroradiol. 2001;22(10):1838–40.
13. Geyik S, Yavuz K, Akgoz A, Koc O, Peynircioglu B, Cil B, et al. The safety and efficacy of the Angio-Seal closure device in diagnostic and interventional neuroangiography setting: a single-center experience with 1,443 closures. Neuroradiology. 2007;49(9):739–46.
14. Jang DK, Stidd DA, Schafer S, Chen M, Moftakhar R, Lopes DK. Monoplane 3D overlay roadmap versus conventional biplane 2D roadmap technique for Neurointervenional procedures. Neurointervention. 2016;11(2):105–13.
15. Mehndiratta A, Rabinov JD, Grasruck M, Liao EC, Crandell D, Gupta R. High-resolution dynamic angiography using flat-panel volume CT: feasibility demonstration for neuro and lower limb vascular applications. Eur Radiol. 2015;25(7):1901–10.
16. Willinsky RA, Taylor SM, TerBrugge K, Farb RI, Tomlinson G, Montanera W. Neurologic complications of cerebral angiography: prospective analysis of 2,899 procedures and review of the literature. Radiology. 2003;227(2):522–8.
17. Ota S, Sekihara Y, Himeno T, Tanaka Y, Ohtonari T. Contrast-less stent placement for vertebral artery origin stenosis. Interv Neuroradiol. 2017;23(1):79–83.

Medical Therapy for Carotid and Vertebral Artery Stenosis

9

Moayd M. Alkhalifah, Paul M. Gadient, and Seemant Chaturvedi

Abbreviations

CHANCE	Clopidogrel in High-Risk Patients With Acute Nondisabling Events
CREST-2	Carotid Revascularization and Medical Management for Asymptomatic Carotid Stenosis Study
ECST	European Carotid Surgery Trial
EPOCH-CAS	Effect of pitavastatin on preventing ischemic complications with carotid artery stenting
ESPRIT	European/Australasian Stroke Prevention in Reversible Ischemia Trial
ESPS2	European Stroke Prevention Study 2
LIPID	Long-term Intervention with Pravastatin in Ischemic Disease
mRS	Modified Rankin Scale
NASCET	North American Symptomatic Carotid Endarterectomy Trial
NIHSS	National Institutes of Health Stroke Scale
PRoFESS	Prevention Regimen for Effectively Avoiding Second Strokes
SAMMPRIS	Stenting and Aggressive Medical Management for Preventing Recurrent Stroke in Intracranial Stenosis
SMART	Second Manifestations of ARTerial disease
SOCRATES	Acute Stroke or Transient Ischemic Attack Treated with Aspirin or Ticagrelor and Patient Outcomes
SPARCL	Stroke Prevention by Aggressive Reduction in Cholesterol Levels
VISSIT	Vitesse Stent Ischemic Therapy
WASID	Warfarin-Aspirin for Symptomatic Intracranial Disease

M. M. Alkhalifah · P. M. Gadient
Vascular Neurology, University of Miami Miller School of Medicine, Miami, FL, USA

S. Chaturvedi (✉)
Vice-Chair for VA Programs, University of Miami Miller School of Medicine, Miami, FL, USA
e-mail: Schaturvedi@med.miami.edu

Antiplatelet Therapy

Antiplatelet therapy is recommended for secondary prevention of noncardioembolic ischemic stroke and TIA. Other antiplatelet medications were later studied for stroke prevention, e.g., clopidogrel, extended-release dipyridamole, cilostazol, and ticagrelor. Several options are recommended for stroke prevention according to guidelines from the American Heart Association/American Stroke Association [1].

Antiplatelet medication effect is achieved through several mechanisms. Aspirin irreversibly

© The Editor(s) (if applicable) and The Author(s) 2018
S. S. Hans (ed.), *Extracranial Carotid and Vertebral Artery Disease*,
https://doi.org/10.1007/978-3-319-91533-3_9

blocks the cyclooxygenase (COX) activity of prostaglandin H synthase 1 and 2 (COX-1 and COX-2). COX-1 inhibition permanently alters the thromboxane A2-dependent platelet functions (platelet aggregation and vasoconstriction). Aspirin is absorbed rapidly and reaches its peak plasma level within 30–40 min. Enteric coated aspirin absorption is slower, but it reduces the gastrointestinal side effects. Dipyridamole and cilostazol are phosphodiesterase inhibitors. They inhibit adenosine reuptake and increase cAMP and gAMP levels which increases platelet survival and causes vasodilation. Clopidogrel, prasugrel, and ticagrelor inhibit the adenosine-dependent platelet aggregation by blocking the P2Y12 receptors. Clopidogrel and prasugrel are prodrugs and need to be activated by cytochrome P-450 enzymes. Conversely, ticagrelor does not need activation and acts rapidly.

The North American Symptomatic Carotid Endarterectomy Trial (NASCET), European Carotid Surgery Trial (ECST), and the Veterans Affairs (VA) carotid stenosis studies were the first-generation studies that evaluated surgical therapy in carotid stenosis. They examined the efficacy of carotid endarterectomy (CEA) compared to medical therapy in symptomatic carotid stenosis of different degrees. CEA resulted in 65% and 45% relative risk reduction of recurrent stroke in patients with ≥70% stenosis in the NASCET and ECST trials, respectively [2, 3]. In NASCET, an aspirin dose of 1300 mg was recommended. NASCET was largely conducted in the pre-statin area, and only about 15% of patients received lipid-lowering medications [2]. There was no formal hypertension management protocol in NASCET.

An alternative regimen to aspirin monotherapy is dual antiplatelet therapy. In the CHANCE trial, dual antiplatelet therapy (DAPT) with aspirin and clopidogrel for 21 days resulted in 32% relative risk reduction of ischemic stroke recurrence at 90 days from the index TIA or minor ischemic stroke (NIHSS ≤ 5) compared to aspirin monotherapy [4]. However, this trial enrolled mostly Asian patients with presumed more intracranial atherosclerosis. In the ESPS-2

and ESPRIT trials, aspirin and extended-release dipyridamole (ASA-ERDP) was superior to aspirin alone in preventing major vascular events [5, 6]. In 2008, the PRoFESS trial showed that ASA-ERDP was not superior to clopidogrel but resulted in more adverse reactions (mostly headache) [7]. The Clopidogrel and Aspirin for Reduction of Emboli in Symptomatic Carotid Stenosis (CARESS) study randomized patients with ≥50% carotid stenosis and transcranial Doppler (TCD) microembolic signals to aspirin or clopidogrel and aspirin [8]. DAPT was superior to monotherapy in reducing TCD microembolic signals 2 and 7 days after randomization. During the first 7 days after randomization, there were no recurrent strokes and four TIAs in the DAPT group compared to four recurrent strokes and seven TIAs in the group that received aspirin alone.

The effect of antiplatelet therapy on specific stroke subtypes was not evaluated in any of the studies mentioned above until the recent SOCRATES trial. SOCRATES is a randomized control trial that evaluated ticagrelor vs aspirin for secondary stroke prevention of noncardioembolic TIA or mild ischemic stroke (NIHSS ≤ 5). Ticagrelor was not superior to aspirin in preventing stroke, MI, or death in the overall trial [9]. But, a subgroup analysis of patients with symptomatic atherosclerotic disease was in favor of ticagrelor over aspirin [10]. At 90 days, ipsilateral stroke, myocardial infarction, or death occurred in 6.7% in the ticagrelor group compared to 9.6% in the aspirin group. There was a 32% reduction in this endpoint with ticagrelor (hazard ratio 0.68 [95% CI 0.53–0.88]; $p = 0.003$).

The optimal dose of aspirin prior to and following CEA has also been studied. The Aspirin and Carotid Endarterectomy (ACE) trial evaluated four doses of ASA (81, 325, 650, and 1300 mg) prior to and for 90 days following CEA. The lower doses (81 and 325 mg) were superior in preventing recurrent stroke, myocardial infarction, or vascular death compared to the higher doses [11]. As a result, current guidelines recommend 81–325 mg of aspirin in patients undergoing CEA [12].

Statins for Carotid Disease

The Stroke Prevention by Aggressive Reduction in Cholesterol Levels (SPARCL) trial is the largest trial to date that has examined the impact of statins on stroke risk [13]. The trial enrolled patients with stroke or TIA within the previous 6 months and with low-density lipoprotein (LDL) cholesterol levels of 100–190 mg per deciliter and with no known coronary heart disease. Subjects were assigned to treatment with 80 mg of atorvastatin per day or placebo. The primary endpoint was a first nonfatal or fatal stroke. Over follow-up of almost 5 years, 11.2% of the atorvastatin group and 13.1% of the placebo group suffered a stroke (5-year absolute reduction in risk, 2.2%; adjusted hazard ratio, 0.84; 95% confidence interval, 0.71–0.99; $P = 0.03$; unadjusted $P = 0.05$). In a subgroup analysis, the effect was found to be similar among all stroke subtypes [14]. While the overall morality was similar between groups, the atorvastatin group did experience a small increase in the incidence of hemorrhagic stroke compared to placebo. A secondary analysis, looking specifically at patients with carotid stenosis, found that when compared with placebo, treatment with atorvastatin was associated with a 33% reduction in the risk of any stroke (hazard ratio [HR] 0.67, 95% confidence interval [CI] 0.47, 0.94; $P = 0.02$) and a 43% reduction in risk of major coronary events (HR 0.57, 95% CI 0.32, 1.00; $P = 0.05$). Carotid revascularization was reduced by 56% (HR 0.44, 95% CI 0.24, 0.79; $P = 0.006$) in the atorvastatin treatment group [15].

Prior treatment with statins may also be beneficial for patients with carotid stenosis. A retrospective analysis found that among acute symptomatic carotid stenosis patients, nonprocedural 7-day stroke risk was 3.8% (CI, 1.2–9.7%) with statin treatment at TIA onset, compared with 13.2% (CI, 8.5–19.8%) in those not statin pretreated ($P = 0.01$; 90-day risks 8.9% versus 20.8% [$P = 0.01$]). Statin pretreatment was associated with reduced stroke risk in patients with carotid stenosis (odds ratio for 90-day stroke, 0.37; CI, 0.17–0.82) but not in patients without stenosis (odds ratio, 1.3; CI, 0.8–2.24; P for interaction, 0.008). This association remained after adjustment for multiple variables [16].

A 2004 systematic review and meta-analysis of randomized trials, testing statin drugs, found that each 10% reduction in LDL was estimated to reduce the risk of all strokes by 15.6% (95% CI, 6.7–23.6) and carotid intima media thickness (IMT) by 0.73% per year (95% CI, 0.27–1.19). Of note, this analysis did not find an association between statin use and intracerebral hemorrhage [17].

A recent multicenter prospective study of patients with large artery atherosclerosis (LAA) found that statin pretreatment was associated with greater neurologic improvement during hospitalization and higher rates of favorable outcomes (FO) (mRS 0–1) in unmatched and matched (odds ratio for FO: 2.44; 95% confidence interval [CI]: 1.07–5.53) analyses. It was also related to lower risk of 1-month mortality and stroke recurrence in unmatched and matched analyses (hazard ratio for recurrent stroke: 0.11, 95% CI: 0.02–0.46; hazard ratio for death: 0.24, 95% CI: 0.08–0.75) [18].

For patients undergoing interventions, prior treatment with statins is also desirable. A 2006 retrospective study examined the effect of statin pretreatment on outcomes in carotid artery stenting (CAS) and found the incidence of cardiovascular events was significantly different between patients with statin pretreatment (4%) and those without pretreatment (15%) ($P < 0.05$). The difference remained after adjustment for age, sex, degree of carotid stenosis, and the use of cerebral protection devices [19].

The multicenter EPOCH-CAS study examined patients with carotid artery stenosis (symptomatic ≥ 50%, asymptomatic ≥ 80%) and a high risk of CEA but without previous statin treatment. Patients were divided into two groups by LDL levels. Patients with LDL ≥ 120 mg/dl received pitavastatin at 4 mg/day. Patients, with LDL <120 mg/dl, did not receive treatment. After 4 weeks, both groups underwent CAS. New ipsilateral ischemic lesions were identified in 25.8% in the pretreatment group and 53.3% among controls ($P = 0.028$) [20]. The Rosuvastatin Pretreatment to Reduce Embolization during Carotid Artery Stenting trial is currently enrolling and will be the largest randomized trial to examine the effect of statin pretreatment on embolization during CAS [21].

The LIPID trial showed that pravastatin use accompanied by low-fat diet, even among patients with average or below average cholesterol levels, resulted in significant reduction in carotid wall thickness when compared to placebo and low-fat diet [22]. Another study demonstrated that attenuation of carotid plaque during statin use was associated with higher high-density lipoprotein (HDL) levels [23].

For patients with symptomatic carotid stenosis, a 4.5-year prospective population-based study in Denmark found that early risk of recurrent stroke in patients with symptomatic significant carotid stenosis is dramatically reduced after urgent aggressive best medical therapy, including statin treatment, in specialized stroke clinics. The rate of early recurrence of neurological symptoms from index event to CEA in symptomatic patients was 1.6% (95% CI 0.5–4%) after best medical therapy and 25% in the 90 days prior to referral to a stroke clinic (95% CI 20–30%, $p < 0.00001$) [24].

Insights regarding the benefits of aggressive medical therapy can also be obtained from studies of intracranial stenosis. An analysis comparing two of the largest trials involving the medical management of intracranial disease (SAMMPRIS and WASID) showed that the better outcomes demonstrated in the medical arm of SAMMPRIS compared to those in WASID were due in large part to the aggressive medical management, including statin use, in SAMMPRIS [25].

A systematic review of the effect of statin use on carotid plaque echogenicity found that statin use was associated with a favorable increase of carotid plaque echogenicity. The effect appears dependent on treatment duration and high-sensitivity C-reactive protein (hs-CRP) change from baseline and independent of changes in LDL and HDL [26].

Blood Pressure Medications and Carotid Disease

There are currently limited data regarding the management of blood pressure in patients with carotid artery stenosis. Studies have generally used <140/90 as a target except in the setting of acute ischemic stroke after which permissive hypertension is allowed for 24–48 h.

The Asymptomatic Carotid Surgery Trial (ACST) enrolled patients as intensive medical management became more popular. The later years of these trials, when more patients were receiving intensive medical therapy, resulted in improved outcomes. Specifically, in the first 5 years of the ACST, medically treated patients had a 1.1% annual risk of stroke. In the final 5 years of the ACST, medically treated patients had a 0.7% risk of stroke per year. The decline in stroke rates from 1995 to 2010 corresponded with increased utilization of statins and antihypertensive medications. As an example, fewer than 10% of patients randomized to medical therapy alone were on lipid-lowering treatment in the first year of the study, and this increased to 82% in the later years of ACST. In addition, diastolic blood pressure improved from 84 mmHg in 1995 to 77.5 mmHg in 2005 [27].

A 2015 study showed that patients whose blood pressure paradoxically increased during sleep (reverse dipper pattern) may be a risk factor for carotid atherosclerosis and play a crucial role in the early formation of carotid plaque [28].

Asymptomatic Carotid Emboli Study (ACES) is a prospective observational study of 477 patients with asymptomatic carotid stenosis [29]. Baseline mean BP weakly predicted any stroke or CVD death ($P = 0.03$). On multivariate analysis, antiplatelets ($P = 0.001$) and lower mean blood pressure ($P = 0.002$) were independent predictors of reduced risk of ipsilateral stroke and transient ischemic attack. Antiplatelets ($P < 0.0001$) and antihypertensives ($P < 0.0001$) were independent predictors of a lower risk of any stroke or cardiovascular death. Antihypertensives predicted a lower risk of ipsilateral stroke or TIA ($P = 0.01$) and any stroke or CVD death ($P < 0.0001$). BP was strongly associated with ipsilateral stroke or TIA and any stroke or CVD death (all $P < 0.0001$). The association of antihypertensives with ipsilateral stroke or TIA was largely mediated via BP control.

In 2003, the Carotid Endarterectomy Trialists' Collaboration compared the relationship between blood pressure (systolic and diastolic blood pressures, pulse pressure) and stroke risk in TIA and stroke patients with documented stenosis of at least one carotid artery (ECST and NASCET) with that in TIA and stroke patients with a low prevalence of carotid disease [United Kingdom Transient Ischemic Attack (UK-TIA) Aspirin Trial]. In ECST and NASCET, investigators also determined the relationship between blood pressure and stroke risk in patients with unilateral carotid occlusion and patients with bilateral ≥70% carotid stenosis. They found that stroke risk on medical treatment increased with blood pressure in ECST and NASCET, but the relationships were less steep than in the UK-TIA trial. The relationship between blood pressure and stroke risk was not affected by the presence of a unilateral carotid occlusion but was significantly affected by the presence of bilateral carotid stenosis ≥70% (interaction: systolic blood pressure, $P = 0.002$; diastolic blood pressure, $P = 0.03$; pulse pressure, $P = 0.003$) [30]. In this group, the relationship was inverted because of the high stroke risks at lower blood pressures. This interaction was not present after carotid endarterectomy and was not present for the risk of myocardial infarction.

Optimal treatment of hypertension may have benefits beyond the carotid artery stenosis. Blood pressure control is especially important in patients with asymptomatic carotid stenosis as about 50% of strokes in patients with asymptomatic carotid stenosis are due to small vessel disease and cardioembolism rather than the stenotic carotid artery [31].

Multimodal Therapy

It is clear that each treatment described above should not be viewed in isolation. Atherosclerosis is a complex disease process, and several treatment modalities are needed to optimize outcomes. Therefore, the concept of "multifaceted" or "multimodal" therapy is now recommended.

Elements of Optimal Medical Therapy for Carotid Stenosis

1. Antiplatelet therapy
2. High potency statins
3. Targeted blood pressure reduction
4. Smoking cessation
5. Guideline-directed treatment of diabetes
6. Increased physical activity (AHA recommendations)
7. Mediterranean diet or AHA DASH diet
8. Evaluation for sleep-disordered breathing

As mentioned above, intracranial stenosis trials have been important in demonstrating the value of multimodal therapy. SAMMPRIS and VISSIT trials evaluated the role of stenting of severe intracranial stenosis compared to aggressive medical therapy [32, 33]. In SAMMPRIS, 12% of the aggressive medical management (AMM) group developed a primary outcome (ipsilateral stroke or death) compared to 22% in the stenting group (the rates were 15% in AMM and 36% in the stenting groups in VISSIT). AMM consisted of dual antiplatelet therapy with aspirin 325 mg daily and clopidogrel 75 mg daily for 90 days followed by aspirin monotherapy indefinitely. Treatment also included aggressive antihypertensive regimen with a goal systolic blood pressure <140 mmHg (≤130 mmHg in diabetics), lipid lowering to a goal LDL <70 mg/dl, smoking cessation, weight loss, and exercise through a specific lifestyle modification program (INTERVENT coaching). The benefits of aggressive medical therapy were seen with the superior outcomes with medical therapy compared to intracranial stenting.

With regard to carotid disease, the use of lipid-lowering medications increased significantly between 1993 and 2003 when the ACST was conducted. The rates of lipid medication use were 17% in the 1993–1996 enrolled patients compared to 58% in those enrolled in 2000–2003 [27].

Three population-based prospective studies of asymptomatic carotid stenosis (Oxford Vascular Study, SMART and London, Ontario study) evaluated the risk of ipsilateral ischemic stroke in medically treated patients with 50–99% asymptomatic carotid stenosis. The annual stroke risk was 0.34–0.5% [34–36]. The lower rate of stroke in these contemporary studies relative to first-generation carotid stenosis suggests that multimodal therapy is having an impact on reducing the stroke rate in patients with asymptomatic carotid stenosis.

Current Clinical Trials

CREST-2 is an ongoing study to evaluate CAS or CEA compared to intensive medical management for asymptomatic carotid stenosis of 70–99% [37]. Medical therapy in CREST-2 includes all the pharmacologic treatments referred to in this chapter [38].

Intensive medical management consists of aspirin 325 mg daily throughout the follow-up period, with CAS patients also receiving clopidogrel in addition to aspirin for 30–90 days. The goal systolic blood pressure is ≤140 mmHg and LDL <70 mg/dl. Secondary risk factors such as smoking, diabetes mellitus, weight, and physical activity will be managed using the INTERVENT program. Statin loading is required for patients undergoing CEA or CAS who were not previously treated with statins. In addition, for patients with hyperlipidemia who are not able to reach the target LDL with high potency statins, treatment with injectable PCSK9 inhibitors is an option. These novel medications have recently been found to reduce cardiovascular events in patients with hyperlipidemia [39].

Conclusion

The landscape of medical management for patients with atherosclerotic disease continues to evolve. In clinical trials and community practice, the rate of cardiovascular events is dropping in conjunction with improvements in medical therapy. Surgeons and interventional physicians should work with medical management physicians to ensure optimal outcomes for patients.

Review Questions

1. Each of the following antiplatelet medications have been proven to reduce stroke except:
   A. Aspirin
   B. Clopidogrel
   C. Aspirin + dipyridamole
   D. Ticagrelor

   Answer: D

2. Which statin was the first to be shown to reduce stroke in patients with previous stroke and no prior coronary artery disease?
   A. Lovastatin
   B. Atorvastatin
   C. Simvastatin
   D. Pravastatin

   Answer: B

3. In current carotid stenosis trials such as CREST-2, the target for LDL lowering is:
   A. <130 mg/dl
   B. <100 mg/dl
   C. <70 mg/dl
   D. <40 mg/dl

   Answer: C

References

1. Kernan WN, Ovbiagele B, Black HR, et al. Guidelines for the prevention of stroke in patients with stroke and transient ischemic attack: a guideline for healthcare professionals from the American Heart Association/American Stroke Association. Stroke. 2014;45:2160–236.
2. Barnett HJM, Taylor DW, Eliasziw M, et al. Benefit of carotid endarterectomy in patients with symptomatic moderate or severe stenosis. N Engl J Med. 1998;339:1415–25.
3. Rothwell PM, Eliasziw M, Gutnikov SA, et al. Analysis of pooled data from the randomised controlled trials of endarterectomy for symptomatic carotid stenosis. Lancet. 2003;361:107–16.
4. Wang Y, Wang Y, Zhao X, et al. Clopidogrel with aspirin in acute minor stroke or transient ischemic attack. N Engl J Med. 2013;369:11–9.
5. Diener HC, Cunha L, Forbes C, et al. European Stroke Prevention Study 2. Dipyridamole and acetylsalicylic

acid in the secondary prevention of stroke. J Neurol Sci. 1996;143:1–13.

6. The Esprit Study Group. Aspirin plus dipyridamole versus aspirin alone after cerebral ischaemia of arterial origin (ESPRIT): randomised controlled trial. Lancet. 2006;367:1665–73.

7. Sacco RL, Diener H-C, Yusuf S, et al. Aspirin and extended-release dipyridamole versus clopidogrel for recurrent stroke. N Engl J Med. 2008;359:1238–51.

8. Markus HS, Droste DW, Kaps M, et al. Dual antiplatelet therapy with clopidogrel and aspirin in symptomatic carotid stenosis evaluated using Doppler embolic signal detection: the Clopidogrel and Aspirin for Reduction of Emboli in Symptomatic Carotid Stenosis (CARESS) trial. Circulation. 2005;111:2233–40.

9. Johnston SC, Amarenco P, Albers GW, et al. Ticagrelor versus aspirin in acute stroke or transient ischemic attack. N Engl J Med. 2016;375:35–43.

10. Amarenco P, Albers GW, Denison H, et al. Efficacy and safety of ticagrelor versus aspirin in acute stroke or transient ischaemic attack of atherosclerotic origin: a subgroup analysis of SOCRATES, a randomised, double-blind, controlled trial. Lancet Neurol. 2017;16:301–10.

11. Taylor DW, Barnett HJM, Haynes RB, et al. Low-dose and high-dose acetylsalicylic acid for patients undergoing carotid endarterectomy: a randomised controlled trial. Lancet. 1999;353:2179–84.

12. Chaturvedi S, Bruno A, Feasby T, et al. Carotid endarterectomy—an evidence-based review: report of the Therapeutics and Technology Assessment Subcommittee of the American Academy of Neurology. Neurology. 2005;65:794–801.

13. SPARCL Investigators. High-dose atorvastatin after stroke or transient ischemic attack. N Engl J Med. 2006;355:549–59.

14. Amarenco P, Benavente O, Goldstein LB, et al. Results of the Stroke Prevention by Aggressive Reduction in Cholesterol Levels (SPARCL) trial by stroke subtypes. Stroke. 2009;40:1405–9.

15. Sillesen H, Amarenco P, Hennerici MG, et al. Atorvastatin reduces the risk of cardiovascular events in patients with carotid atherosclerosis: a secondary analysis of the Stroke Prevention by Aggressive Reduction in Cholesterol Levels (SPARCL) trial. Stroke. 2008;39:3297–302.

16. Merwick Á, Albers GW, Arsava EM, et al. Reduction in early stroke risk in carotid stenosis with transient ischemic attack associated with statin treatment. Stroke. 2013;44:2814–20.

17. Amarenco P, Labreuche J, Lavallée P, Touboul P-J. Statins in stroke prevention and carotid atherosclerosis: systematic review and up-to-date meta-analysis. Stroke. 2004;35(12):2902–9.

18. Tsivgoulis G, Katsanos AH, Sharma VK, et al. Statin pretreatment is associated with better outcomes in large artery atherosclerotic stroke. Neurology. 2016;86:1103–11.

19. Groschel K, Ernemann U, Schulz JB, et al. Statin therapy at carotid angioplasty and stent placement: effect on procedure-related stroke, myocardial infarction, and death. Radiology. 2006;240:145.

20. Takayama K, Taki W, Toma N, et al. Effect of pitavastatin on preventing ischemic complications with carotid artery stenting: a multicenter prospective study—EPOCH-CAS study. Cardiovasc Intervent Radiol. 2014;37:1436–43.

21. De Carlo M, Cortese B, Pennesi M, et al. Design of the rosuvastatin pretreatment to reduce embolization during Carotid Artery Stenting trial. J Cardiovasc Med (Hagerstown). 2014;15:595–600.

22. MacMahon S, Sharpe N, Gamble G, et al. Effects of lowering average or below-average cholesterol levels on the progression of carotid atherosclerosis. Results of the LIPID atherosclerosis substudy. Circulation. 1998;97:1784–90.

23. Okumura K, Tsukamoto H, Tsuboi H, et al. High HDL cholesterol level after treatment with pitavastatin is an important factor for regression in carotid intima-media thickness. Heart Vessel. 2015;30:154–61.

24. Shahidi S, Owen-Falkenberg A, Hjerpsted U, et al. Urgent best medical therapy may obviate the need for urgent surgery in patients with symptomatic carotid stenosis. Stroke. 2013;44:2220–5.

25. Chaturvedi S, Turan TN, Lynn MJ, et al. Do patient characteristics explain the differences in outcome between medically treated patients in SAMMPRIS and WASID? Stroke. 2015;46:2562–7.

26. Ibrahimi P, Jashari F, Bajraktari G, et al. Ultrasound assessment of carotid plaque echogenicity response to statin therapy: a systematic review and meta-analysis. Int J Mol Sci. 2015;16:10734–47.

27. Halliday A, Harrison M, Hayter E, et al. 10-year stroke prevention after successful carotid endarterectomy for asymptomatic stenosis (ACST-1): a multicentre randomised trial. Lancet. 2010;376:1074–84.

28. Yan B, Peng L, Han D, et al. Blood pressure reverse-dipping is associated with early formation of carotid plaque in senior hypertensive patients. Medicine (Baltimore). 2015;94:e604.

29. Markus HS, King A, Shipley M, et al. Asymptomatic embolisation for prediction of stroke in the Asymptomatic Carotid Emboli Study (ACES): a prospective observational study. Lancet Neurol. 2010;9:663–71.

30. Rothwell PM, Howard SC, Spence JD. Relationship between blood pressure and stroke risk in patients with symptomatic carotid occlusive disease. Stroke. 2003;34:2583–90.

31. Inzitari D, Eliasziw M, Gates P, et al. The causes and risk of stroke in patients with asymptomatic internal-carotid-artery stenosis. N Engl J Med. 2000;342:1693–701.

32. Chimowitz MI, Lynn MJ, Derdeyn CP, et al. Stenting versus aggressive medical therapy for intracranial arterial stenosis. N Engl J Med. 2011;365:993–1003.

33. Zaidat OO, Fitzsimmons B, Woodward B, et al. Effect of a balloon-expandable intracranial stent vs medical therapy on risk of stroke in patients with symptomatic intracranial stenosis: the VISSIT randomized clinical trial. JAMA. 2015;313:1240–8.

34. Marquardt L, Geraghty OC, Mehta Z, Rothwell PM. Low risk of ipsilateral stroke in patients with asymptomatic carotid stenosis on best medical treatment: a prospective, population-based study. Stroke. 2010;41:e11–7.

35. den Hartog AG, Achterberg S, Moll FL, et al. Asymptomatic carotid artery stenosis and the risk of ischemic stroke according to subtype in patients with clinical manifest arterial disease. Stroke. 2013;44:1002–7.

36. Spence JD, Coates V, Li H, et al. Effects of intensive medical therapy on microemboli and cardiovascular risk in asymptomatic carotid stenosis. Arch Neurol. 2010;67:180–6.

37. Chaturvedi S, Chimowitz M, Brown RD, et al. The urgent need for contemporary clinical trials in patients with asymptomatic carotid stenosis. Neurology. 2016;87:2271.

38. Howard VJ, Meschia JF, Lal BK, et al. Carotid revascularization and medical management for asymptomatic carotid stenosis: protocol of the CREST-2 clinical trials. Int J Stroke. 2017;12(7):770–8.

39. Sabatine MS, Giugliano RP, Keech AC, et al. Evolocumab and clinical outcomes in patients with cardiovascular disease. N Engl J Med. 2017;376:1713–22.

Carotid Endarterectomy

10

Sachinder Singh Hans

Introduction

Stroke is the fifth leading cause of death and is the principal cause of disability in the United States of America. Approximately 700,000 strokes occur per year; 25% die within the first year following stroke. Approximately 85% of strokes are ischemic, and 10–15% are due to intracerebral hemorrhage [1–7]. Extracranial atherosclerosis is accountable for 10–20% of all ischemic strokes [1–7]. Clinical trials have demonstrated that carotid endarterectomy (CEA) reduces the incidence of stroke in patients with symptoms of focal transient ischemic attack and transient mono-ocular blindness and in patients with recent stroke [1–7]. Patients, presenting with focal transient ischemic attack (TIA) lasting for more than 10 min, age greater than 60, and those with diabetes mellitus, have greater risk of stroke; the risk is greatest within the first few days of TIA [6]. Eliasziw et al. reported that for patients with a first recorded hemisphere

TIA, the 90-day risk of ipsilateral stroke was 20%, higher than the 2.3% for patients with a hemispheric stroke [5]. Carotid endarterectomy (CEA) is one of the most common vascular operations, secondary only to coronary artery bypass grafting, though the number of carotid endarterectomies has decreased due to improvements in medical management and the introduction of carotid artery stenting (CAS). The rate of CEA varies with geographic location, gender, and ethnicity in the United States. The rate of CEA among men is approximately 1.9 times as compared to women [8]. The SAPPHIRE (Stenting and Angioplasty with Protection in Patients at High Risk for Endarterectomy) trial demonstrated non-inferiority of carotid artery stenting for both asymptomatic and symptomatic patients [9]. The CREST study (Carotid Revascularization Endarterectomy vs. Stenting Trial) enrolled both asymptomatic and symptomatic patients. There was no statistically significant difference between CEA and CAS in the primary composite end point of stroke, MI, or death from any cause or ipsilateral stroke within 4 years after randomization. However, stroke rate was higher in the CAS group, but MI with associated mortality was higher in the CEA group [10, 11].

The original version of the chapter was revised. A correction to this chapter can be found at https://doi.org/10.1007/978-3-319-91533-3_25

S. S. Hans
Medical Director of Vascular and Endovascular Services, Henry Ford Macomb Hospital, Clinton Township, MI, USA

Chief of Vascular Surgery, St. John Macomb Hospital, Warren, MI, USA

Department of Surgery, Wayne State University School of Medicine, Detroit, MI, USA

Pathophysiology

As the plaque burden increases at the origin of internal carotid artery due to low wall shear stress, flow separation, and loss of unidirectional flow, it results in prolonged exposure of the plasma binding to the vessel wall. The plaque may develop intraplaque hemorrhage, resulting in plaque rupture with ulceration, and collection of platelets with embolization into the branches of MCA, rarely to ACA, and to the branches of central artery of retina resulting in transient focal weakness of upper/lower extremity and transient loss of vision, respectively. If the embolus is large, it can cause major arterial occlusion intracranially resulting in cerebral infarction with hemiplegia or retinal infarct with blindness.

A high-grade stenosis of the ICA (>70%) may reduce blood flow to the brain and results in temporary or permanent neurological deficit. Acute thrombosis superimposed on the pre-existing high grade stenosis in the ICA may be asymptomatic and cause temporary eye symptoms, mild stroke, or major stroke depending upon the collateral flow to the brain. It is well established that patients with symptoms of TIA, or crescendo TIAs, are potentially at a high risk for developing major stroke in the presence of significant ipsilateral extracranial ICA stenosis.

Indications

1. Patients with recent minor to moderate stroke (NIH Stroke Scale <15) in the distribution of MCA (rarely anterior cerebral artery) in whom the neurological deficit has plateaued. CEA is rarely performed as an emergency in patients with recent stroke as medical optimization and edema around the area of infarct should subside before the operation. The risk of perioperative stroke in this group of patients is not increased if CEA is undertaken within 2 weeks of the event. Previous published trials reported greatest benefit of CEA within 2 weeks of the last event, and after 12 weeks, the benefit of CEA is considerably reduced [1].
2. Transient contralateral motor or sensory deficit or speech involvement with spontaneous recovery. Transient loss of vision (amaurosis fugax) which may be complete or partial. Typically the symptoms last for a few minutes and at the most 1 h [7]. There is no evidence of infarction on MRI of the brain.

3. Asymptomatic high-grade ICA stenosis (>70%) in selected patients who are at good risk for the procedure and have at least 5 years of life expectancy.

It is important to know the symptomatic nature of the lesion as well as the plaque morphology in consideration for intervention in the form of CEA or CAS. For example, in an asymptomatic patient above the age of 80 with heavily calcified plaque causing 80% stenosis, carotid endarterectomy is probably not the best option. On the other hand, in an 80-year-old patient with focal TIA symptoms or recent mild stroke with a 60% stenosis but primarily with a soft (hypoechoic) plaque, the procedure should be given a strong consideration. Demonstration of infarct on brain imaging and intracerebral stenosis double the risk of stroke in patients with hemispheric TIA [5]. There have been advances in the medical management of carotid artery stenosis (see Chap. 9). CEA is strongly indicated in prevention of stroke in patients with crescendo TIAs or following mild stroke [1–7]. Syncope, dizziness, and vertigo are usually not associated with carotid stenosis, and thorough workup with detailed clinical history, cardiac evaluation, tilt-table test, and, in some instances, consultation with ENT surgeon should be undertaken.

Following clinical evaluation, patients should undergo carotid duplex imaging and non-contrast CT scan of the head followed by CT angiography of the neck/head. MRI/MRA of the brain is often necessary for further evaluation in patients who exhibit focal neurological symptoms and or positive neurological findings.

Anesthesia

Regional (cervical block anesthesia) versus general anesthesia (GA) has been debated over many years as the best anesthetic for patients undergoing CEA. Recent results from GALA trial have not shown any superiority in the outcome following CEA for either CBA or GA [12]. Since 2003, the author has preferred CBA except in patients with high plaque (upper end of the plaque at the level of second cervical vertebrae), those with an anxiety disorder, patients with hearing loss, or poor command of English language, for whom GA is preferred.

Positioning and Incision

A roll is placed between the scapulae to hyperextend the neck with occipital support. The neck is turned laterally to contralateral side. In patients with "short neck," the shoulder is slightly pulled downward with a wide tape attached to the shoulder with Mastisol adhesive (Eloquest, Ferndale, Michigan), and tape is then stretched and temporarily attached to the railing on the side of the table near its distal end.

Incision

Three incisions are commonly used:

1. Vertical with slight angulation anteriorly at the lower end.
2. Oblique (starting 2 cm behind the sternomastoid at the upper end and ending 2 cm in front of the sternomastoid) (Fig. 10.1).
3. Transverse incision.

Vertical incisions leave an unsightly scar, and transverse incisions may limit the exposure in the event the plaque extends for a considerable distance superiorly or inferiorly. The length of incision is determined by the level of carotid bifurcation in relation to the cervical vertebrae and the extent of the plaque in the internal carotid artery and the common carotid artery as determined by preoperative CT angiography. After dividing the platysma, the external jugular vein is ligated and divided. In the upper portion of the incision, the greater auricular nerve is preserved and mobilized posteriorly and superiorly. Division of the greater auricular nerves results in temporary sensory loss in the corresponding lobule of the ear. Dissection plan is continued along the anteromedial border of the sternocleidomastoid muscle. Following which, the dissection plane is developed among the medial border of the internal jugular vein and

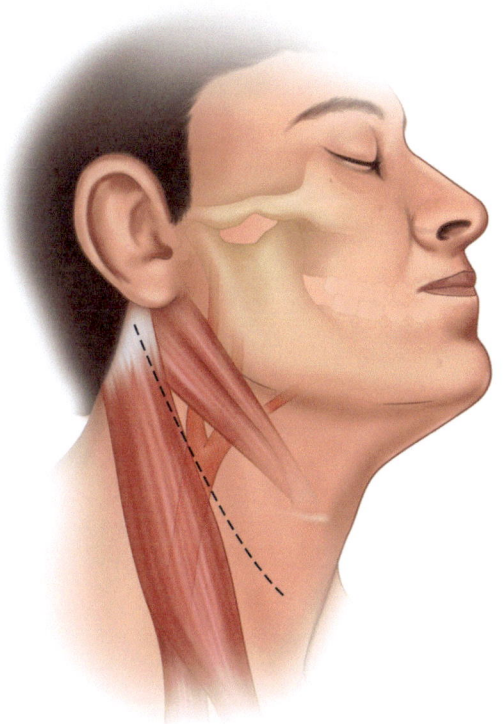

Fig. 10.1 Line of skin incision

is continued cephalad. Common facial vein is encountered and ligated and divided, and upper deep cervical lymph nodes are mobilized posteriorly. As the carotid sheath is opened, vagus nerve is visualized posterolaterally between the artery and the vein. Vagus nerve may descend anteriorly as it courses inferiorly. External carotid artery is looped with a silastic loop which is then pulled caudally and held with a hemostat on the drapes near the chest wall. Ansa cervicalis is seen in the upper part of the dissection and is mobilized anteriorly. In the exposed area above the confluence of the common facial vein to the internal jugular vein, small unnamed veins joining the internal jugular vein are ligated and divided followed by division of the sternocleidomastoid branch of the occipital artery, and this helps to mobilize the hypoglossal nerve cephalad. Local anesthetic (1% lidocaine) is infiltrated in the area of the carotid body to prevent bradycardia. Intravenous heparin (100 units/kg m) is administered by the anesthesia team with ACT monitoring.

Fig. 10.2 Measurement of carotid stump pressure

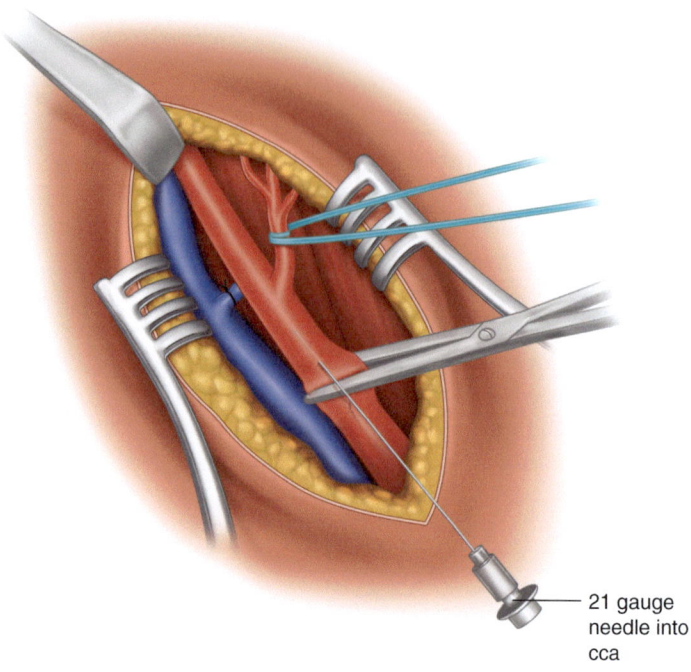

21 gauge
needle into
cca

Shunt Placement

There are three approaches regarding the use of shunt to maintain cerebral perfusion during carotid cross clamping.

1. Routine use of shunt
2. Selective use of shunt
3. Carotid endarterectomy without shunt

Surgeons using routine indwelling shunt generally perform the procedure under GA and do not need measurement of SP and EEG monitoring to access cerebral perfusion, but flow through the shunt should be documented by the arterial Doppler. The disadvantages of routine use of the shunt include that shunt may interfere with the visualization of the distal end of the plaque at the distal end of the arteriotomy. In addition, shunt may cause intimal injury, dissection, and athero-embolization from the proximal common carotid artery.

For surgeons using selective shunt under GA, stump pressure monitoring can be performed by an insertion of a 21 gauge needle and clamp-ing the common and external carotid arteries. Measurement of back pressure (stump pressure) is then performed with the help of a monitor from the anesthesia team (Fig. 10.2). In general, patients with stump pressure of 40 mmHg or above do not need placement of indwelling shunt during carotid endarterectomy unless they become hypotensive during the procedure. Transcranial Doppler with measurement of peak systolic velocity of middle cerebral artery can be used to determine the need for the shunt but is somewhat cumbersome and is not used by majority of the surgeons performing carotid endarterectomy in the United States. EEG monitoring with measurement of median nerve evoked potentials is useful in determining the need for the shunt in patients undergoing CEA under GA.

Under CBA, continuous neurological assessment can be performed by having the patient squeeze with his contralateral hand with a toy that makes a "squeaky" noise. If a patient develops contralateral weakness or becomes unresponsive on clamping off the CCA, a shunt is immediately placed [13–15].

Under GA with EEG monitoring, shunt usage is reported to be in 12–18% of patients, and under regional anesthesia about 10% of patients need shunt placement [12, 14].

Normal cerebral blood flow is about 50 ml/100 g/min, and cerebral ischemia resulting in unresponsive state occurs when the flow is less than 20 ml/100 g/min, and if cerebral ischemia is not prolonged, brain function will return if cerebral perfusion is restored. Ischemic EEG changes during carotid cross clamping under GA overestimate the need for shunt. There are minority of surgeons who perform CEA without shunt and have reported excellent results [16, 17] (Robb, 1980, personal communication). Their excellent results are probably due to careful technique to avoid embolization during CEA as the latter is the most common cause of postoperative neurological deficit. A techniquely satisfactory CEA is very important as any distal flap will lead to thrombosis at the endarterectomy site which may result in a major neurological deficit.

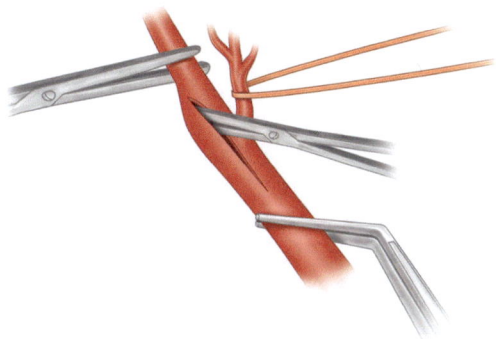

Fig. 10.3 Arteriotomy into distal CCA and proximal ICA

Types of Shunts

One of the original shunts used in carotid artery surgery is Javid™ shunt (Bard, Tempe AZ). The author prefers Sundt™ shunt (Integra, Plainsboro, NJ) because of its flexibility and ease of insertion. Some surgeons prefer small caliber Pruitt-Inahara® (LeMaitre Vascular, Burlington, MA) shunt with balloon occlusion proximally and distally. Argyl carotid shunt [Cardinal Health Dublin, OH] is also used by some surgeons.

Insertion of Indwelling Shunt

Following placement of an angled vascular clamp to CCA and a Kitzmiller clamp distally into the ICA, an arteriotomy incision is made into the distal CCA and extending into the proximal internal carotid artery by angled Potts scissors (Fig. 10.3). The smaller end of the shunt is inserted into the ICA, and a small Javid clamp is applied, and retrograde bleeding occurs through the larger end of

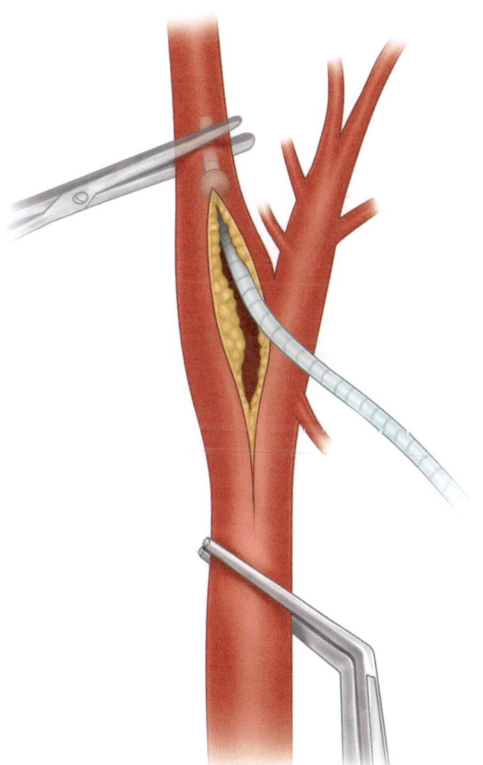

Fig. 10.4 Insertion of distal end of shunt into ICA

the shunt (Fig. 10.4). This end of the shunt is then inserted proximally into the CCA and large Javid clamp is applied. It is to be noted, silastic vessel loop has already been applied to the CCA and that can be tightened around the CCA along with the larger Javid clamp (Fig. 10.5). Unless there

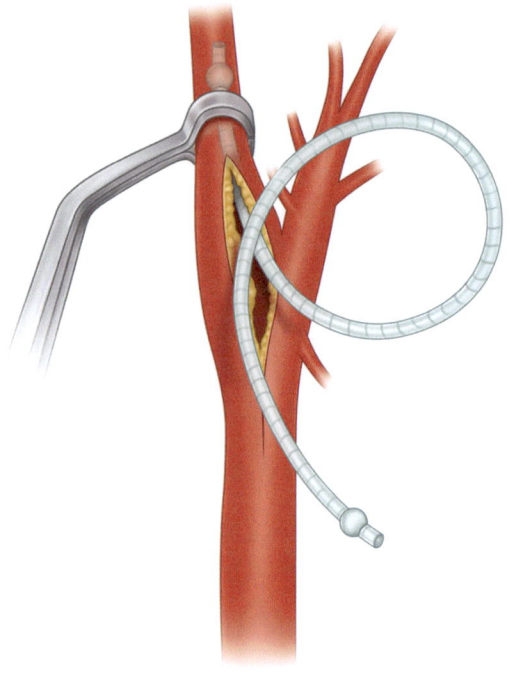

Fig. 10.5 Distal end of shunt secured by Javid clamp

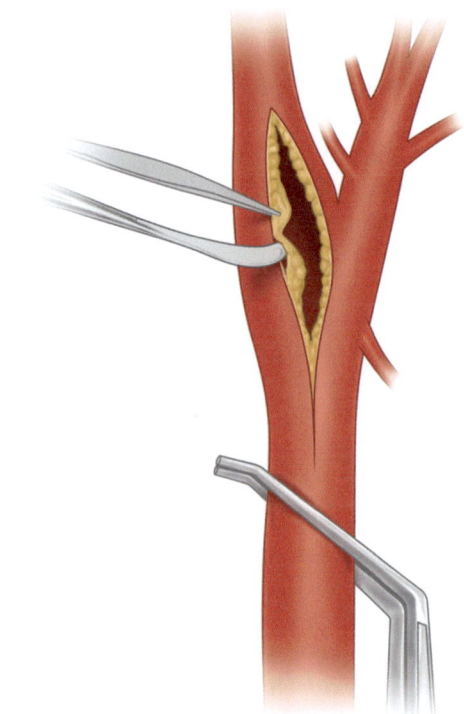

Fig. 10.6 Plaque dissection

are technical difficulties, the cerebral ischemia time during insertion of the shunt should be less than 2–3 min. In patients in whom mid CCA is found to have significant plaque with possibility of ulceration, it is better to insert the larger end of the shunt first into the CCA and to extrude any plaque or debris and then clamp the shunt with a Fogarty softjaw clamp before inserting the distal end into the ICA to prevent plaque embolization.

Plaque is dissected with a Freer-type of elevator at the thickest portion of the plaque and continued cephalad until the plaque thins out at its feathery end (Fig. 10.6). Plaque is sharply divided proximally in the CCA. In patients in whom the distal end of the plaque is not firmly adherent to the arterial wall, a tacking suture is applied in a U-shaped manner.

Unless the diameter of the distal ICA is greater than 5 mm, arteriotomy should preferably be closed with a patch graft (bovine pericardium PTFE or Dacron patch) (Fig. 10.7). Heparin should be reversed with protamine sulfate depending upon the results of ACT.

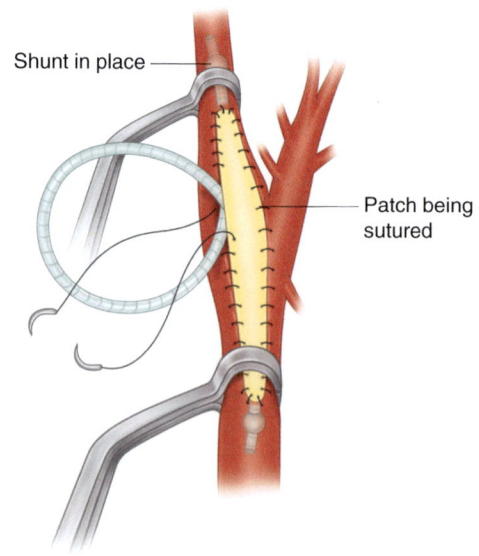

Shunt in place

Patch being sutured

Fig. 10.7 Patch closure with shunt in place

Postoperative Care

The patient should be kept on antiplatelet medications in the form of aspirin and continue statins and judicious use of antihypertensives unless the patient's blood pressure is low in the recovery room.

Complications

Hematoma of the Neck

Small hematoma in the neck is common and resolves spontaneously in most patients within a few days to 1 week. However, large hematoma causing extrinsic compression of the trachea and esophagus should be evacuated in the operating room as an emergency. It may be difficult to perform oral tracheal intubation in a patient with large hematoma of the neck because of the tracheal deviation, and it is often preferable to evacuate the hematoma by removing the sutures and staples to relieve the pressure on the trachea before attempting intubation. In majority of instances, the bleeding is from the venous branches; however, occasionally the bleeding is from the suture line for which additional suturing may be required.

Hemodynamic Instability

Patients may experience hypotension and bradycardia within the first few hours following CEA. This is usually due to carotid sinus nerve stimulation and can be prevented by blocking the carotid body by injecting local anesthetic in the form of 1% lidocaine. Intraoperative hypertension or hypotension in the recovery room while the patient is waking up from general anesthesia is quite frequent and is more common in patients in whom the blood pressure was not well-controlled preoperatively. These patients should be treated with intravenous labetalol or hydralazine. We and others have reported fewer fluctuations in blood pressure in patients undergoing CEA under CBA.

Cranial Nerve Palsy

Hypoglossal nerve is the most common cranial nerve injured during CEA. Temporary hypoglossal nerve palsy with deviation of the tongue to the ipsilateral side and injury to vagus nerve (causing hoarseness) are not uncommon following CEA. Vagus nerve injury occurs during the application of vascular clamp to the common carotid artery. If there is no recovery in 3 months, permanent damage should be suspected. Hoarseness secondary to vagus nerve injury tends to improve as the opposite vocal cord compensates by its moving to the opposite side. Glossopharyngeal nerve injury, though uncommon, may occur during CEA for high plaque and results in loss of sensation in the posterior one-third of the tongue, and the patient may need a PEG tube. If hoarseness persists following CEA, contralateral CEA if necessary should not be performed unless vocal cord function assessment is performed by an ENT surgeon, as bilateral vagus nerve injury will necessitate tracheotomy. Injury to external laryngeal nerve results in the loss of pitch in the voice. Injury to the spinal accessory nerve results in winging of the scapula.

Postoperative Stroke

Postoperative stroke is the most serious complication of the CEA and occurs in 1–5% of patients undergoing CEA [18]. It usually manifests as a contralateral motor weakness of the upper and lower extremities with speech involvement in right-handed individuals if endarterectomy is performed on the left side. Embolization occurs during the operation or in the very early postoperative period. Patient may develop thrombosis at the endarterectomy site usually due to residual intimal flap which may manifest with a neurological deficit following a normal neurological function after the completion of CEA. Cerebral ischemia caused by lack of use of shunt in a patient who has inadequate collateral flow or malfunction of the shunt may be responsible for stroke in less than 10% of individuals. If the patient wakes up with a neurological deficit in the operating

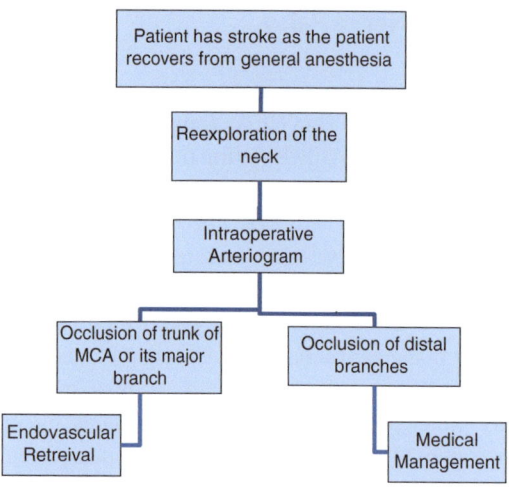

Fig. 10.8 Flow chart for managing intraoperative stroke after CEA

room, the CEA site should be reexplored, and a completion arteriogram should be performed (Fig. 10.8). If patient develops neurological deficit in the recovery room or later (typically 30 min to 12 h after CEA), the patient should undergo emergency non-contrast CT scan of the head to rule out intracerebral hemorrhage which is exceedingly uncommon at this early stage. Once intracerebral hemorrhage is ruled out, the patient should undergo CT angiography of the neck and head as the patient is still in the CT department. If the patient has thrombosis of the ICA with associated MCA (M1 or M2 occlusion), the patient should undergo CEA site thrombectomy and neurovascular intervention for retrieval of the embolic occlusion during the window of 6–8 h following stroke. If there is embolic occlusion in the peripheral branches of MCA, neurovascular intervention is not helpful. Patient should be managed medically and undergo physical, occupational, and speech therapy. Reexploration of the endarterectomy site for suspected thrombosis may be helpful in about 40–50% of patients, but in patients with simultaneous occlusion of the MCA, operative thrombectomy at the endarterectomy site will not improve neurological function in majority of instances (Fig. 10.9). Following left CEA, a patient woke up from GA with right-sided weakness and aphasia in the operating room. Neck incision was reopened, and arteriogram was performed which showed occlusion of M1 segment of MCA. Patient underwent neurosurgical retrieval by Solitaire device (EV3 Irvine, CA) and had a complete recovery (Figs. 10.10, 10.11, and 10.12).

For patients with postoperative intracerebral hemorrhage, neurosurgical consultation should be obtained, and in some instances (hemorrhage in frontal lobe), craniotomy and evacuation of the cerebral hemorrhage may help in neurological recovery (Figs. 10.1 and 10.2). Intracerebral hemorrhage is often due to cerebral hyperperfusion and is often associated with CEA for high-grade ipsilateral carotid stenosis with severe contralateral ICA disease in the form of high-grade stenosis or occlusion. Hyperperfusion syndrome in its mild form presents as post CEA headache and, in its more severe form, as seizures or as intracerebral hemorrhage. It is important to maintain satisfactory blood pressure control following CEA, but this complication is often unavoidable.

Postoperative Myocardial Infarction and Cardiac Arrhythmias

Postoperative myocardial infarction and cardiac arrhythmias may occur following CEA as patients often have associated coronary artery disease. Serum troponin and 12-lead ECG should be performed in patients with unexplained postoperative hypotension, and cardiology consultation should be obtained. It should be noted that annual cardiac event rate was 8.2% and death rate of 6.5% of patients with greater than 75% ICA stenosis [19].

Patch Graft Infection

Synthetic patch graft infection following CEA is rare but a serious complication of CEA and requires removal of the patch and an autogenous reconstruction using interposition greater

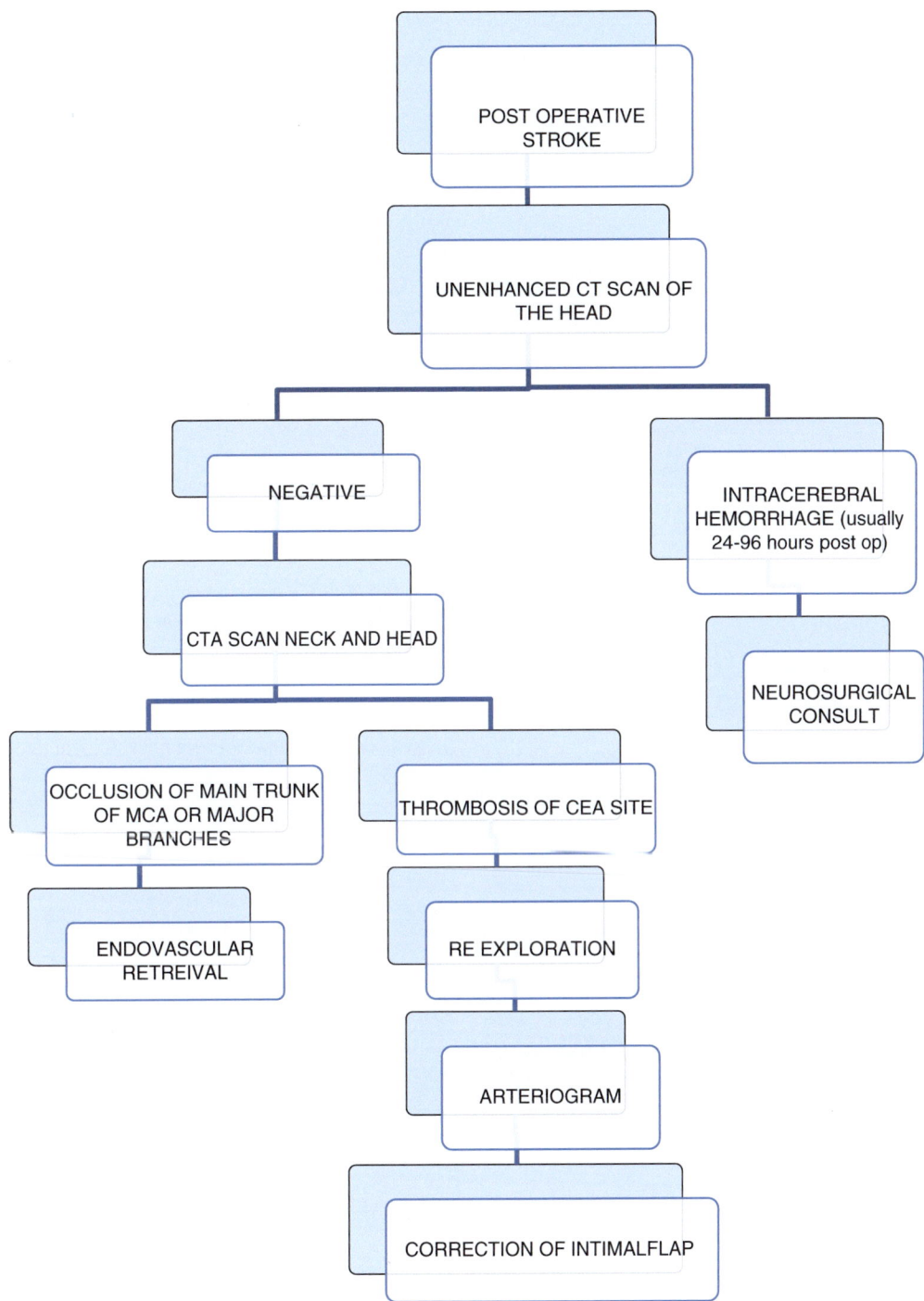

Fig. 10.9 Flow chart for managing postoperative stroke following CEA

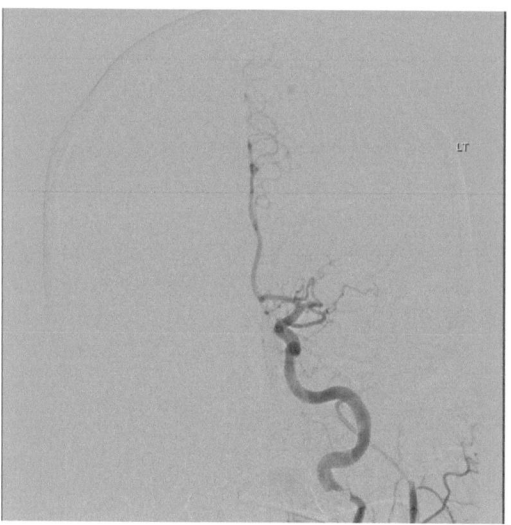

Fig. 10.10 MCA occlusion by the plaque

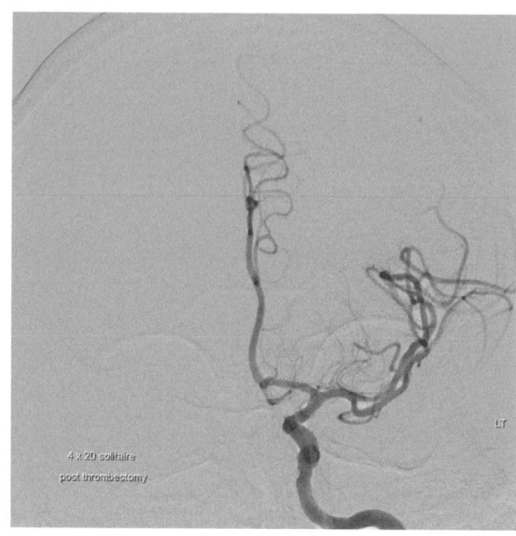

Fig. 10.12 Completing filling of MCA

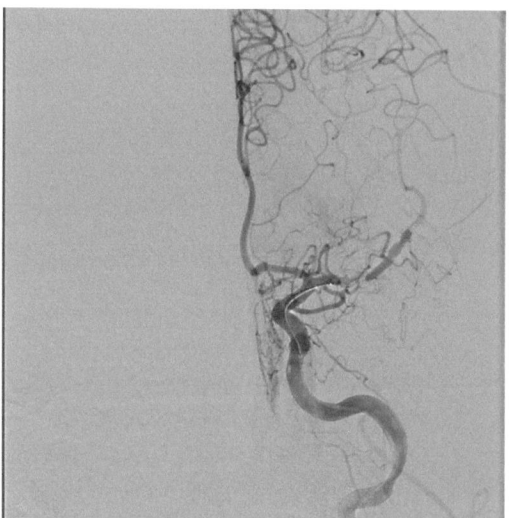

Fig. 10.11 Retrieval of plaque by neuroendovascular Solitaire™ device

saphenous vein graft. If there is extensive induration of tissues around the CEA site, a myocutaneous flap may be required in consultation with plastic surgery. Carotid pseudoaneurysm is an uncommon complication of CEA and can be treated with endovascular techniques if infected pseudoaneurysm is ruled out (covered stent). However, patient may require open repair with interposition vein graft if the aneurysm is accessible from the neck and general condition of the patient is satisfactory.

In the author's experience of over 3000 carotid endarterectomies, the incidence of new neurological deficit following CEA was 2.4%. One-third of these deficits were temporary and resolved within a few days to a few weeks. However, 1.7% of patients developed permanent neurological deficit.

Review Questions
1. Carotid endarterectomy in patient with >70% stenosis of ICA with mild to moderate stroke:
    A. Should have a waiting period of 6–8 weeks
    B. CEA within 2 weeks of stroke
    C. CEA is contraindicated in patient with recent stroke
    D. Carotid stenting is a better option in patients with recent mild to moderate stroke

Answer: B

2. The percentage of patients requiring shunt placement during CEA under cervical block anesthesia (awake) is:
    A. Less than 5%
    B. Approximately 10%
    C. Approximately 20%
    D. Approximately 30%

Answer: B

3. A patient undergoing CEA under cervical block anesthesia (CBA), as compared to general anesthesia (GA), has:
   A. A lower incidence of perioperative neurological complications
   B. A decreased incidence of neck hematoma
   C. Early discharge
   D. More stable hemodynamics during and immediately after CEA

   Answer: D

4. Patient undergoing CEA under GA with EEG monitoring awakening from anesthesia has significant contralateral neurological deficit. CTA of the head and neck shows normal CEA site but occlusion of the main trunk of the MCA. The next best management option is:
   A. Immediate carotid reexploration in the neck
   B. Neurovascular retrieval by interventional neurosurgeon or neurointerventionalist
   C. Intravenous heparin therapy
   D. Initiate TPA infusion into the ICA

   Answer: B

5. The most common nerve injured during CEA is the:
   A. Ramus mandibularis
   B. Hypoglossal nerve
   C. Glossopharyngeal nerve
   D. Vagus nerve

   Answer: B

6. Synthetic patch site infection following CEA is best treated with:
   A. Debridement, removal of patch, autogenous reconstruction, and antibiotics
   B. Interposition synthetic graft, debridement, and antibiotics
   C. Ligation of ICA and antibiotics
   D. Antibiotics alone

   Answer: A

7. A 72-year-old male undergoes carotid endarterectomy for >80% of right ICA with contralateral ICA occlusion. After 72 h, patient wakes up with headache and contralateral weakness. CT of head reveals a frontal lobe hemorrhage without midline shift. The next step in management of this patient is:
   A. Continue medical management
   B. Urgent neurosurgical consult for possible craniotomy
   C. Insert ventriculojugular shunt
   D. This complication could have been avoided if CAS was performed

   Answer: B

References

1. Barnett HJM, Taylor DW, Eliasziw M, et al. Benefits of carotid endarterectomy in patients with symptomatic moderate or severe stenosis. N Engl J Med. 1998;339:1415–25.
2. Rothwell PM, Eliasziw M, Gutnikov SA, Warlow CP, Barnett HJM. Endarterectomy for symptomatic carotid stenosis in related to clinical subgroup and timing of surgery. Lancet. 2004;363:915–24.
3. Rothwell PM, GIles MF, Flossmann E, Lorelock CE, Redgrave JN, Warlon CP, et al. A simple curve (ABCD) to identify individuals at high early risk of stroke after transient ischemic attack. Lancet. 2005;336:29–36.
4. Johnston SC, Sidney S. Validation of a 4-point predication rule to stratify short term stroke risk after TIA. Stroke. 2005;36:430.
5. Eliasziw M, Kennedy J, Hill MD, Buchan AM, Barnett HJM. Early risk of stroke after a transient ischemic attack in patients with internal carotid disease. CMAJ. 2004;170(7):1105–9.
6. Hill MD, Gladstone DJ. Patients with transient ischemic attack or minor stroke should be admitted to the hospital. Stroke. 2006;37:1137–8.
7. Caplan LR. Curr Atheroscler Rep. 2006;8:276–80.
8. Sheikh K, Bullock C. Variation and changes in state-specific carotid endarterectomy and 30-day mortality rates, Unitsed States, 1991-2000. J Vasc Surg. 2003;38(4):779–84.
9. Yadev JS, Wholey MH, Kuntz RE, Foyad P, et al. Protected carotid artery stenting versus endarterectomy in high risk patients. N Engl J Med. 2004;351:1493–501.

10. Silver FL, Mackey A, Clark WM, Brooks W, et al. Safety of stenting and endarterectomy by symptomatic status in the Carotid Revascularization Endarterectomy Versus Stenting Trial (CREST). Stroke. 2011;42:675–80.

11. Brott TG, Hobson RW, Howard G, Roubin GS, The Crest Investigators, et al. Stenting versus endarterectomy for treatment of carotid artery stenosis. N Engl J Med. 2006;355:1600–11.

12. General anesthesia versus local anesthesia for carotid surgery (GALA): a multicentre, randomized controlled trial. Lancet. 2008;372:2132–42.

13. Schneider JD, Droste JS, Schindler N, Golan JP, Bernstein LP, Rosenberg RS. Carotid endarterectomy with routine electroencephalography and selective shunting. J Vasc Surg. 2002;35:1114–22.

14. Calligaro KD, Dougherty MJ. Correlation of carotid artery stump pressure and neurological changes during 474 carotid endarterectomies performed in awake patients. J Vasc Surg. 2005;42:684–9.

15. Hans SS, Jareunpoon O. Prospective evaluation of electroencephalography, carotid artery stump pressure and neurological changes during 314 consecutive carotid endarterectomies performed in awake patients. J Vasc Surg. 2007;45:511–5.

16. Berguer R. Operations on internal carotid artery. In: Function and surgery of carotid and vertebral arteries. Philadelphia: Wolters Kluwer; 2014.

17. Baker WH, Littooy FN, Hayes AC, Dorner DB, Stubbs D. Carotid endarterectomy without a shunt: the control series. J Vasc Surg. 1984;1(1):50–6.

18. Goodney PP, Likosky DS, Cronenwett JL. Factors associated with stroke or death after carotid endarterectomy in Northern New England. J Vasc Surg. 2008;48:1139–45.

19. Norris JW, Zhu CZ, Bornstein NM, Chamber BR. Vascular risks of asymptomatic carotid stenosis. Stroke. 1991;22:1485–90.

Carotid Endarterectomy for High Plaque

11

Sachinder Singh Hans

During carotid endarterectomy (CEA), the distal end of the plaque may extend cephalad for a considerable distance and will need a distal exposure than is necessary during routine carotid endarterectomy (CEA). This difficulty in exposure may be complicated by a high carotid bifurcation in obese patients with a "short neck." With a high-quality CTA (axial, coronal, and sagittal cuts with reconstruction), the relationship of the upper end of plaque in relation to the body of the cervical vertebra can be determined.

For practical purposes, the extracranial portion of ICA can be divided into three segments (zones) in planning for CEA. The usual location of carotid bifurcation is at the level of C3–C4 vertebral body, and plaque extends to Zone 1 (upper end of C3) in the vast majority of patients. Zone 2 extends from upper end of C3 to upper end of C2, and typically a high plaque often extends to this level. Zone 3 is extremely uncommon for plaque to extend to a level higher than the C2 vertebral body (Fig. 11.1). In some patients, CTA imaging may fail to detect the distal feathery end of the plaque; high plaque may be

an unexpected finding as the plaque is dissected during CEA. In majority of patients with high plaque, general anesthesia is required as patient may become uncooperative due to distal dissection under cervical block anesthesia (CBA). In some patients with high plaque, carotid artery stenting (CAS) should be considered as an alternative to CEA.

In order to gain distal exposure, sternocleidomastoid branch of the occipital artery or the occipital artery itself is ligated and divided freeing up to the hypoglossal nerve which then can be retracted upward with a silastic vessel loop carefully. In many instances, venous tributaries are crossing this area and should be carefully ligated and divided (Fig. 11.2). Posterior belly of the digastric muscle is either retracted upward after careful mobilization or may have to be divided (Figs. 11.3 and 11.4). If the distal termination of the plaque does not terminate as a feathery distal end, we place 3.5 mm or 4.5 mm arterial dilator (Teleflex Medical, Morrisville, NC) into the ICA for dissecting the distal intimal end around the dilator. Another option would be to place a distal Pruitt® balloon occlusion catheter (LeMaitre Vascular, Burlington, MA) in the ICA at the base of the skull. Other options include:

1. Transposing the ICA in front of the XII nerve by dividing the ICA at its origin and transposing in front of the XII nerve. This technique is often necessary during eversion carotid endarterectomy when the plaque is high.

S. S. Hans
Medical Director of Vascular and Endovascular Services, Henry Ford Macomb Hospital, Clinton Township, MI, USA

Chief of Vascular Surgery, St. John Macomb Hospital, Warren, MI, USA

Department of Surgery, Wayne State University School of Medicine, Warren, MI, USA

© The Editor(s) (if applicable) and The Author(s) 2018
S. S. Hans (ed.), *Extracranial Carotid and Vertebral Artery Disease*,
https://doi.org/10.1007/978-3-319-91533-3_11

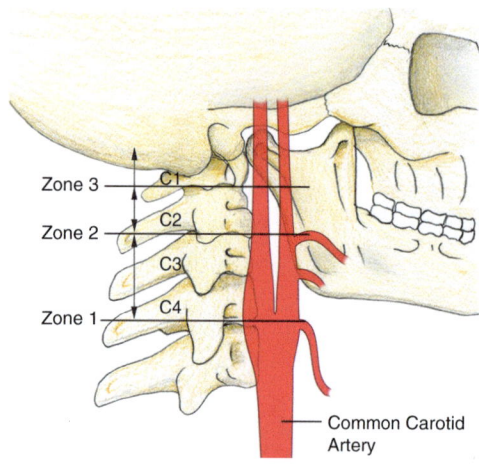

Fig. 11.1 Zones of neck in relation to the plaque. From: Hans SS, Shepard AD, Weaver MR, Bove P, Long GW. Endovascular and Open Vascular Reconstruction: A Practical Approach. Copyright © 2017, CRC Press, reproduced by permission of Taylor & Francis Books UK

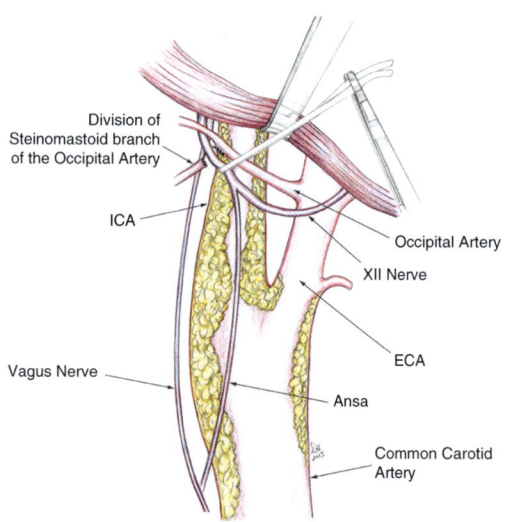

Fig. 11.2 Distal exposure of ICA by division of occipital artery and its branch. From: Hans SS, Shepard AD, Weaver MR, Bove P, Long GW. Endovascular and Open Vascular Reconstruction: A Practical Approach. Copyright © 2017, CRC Press, reproduced by permission of Taylor & Francis Books UK

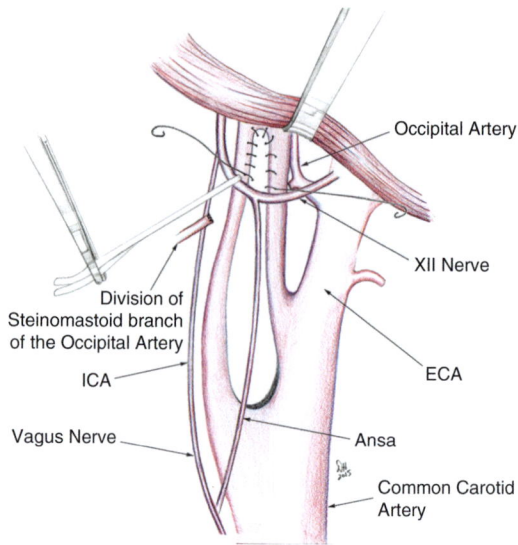

Fig. 11.3 Retraction or division of the posterior belly of digastric. From: Hans SS, Shepard AD, Weaver MR, Bove P, Long GW. Endovascular and Open Vascular Reconstruction: A Practical Approach. Copyright © 2017, CRC Press, reproduced by permission of Taylor & Francis Books UK

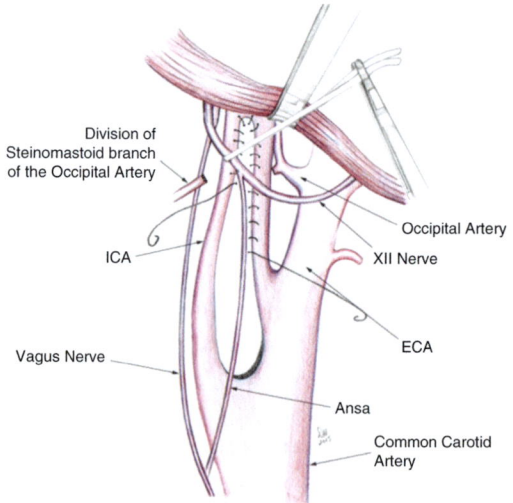

Fig. 11.4 Patch brought under the hypoglossal nerve after removal of the plaque. From: Hans SS, Shepard AD, Weaver MR, Bove P, Long GW. Endovascular and Open Vascular Reconstruction: A Practical Approach. Copyright © 2017, CRC Press, reproduced by permission of Taylor & Francis Books UK

Following endarterectomy, the ICA is then sutured at the origin of the ICA near the CCA bifurcation.

2. Retrojugular approach to ICA—the upper end of the incision is extended posteriorly behind the ear, and internal jugular vein is mobilized anteriorly. Spinal accessory nerve is identified and vagus nerve is mobilized anteriorly. Hypoglossal nerve is not seen as it is not in the

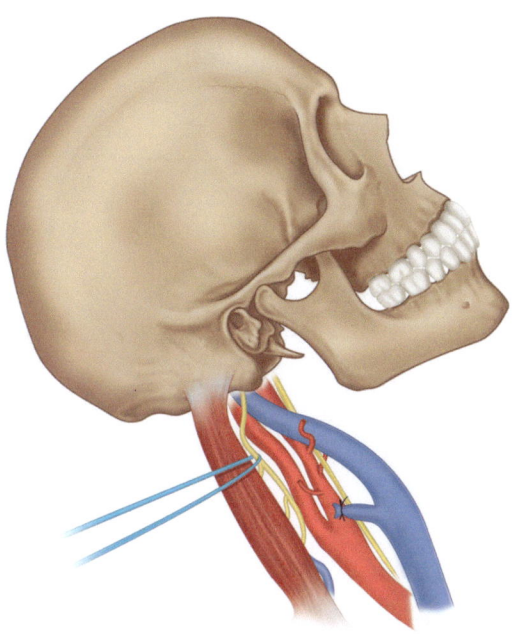

Fig. 11.5 Retrojugular approach for CEA

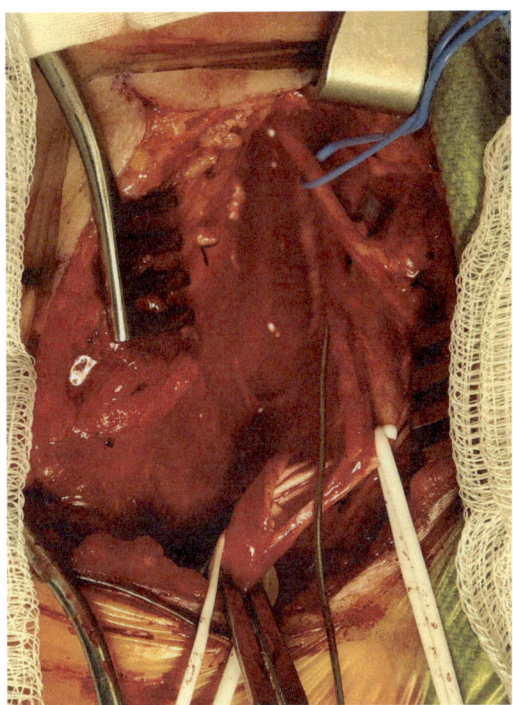

Fig. 11.6 Operative picture in a patient with CEA for high plaque with a blue loop around the hypoglossal nerve and arterial dilator in the distal ICA

operative field. Distal portion of extracranial ICA can now be exposed (Fig. 11.5).

3. For lesions extending to the junction of upper border of C2 and lower end of C1 (patients not candidates for carotid stenting due to heavy calcification), mandibular subluxation by an ENT surgeon/oral maxillofacial surgeon should be performed; in those cases nasotracheal intubation should be performed by anesthesiologist. The mandible is kept in place by a wire through the anterior nasal spine and through the mandible. In patients with high plaque extending at the level of the upper portion of the body of the C2 (following division of the posterior belly of the digastric muscle), one can palpate the tip of the styloid process which should be carefully removed by a rongeur as the glossopharyngeal nerve is in close approximation to the styloid process.

Intraoperative Carotid Stenting

If the operating surgeon is not certain about the end point of CEA, intraoperative carotid stenting (CAS) should be considered. Some plaques are soft and feathery at its distal end making the determination of their ending difficult on CTA neck images. Intraoperative CAS is performed by extending the lower end of the incision toward the base of the neck with division of the inferior belly of omohyoid using micropuncture technique. 7Fr sheath is inserted into CCA just above the base of the neck. A carotid/cerebral arteriogram is performed in the OR by injecting 8 cc of diluted contrast through the sheath using a 0.014 mm guidewire (CHOICE™ PT, Boston Scientific Corporation Marlborough, MA, USA) and advancing it under fluoroscopy into the intracranial portion of the ICA, and 6 mm × 4 cm self-expanding stent is deployed. Post-angioplasty is performed by an appropriately sized angioplasty catheter.

Distal exposure of ICA for removal of high plaque with arterial dilator in the ICA controlling retrograde bleeding and a blue loop around the hypoglossal nerve is shown in Fig. 11.6.

Complications

The majority of the complications of carotid end-arterectomy for high plaque are similar to those performed for carotid endarterectomy except there is higher incidence of cranial nerve palsy (hypoglossal, glossopharyngeal, and spinal accessory nerve), and these nerves should be carefully preserved. In my personal series of 120 carotid endarterectomies for high plaque, four patients developed postoperative stroke, one mild and three major strokes with an incidence of 3.3%. One patient developed glossopharyngeal nerve injury with PEG tube placement for 3 months, and two patients developed temporary hypoglossal nerve palsy.

Review Questions

1. During CEA for high plaque, the distal end of the intimal flap could be ascertained. You complete the CEA with patch grafting.
   A. No further study is indicated.
   B. Perform completion carotid arteriogram.
   C. Continuous wave Doppler analysis of the CEA site.
   D. Transcranial Doppler study.

   Answer: B

2. The most commonly injured nerve during distal exposure of ICA accompanied by division of the stylohyoid muscle and styloid process is?
   A. Hypoglossal nerve
   B. Spinal accessory nerve
   C. Vagus nerve
   D. Glossopharyngeal nerve

   Answer: D

3. Anesthesia of choice for a carotid endarterectomy for a high plaque is?
   A. General
   B. Cervical block anesthesia (superficial cervical block)
   C. Anesthesia using laryngeal mask airway (LMA)
   D. Cervical block anesthesia with deep cervical block

   Answer: A

4. A patient with focal neurological symptoms associated with a heavy calcified plaque resulting in >70% stenosis with plaque ending at the level of the second cervical vertebra should undergo?
   A. Carotid stenting (CAS)
   B. CEA with high distal exposure
   C. Carotid ligation
   D. Medical management

   Answer: B

5. The incidence of cranial nerve injury in patient undergoing CEA for high plaque is:
   A. Similar to conventional CEA.
   B. Higher than conventional CEA.
   C. The incidence of cranial nerve injury is so high that CEA should not be performed.
   D. Cranial nerve injury repair has excellent result.

   Answer: B

Suggested Reading

Berguer R. Operations on the internal carotid artery in function and surgery of the carotid and vertebral arteries. Dordecht: Wolters Kluwer; 2014. p. 90–119.

Dossa C, Shepard AD, Wolford DG, Reddy DJ, Ernest CB. Distal internal carotid exposure: a simplified technique for temporary mandibular subluxation. J Vasc Surg. 1990;12:319–25.

Hans SS, Shah S, Hans BA. Carotid endarterectomy for high plaques. Am J Surg. 1989;157(4):431–4.

Ross CB, Ranval TJ. Intraoperative use of stents for the management of unacceptable distal internal carotid artery end points during carotid endarterectomy: short-term and midterm results. J Vasc Surg. 2000;32(3):420–7. 427–8.

Eversion Carotid Endarterectomy: Indications, Techniques, Pitfalls, and Complications

12

Judith C. Lin

Indications

Since its introduction nearly 75 years ago, there have been few modifications to the technical approach of standard carotid endarterectomy (CEA). Indications for carotid stenosis to reduce the risk of stroke and other neurologic complications in selected patients have been published in large randomized studies [1, 2]. In 2008, the Society for Vascular Surgery (SVS) summarized evidence-based clinical practice recommendations for the management of carotid stenosis [3]. Carotid duplex ultrasonography is currently the preferred imaging modality for the diagnosis of carotid artery stenosis due to its safety, availability, and reliable results. However, duplex ultrasound is highly operator-dependent. Thus, computed tomography angiography (CTA), magnetic resonance angiography (MRA), and conventional angiography can be used to detect plaque morphology, identify technically difficult lesions, and plan for standard CEA, eversion CEA, or carotid stenting.

Conventional CEA with patch angioplasty has been the most widely practiced technique and the standard to which the approach of eversion CEA (ECEA) is compared. Any closure of standard CEA is associated with appreciable rates of persistent or recurrent stenosis [4]. Management of the end point may be tedious, and closure of the arteriotomy may be problematic. Eversion endarterectomy with reimplantation is preferred if the internal carotid artery is elongated, is less than 4 mm wide, and occurs in women [5]. As medical management of atherosclerotic risk factors and perioperative care improves, the outcome differences attributed to these small but significant technical details embody the "holy grail" of carotid atherosclerosis surgery. The contemporary method of ECEA is an alternative technique to facilitate the removal of plaque isolated to the carotid bulb and proximal internal carotid artery (ICA). Advantages of eversion versus standard endarterectomy include the ability to shorten a redundant ICA, better visualized end point and easier detection of intimal flaps, faster closure by simple anastomosis of the ICA to the carotid bulb, an all-autogenous reconstruction, and decreased restenosis rates in women.

Techniques

Anesthetic choice, cerebral monitoring, and neuroprotection are identical for both methods of CEA. During the case, neurologic monitoring is routine. The use of shunting and/or monitoring of cerebral functions is determined by the attending surgeon and anesthesiologist.

J. C. Lin
Department of Surgery, Division of Vascular Surgery, Henry Ford Hospital, Detroit, MI, USA
e-mail: jlin1@hfhs.org

© The Editor(s) (if applicable) and The Author(s) 2018
S. S. Hans (ed.), *Extracranial Carotid and Vertebral Artery Disease*,
https://doi.org/10.1007/978-3-319-91533-3_12

Electroencephalographic (EEG) monitoring is used for patients under general anesthesia, while continuous neurological assessment is used for patients undergoing CEA under cervical block anesthesia. Most patients undergoing CEA do not require intraoperative shunt placement. If shunting is needed during ECEA, insertion of the shunt is performed after everting and removing the bulk of the ICA plaque. We prefer to use the short Sundt (internal shunt) with non-reinforced segment, 3 mm × 4 mm (Integra NeuroSciences™, Plainsboro, NJ). Shunt insertion is performed distally into the ICA and held in place with a shunt clamp. An extension of the common carotid arteriotomy may be needed to expose the open lumen prior to shunt insertion into the common carotid artery (CCA). Eversion endarterectomy is the preferred procedure for ICA carotid kinks or loops. After transection, redundant ICA may be resected and anastomosis completed to a more distal portion of the ICA. Initial neck dissection and isolation of the carotid artery are similar to the conventional CEA technique. Dissection and mobilization of the carotid bulb and proximal ICA are more extensive with ECEA than standard CEA. The need for more extensive dissection for ECEA has not caused an increase in vagus nerve injury. Some surgeons mark the level of the carotid bulb with ultrasound prior to skin incision to minimize the length of the incision.

The patient is placed supine on the operating table with a shoulder roll and the head rotated to the opposite side. The neck is prepped and draped to expose the mastoid process, angle of the mandible, sternal notch, and cervical incision. An incision is made along the anterior border of the sternocleidomastoid muscle (SCM) over the carotid bifurcation. We prefer a longitudinal incision over a transverse incision due to better exposure of the distal ICA. After the platysma muscle is divided, dissection is made along the anterior border of the SCM to identify the confluence of the internal jugular and facial veins. The facial vein is suture ligated and divided to expose the underlying carotid artery medially. The carotid artery is exposed circumferentially to isolate the ICA and the carotid bulb. Within the carotid sheath, the vagus nerve lies posteriorly between the CCA medially and internal jugular vein laterally. If sinus bradycardia occurs, 1–2 ml of 1% lidocaine without preservatives may be administered topically between the ICA and ECA to block nerve conduction to the carotid sinus.

After dissection of the common carotid artery (CCA), ICA, and external carotid artery (ECA), intravenous heparin is administered to achieve an activated clotting time (ACT) >250 s. The ICA is clamped first, followed by the CCA, and finally the ECA. At this time, the ICA is transected obliquely by dividing the crotch of the carotid bulb from carotid bifurcation to a point more proximal on the lateral side of the CCA (Fig. 12.1a). Generally, an opening of 10–15 mm can be obtained without extending the arteriotomy at either end as long as the transection line is beveled enough (Fig. 12.2). Otherwise, the arteriotomy on the lateral wall of the CCA may be extended caudally, and the arteriotomy medial wall of the ICA extended cephalad to a similar length to facilitate later anastomosis of the arteries (Fig. 12.1b). An extended arteriotomy on the CCA also allows for removal of a more proximal plaque in the CCA.

Eversion CEA is performed by circumferentially elevating the plaque with a Penfield plaque elevator from the arterial wall to remove both the intima and media; the adventitia is grasped with two fine forceps, while the assistant holds the plaque (Fig. 12.1c). The adventitia with its outer layer of media is everted, and the atheromatous core is held away in tension until the end of the plaque is reached in the distal ICA. After removal of the plaque, the surgeon may inspect the entire circumference of the end point, remove loose fragments, and make sure the distal intima is adherent with no loose pieces. If a loose flap is found, it may be peeled off or alternatively "tacked" down using 7-0 double-armed polypropylene sutures from the luminal aide and tied externally (Fig. 12.1d).

After the end point is secured, the ICA is unrolled and the luminal surface inspected for loose debris with irrigation of heparinized saline (Fig. 12.3). Any loose fragment should be removed and the entire circumference of the end point inspected. Any persistent plaque or flap is

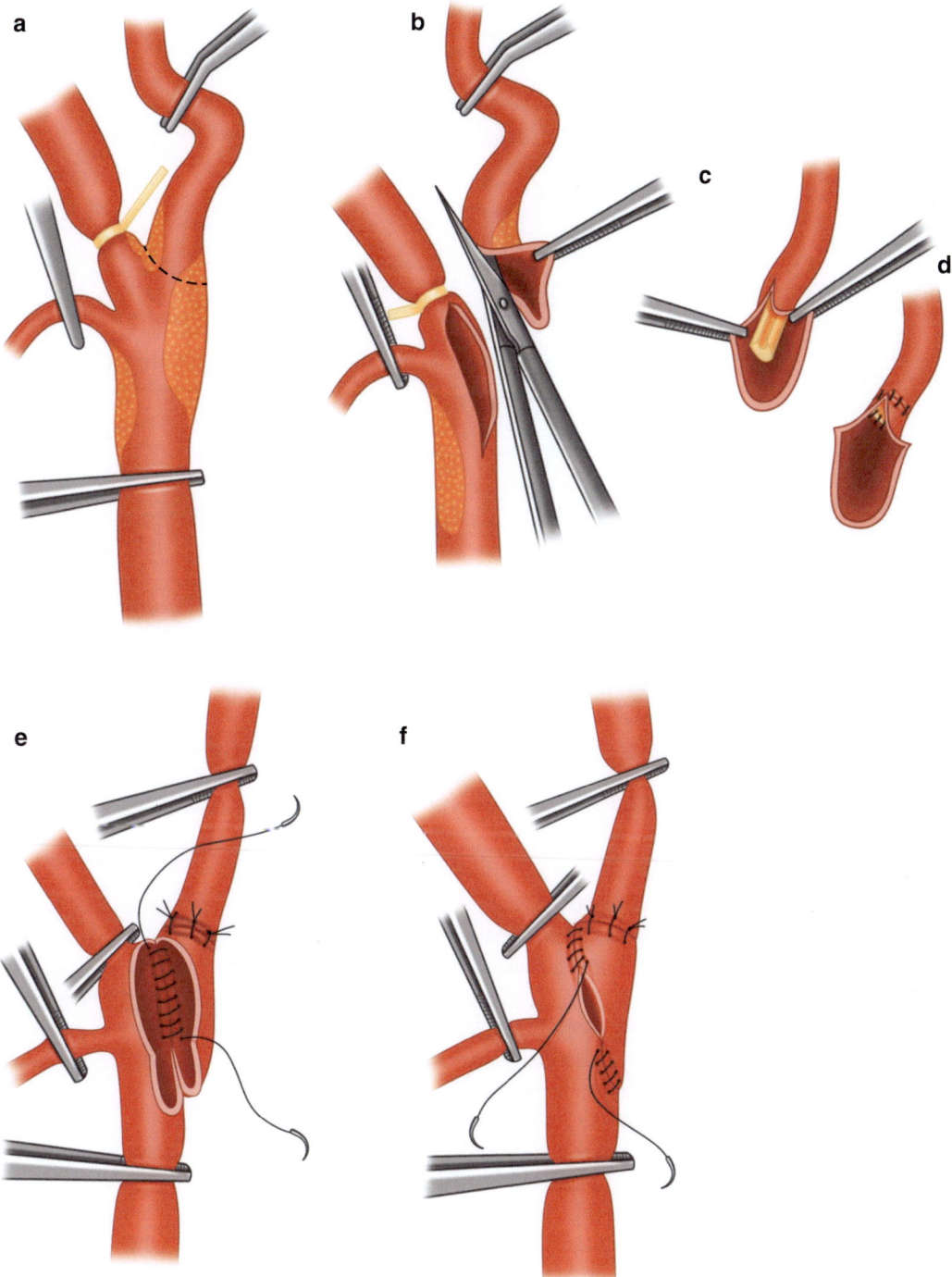

Fig. 12.1 (**a–d**) Schematics of eversion carotid endarterectomy. (**e**, **f**) Schematics of anastomosis

identified and corrected prior to re-anastomosis. To shorten an elongated or kinked ICA at the carotid bifurcation, spatulated ICA is then pulled down to straighten the carotid kink. Once the endarterectomy of the ICA is completed, the distal CCA and the ECA are inspected for plaque removal. The plaque is elevated in the bulb and carried up the ECA and proximally into the

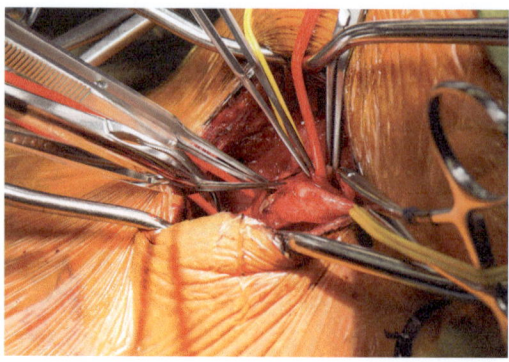

Fig. 12.2 Oblique transection of internal carotid artery from the carotid bifurcation

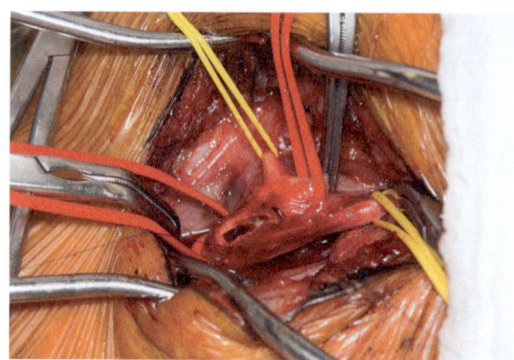

Fig. 12.4 Running suture completed posteriorly and then anteriorly

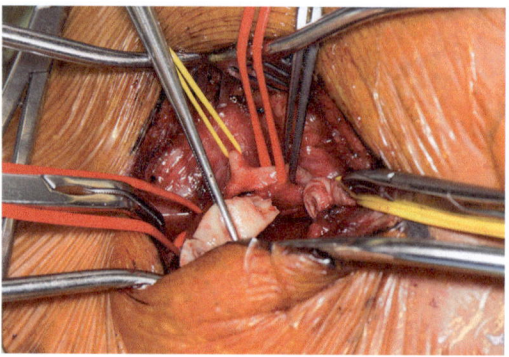

Fig. 12.3 Plaque elevation and removal after eversion carotid endarterectomy

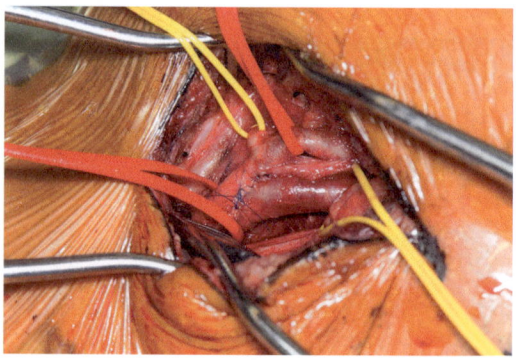

Fig. 12.5 Completion of the anastomosis

CCA. Endarterectomy of the ECA and CCA may be performed with direct elevation of the exposed plaque and proximal eversion of a more extensive plaque.

The arteriotomy is irrigated with heparinized saline to remove loose fragments and with low molecular weight dextran to inhibit platelet adhesion. Primary anastomosis between the ICA and CCA is performed using continuous 6-0 monofilament suture, starting at the most cephalad portion of the internal carotid arteriotomy (Fig. 12.1e). The back wall of the anastomosis is usually sewn from the inside of the artery which provides the best visualization (Fig. 12.1f). The running suture is completed posteriorly then brought anteriorly where it is tied to the other end (Fig. 12.4). After completion of the anastomosis, blood flow is restored in the usual sequence—temporarily opening the ICA first to allow backfilling of the

bulb, then unclamping the ECA to allow back filling, then opening the CCA to allow forward blood flow into the ECA, and finally opening the ICA (Fig. 12.5). Hemostasis is obtained. The effect of intravenous heparin is reversed by protamine sulfate to reduce the risk of postoperative hematoma.

Pitfalls

Care must be taken to avoid beginning different planes of dissection for plaque removal. The distal end point of the plaque in the ICA is visualized and disengaged from the underlying media. Demonstration of the plaque shows a feathered end superficial to the internal elastic lamina. This natural transition and termination for plaque allows for a taper end of the carotid occlusive disease. If the transition endpoint of the ICA is unobtainable or the plaque extended distally, ICA replacement by a graft may be necessary with an interposition saphenous or PTFE graft. During the eversion endarterectomy, an internal carotid shunt placement is limited, and a CCA to ECA shunt may be used for cerebral protection.

Postoperative care is routine with blood pressure control and assessment of neurologic deficits. Postoperative complications of ECEA are similar as standard CEA: stroke, transient ischemic attack (TIA), cranial nerve injury, hematoma in the neck, and cardiac morbidity. Cranial nerve injury includes the hypoglossal, vagus, pharyngeal and laryngeal branches of vagus, and the glossopharyngeal nerves.

Complications

Results of the EVEREST (EVERsion carotid Endarterectomy versus Standard Trial) validated the short- and long-term safety and efficacy of ECEA for ICA. This prospective, multicenter, randomized trial compared rates of carotid occlusion, restenosis rate, major stroke, and death among standard CEA (n = 675) and ECEA (n = 678) patients. Long-term results showed a significantly lower restenosis rate in the eversion group (2.7% vs. 5.6%, p = 0.01) at a mean follow-up of 33 months. Eversion CEA was found to be an independent predictor of carotid patency, in that the eversion population of patients was three times less likely to have restenosis than were patients who had standard CEA with either patch or primary closure [6].

Several single-institution studies have provided a consensus that there is no significant difference between eversion and standard techniques in early (<30 days) postoperative complications [7]. Among its advantages, the ECEA is associated with decreased operative times and shorter cross-clamp times due to a single anastomosis. Schneider et al. compared results of 2635 ECEA and 17,155 standard CEA. Early perioperative morbidity including ipsilateral stroke and TIA were equivalent, although eversion CEA showed significantly less operative time (median 99 vs.

114 min, p < 0.001) but a higher incidence of return to the operative suite for bleeding (1.4% vs. 8%, p = 0.002) [8].

The decline in perioperative morbidity and mortality over the past decade can be explained by improved surgical techniques, preoperative evaluation, and treatment with statin therapy. Better surgical skills and optimal medical therapy also have resulted in lower rate of ICA restenosis, ICA occlusion, and cranial nerve injury. In a study of 9897 patients who underwent ECEA, early postoperative complications included surgical bleeding (1.7%), contralateral neurological deficit (0.92%), cranial nerve injury (0.8%), reperfusion injury (0.48%), and ICA thrombosis (0.38%); the overall mortality is 1.32% and stroke-related mortality 0.52%. Due to the shorter clamping time (11.9 ± 3.2 min), shunting has become almost unnecessary during ECEA and dropped to 0.5% of their patients in recent years [9].

Antonopoulos et al. pooled randomized and nonrandomized studies in a meta-analysis that favored ECEA in both short- and long-term outcomes among 16,251 CEA procedures. Eversion CEA was associated with significant reduction in perioperative stroke [odds ratio (OR) = 0.46; 95% confidence interval (CI), 0.35 0.62; numbers needed to treat (NNT) = 68; 95% CI, 56–96], death (OR = 0.49; 95%CI, 0.34–0.69; NNT = 100; 95% CI, 85–185), and stroke-related death (OR = 0.40; 95% CI, 0.23–0.67; NNT = 147; 95% CI, 115–270); the results were replicated at the sub-analysis on patch CEA. With regard to long-term outcomes, ECEA was associated with a significant reduction in late carotid artery occlusion (OR = 0.48; 95% CI, 0.25–0.90; NNT = 143; 95% CI, 100–769) and late mortality (OR = 0.76; 95% CI, 0.61–0.94; NNT = 40; 95% CI, 25–167); sub-analysis of patched CEA replicated only the finding on late mortality [10].

In the longest follow-up published to date, Black et al. reported a restenosis rate of 4.1% (n = 20/534) within a mean follow-up period of 8.86 years (95% CI: 6.56–9.16). The mean time to recurrence was 4.4 years, following no predilection for anatomic distribution; suggesting these occurrences represent systemic atherosclerotic disease rather than neo-intimal hyperplasia of the single eversion CEA suture line [11]. Current Level I evidence studies and meta-analyses comparing eversion and standard CEA have validated excellent results of both techniques. Although the eversion method has not shown superior results conclusively, eversion CEA does allow for another reliable technique that should be in every vascular surgeon's armamentarium for the treatment of high-grade, carotid occlusive disease.

Review Questions

1. Which of the following is demonstrated from the eversion carotid endarterectomy versus standard trial (EVEREST)?
   A. Eversion CEA and patch angioplasty had significantly lower restenosis rates when compared with primary closure CEA.
   B. Eversion CEA had no difference in restenosis rates when compared with primary closure CEA.
   C. Eversion CEA had significantly higher restenosis rates when compared with patch angioplasty closure after conventional CEA.
   D. Eversion CEA had significantly lower restenosis rates when compared with primary closure after CEA and patch angioplasty after conventional CEA.

   Answer: A

2. A Cochrane review of the literature that included close to 2500 patients from 5 controlled clinical trials found that:
   A. There is higher rate of perioperative stroke and perioperative mortality of eversion CEA when compared with patch angioplasty CEA.
   B. There is no significant difference between eversion CEA and patch angioplasty CEA with respect to the rate of perioperative stroke and perioperative mortality.
   C. There is lower rate of perioperative stroke and perioperative mortality of eversion CEA when compared with patch angioplasty CEA.
   D. None of the above.

   Answer: B

3. The choice of surgical technique for the treatment of carotid artery stenosis should depend on following criteria:
   A. Clinical judgment
   B. Prior experience
   C. Preference of the surgeon
   D. All of the above

   Answer: D

References

1. North American Symptomatic Endarterectomy Trial Collaborators. Beneficial effect of carotid endarterectomy in symptomatic patients with high-grade carotid stenosis. N Engl J Med. 1991;325:445–53.
2. Executive Committee for the Asymptomatic Carotid Atherosclerosis Study. Endarterectomy for asymptomatic carotid artery stenosis. JAMA. 1995;273:1421–8.
3. Hobson RW 2nd, Mackey WC, Ascher E, Murad MH, Calligaro KD, Comerota AJ. Management of atherosclerotic carotid artery disease: clinical practice guidelines of the Society for Vascular Surgery. J Vasc Surg. 2008;48(2):480–6.
4. Cao PG, De Rango P, Zannetti S, Giordano G, Ricci S, Celani MG. Eversion versus conventional carotid endarterectomy for preventing stroke (review). Cochrane Libr. 2008;3:1–36.
5. Kieny R, Hirsch D, Seiller C, Thiranos JC, Petit H. Does carotid eversion endarterectomy and reimplantation reduce the risk of restenosis? Ann Vasc Surg. 1993;7:407–13.
6. Cao P, Giordano G, De Rango P, Zannetti S, Chiesa R, Coppi G, et al. Eversion versus conventional

carotid endarterectomy: late results of a prospective multicenter randomized trial. J Vasc Surg. 2000; 31:19–30.

7. Ben Ahmed S, Daniel G, Benezit M, Ribal JP, Rosset E. Eversion carotid endarterectomy without shunt: concerning 1,385 consecutive cases. J Cardiovasc Surg. 2017;58(4):543–50.

8. Schneider JR, Helenowski IB, Jackson CR, Verta MJ, Zamor KC, Ptel NH, Kim S, Hoel AW. A comparison of results with eversion versus conventional carotid endarterectomy from the Vascular Quality Initiative and the Mid-American Vascular Study Group. J Vasc Surg. 2015;61:1216–22.

9. Radak D, Tanaskovic S, Matic P, Babic S, Aleksic N, Ilijevski N. Eversion carotid endarterectomy—our experience after 20 years of carotid surgery and 9897 carotid endarterectomy procedures. Ann Vasc Surg. 2012;26:924–8.

10. Antonopoulos CN, Kakisis JD, Sergentanis TN, Liapis CD. Eversion versus conventional carotid endarterectomy: a meta-analysis of randomised and non-randomised studies. Eur J Vasc Endovasc Surg. 2011;42(6):751–65.

11. Black JH 3rd, Ricotta JJ, Jones CE. Long-term results of eversion carotid endarterectomy. Ann Vasc Surg. 2010;24(1):92–9.

Natural History and Contemporary Management of Recurrent Carotid Stenosis

13

Jeffrey R. Rubin and Yevgeniy Rits

Introduction

Duplex ultrasound surveillance of patients following carotid artery intervention has increased the identification of recurrent disease in this patient population. Carotid artery restenosis (RCAD) following both carotid endarterectomy (CEA) and stenting averages 4–10% nationally (ranging from 1% to 20%) [1–3]. Recommended treatment of primary carotid stenosis carries very strong evidence based upon multiple randomized trials; however, evidence for treatment of recurrent disease is mostly based upon retrospective reviews, and it is unclear if it has the same risk of stroke as primary lesion treatment. The approach to recurrent carotid disease has to be individualized. Restenosis poses a clinical dilemma for many physicians since they face several options: (1) redo endarterectomy, (2) carotid artery angioplasty with and without stenting, or (3) carotid bypass. There is currently no consensus as to which treatment method provides the safest and best long-term outcomes for treating recurrent carotid artery disease [4–6]. This chapter summarizes the pathophysiology and therapy for redo CEA (RCEA) for restenosis.

J. R. Rubin (✉) · Y. Rits
Vascular Surgery, Detroit Medical Center,
Detroit, MI, USA
e-mail: jrubin@dmc.org

Pathogenesis

Recurrent carotid disease after endarterectomy can be separated into three different categories: residual disease and/or technical problem, early recurrent stenosis, and late recurrent stenosis.

Very early on, recurrent carotid stenosis is usually due to technical problems with the initial repair. There may be residual disease in up to 1/3 of the cases, and this is due to the inadequacy of the endarterectomy. Failure to adequately remove the proximal common carotid artery plaque is not uncommon, especially when surgeons do not carefully examine the duplex scan, thus missing a potentially large proximal segment of disease. Also not identifying and treating distal internal carotid artery kinks or coils with significant stenoses, will result in postoperative velocity elevations and, therefore, residual disease. This can be avoided with preoperative planning, meticulous surgical technique, and intraoperative imaging. The authors routinely use intraoperative post-endarterectomy completion angiography to identify any potential repair defects that need to be dealt with prior to wound closure.

There is consensus that the routine use of patch angioplasty rather than primary closure results in decreased risk of ipsilateral stroke during the perioperative period and in long-term follow-up. A decreased restenosis rate has also been noted in follow-up for patients who have had patch angioplasty arterial closure. There is no absolute consensus on which patch material, vein, bovine pericardium, PTFE, or Dacron, has better results [7, 8].

Recurrent carotid stenosis following angioplasty and stenting may be found in the stented area of the artery, proximal to the stent, distal to the stent, or in a combination of both. The frequency of severe post-stent recurrence varies significantly, ranging from 2% to 14% [9] in the CAVATAS study [10].

It is generally thought that in-stent restenosis (ISR) is likely due to vessel wall (intimal and medial) injury. This is followed by an inflammatory response and then a proliferative cellular response. Intraluminal remodeling then occurs which may result in a hyperplastic restenosis. This has nothing to do with progressive atheromatous changes which are a separate process, not related to the angioplasty and/or stenting.

In-stent restenosis has been identified more commonly in patients of advanced age and females and in cases requiring multiple stents or if stent sizing and/or deployment techniques are not done appropriately. Oversizing the balloons and/or stents has been experimentally related to arterial injury [11].

Restenosis that develops within the first 24 months of endarterectomy is most likely due to the myointimal hyperplasia (MIH). This is a concentric smooth/fibrotic thickening which is firmly adherent to the arterial surface. MIH is usually apparent by 6 months after CEA [12]. It is generally a smooth fibrous lesion with low embolic potential, and it may be easily identified on duplex ultrasound. It is usually located at the site of the previous endarterectomy and is characterized by a smooth muscle cell proliferation throughout this area.

Hyperplastic restenosis may also occur at areas of the artery where clamps were applied. This is referred to as "clamp trauma" or "clamp fibrosis" [13]. Iatrogenic clamp injury is also noted to be an accelerator of the atherosclerotic cascade, proximal and/or distal to the endarterectomy site. Early recurrence is more common in women, and no clear explanation has been ascertained, although smaller artery size has been implicated. The incidence of early recurrence

may be decreased by using patch angioplasty rather than primary repair.

After 24 months, late RCS is usually due to recurrent, progressive, or *de novo* atherosclerosis, and it may be asymptomatic or symptomatic, smooth, heterogenous, complex, irregular, and/or ulcerated. Risk factors such as hypertension, continued smoking, hypercholesterolemia, and diabetes have all been implicated.

Plaque has been noted to occur in no specific area of the carotid artery [5]. We have found recurrent lesions in the proximal common carotids, in the area of the endarterectomy, and distal to the endarterectomy site. Most late recurring plaques are atherosclerotic in their composition, as opposed to hyperplastic.

When patients are referred for RCS requiring intervention, it is the responsibility of the surgeon to determine the best treatment modality. Factors that enter into the equation include plaque morphology, anticipated neck "hostility," location of the recurrent lesion, and the patient's overall health and anticipated life expectancy. Finally, the open and endovascular operative skill sets of the treating surgeon need to be weighed when determining the best approach. The decision to intervene and the type of intervention should be balanced among the risk of intervention, operator's personal experience, and the risk of stroke with medical therapy alone.

The authors do not have adequate information from their own experience to determine whether stenting is appropriate for the treatment of RCS. However, the good long-term results achieved by open intervention for RCEA has led them to recommend this treatment for the vast majority of their patients [6].

Indications

Indications for RCEA are identical to those for the initial CEA and include asymptomatic severe carotid artery stenosis (>60%), asymptomatic or symptomatic stenosis with large or multiple plaque ulcerations, a soft lipid core or intraplaque hemorrhage, symptomatic carotid stenosis <60%, crescendo transient ischemic attacks (TIAs) or stroke in evolution with high-grade carotid stenosis, and/or >50% ipsilateral carotid artery stenosis associated with a contralateral occlusion.

Contraindications

Contraindications to RCEA include patients with significantly reduced life expectancy and when the risk of RCEA outweighs the anticipated benefits of intervention.

Preoperative Evaluation

With a few exceptions, patient preoperative evaluation should not differ from that performed on the patients being considered for primary CEA. Surgical risk evaluation and cardiac assessment should be performed with special emphasis on blood pressure management.

If possible, the operative report from the original operation should be obtained since it may provide helpful information about the preceding endarterectomy(ies). This would include intraoperative difficulties and complications, and whether the artery was patched or closed primarily.

Carotid Duplex scanning by an Intersocietal Accreditation Commission-accredited Vascular Laboratory (ICAVL) is the authors' diagnostic modality of choice and is the only noninvasive test performed in most patients. The technician must pay particular attention to the level of the bifurcation, plaque morphology, and the presence of disease in the proximal common carotid artery (CCA). The presence or absence of internal carotid artery coils and/or kinks should be noted.

If duplex ultrasonography does not provide adequate information for operative planning, CT angiography is frequently useful. Rarely is carotid angiography required.

Routine cardiac and pulmonary evaluation are recommended. If a patient has a history of head and neck cancer, discussion with the medical and surgical oncologists is essential for operative planning.

Indirect laryngoscopy should routinely be performed preoperatively to evaluate cord function.

This is especially important in patients who have had previous cranial nerve injury, preoperative neck radiation, previous neck surgery exclusive of CEA, and with known head and neck cancer. Patients with a history of TIAs and/or stroke should undergo head CT scanning or magnetic resonance imaging to ascertain whether there is a pre-existing infarction, since this may affect the need for intraoperative shunting.

Patients should be well hydrated preoperatively. A minimal hemoglobin in the 8.0–8.5 g/dL range is desirable. Of critical importance is the patient's blood pressure, which should be stabilized preoperatively and should be maintained at the patient's presenting pressure or slightly higher. If the patient is significantly hypertensive before the operation and emergent surgery is not required, the authors prefer outpatient blood pressure stabilization before intervention. It is not appropriate to aggressively reduce blood pressure immediately before the operation, intraoperatively, or postoperatively. Blood pressure control, however, is of paramount importance during the operation, and wide fluctuations are to be avoided. The anesthesia team should have vasopressors and antihypertensive agents ready to be infused if necessary.

They should also have atropine available in case carotid bulb handling results in bradycardia and subsequent hypotension. The authors prefer to inject the carotid sinus (nerve of Herring) at the carotid bulb with lidocaine 1% if problems arise during dissection in this area. If bradycardia continues, intravenous atropine should be used. The type of anesthesia used for RCEA depends upon the comfort level of the patient, surgeon, and anesthesiologist; however, because RCEA takes longer than a *de novo* CEA, general anesthesia is generally preferred. For the same reason, a Foley catheter is inserted at the beginning of all cases.

Consultation with appropriate oral maxillofacial surgery service preoperatively is essential when mandibular subluxation is anticipated. Nasotracheal intubation should also be performed in these cases. We also recommended evaluation of the saphenous venous system in case an interpositional vein bypass graft is needed.

Procedure

Following intubation, the patient is positioned with a scapular roll and extension and rotation of the head to the contralateral side. Excessive head extension and rotation should be avoided to prevent possible kinking of the vertebral arteries and muscle strain. The bed is generally placed in a relaxed, semi-Fowler's position with slight head elevation. The authors recommend prepping one of the thighs for saphenous vein or superficial femoral artery (SFA) harvesting in cases where interposition grafting is anticipated.

The authors prefer an oblique incision, anterior to the sternocleidomastoid muscle. Preexisting transverse incisions are modified to gain more distal exposure; otherwise, the previous neck incision is reopened in its entirety. Dissection is deliberate if not tedious. Knowledge of normal anatomy and common variants is essential. Exposure of the internal (ICA), external (ECA), and common carotid (CCA) arteries is usually begun either as far distal or as far proximal as possible, attempting to find an artery that has not been previously dissected. The author avoids dissection around the area of recurrent disease (usually the carotid bulb) and obtains proximal and distal control first. Excessive "Weitlaner" retraction can cause a traction injury to the vagus nerve and should be avoided. Dissection should be carried out directly on the anterior surfaces of the arteries to avoid nerve injury. The vagus nerve and jugular vein are carefully dissected free from the carotid artery to avoid clamp and retractor injury. Distal dissection of the ICA needs to proceed cautiously. The hypoglossal nerve is frequently indistinguishable from surrounding scar tissue crossing the ICA. Dissection in unusual planes and increased retraction for "better exposure" may result in nerve trauma. Vagal, marginal mandibular, superior laryngeal, glossopharyngeal, recurrent laryngeal, hypoglossal, and other nerve injuries are more common following RCEA than primary CEA and are to be avoided [5].

Distal control of the ICA should be obtained above the previous endarterectomy site. It is not unusual to need to divide the digastric muscle, which is best accomplished with a right angle clamp and electrocautery. Dissection along the lateral aspect of the hypoglossal nerve may provide additional mobility and allow for gentle vessel loop retraction of the nerve. Strong retraction on the mandible is occasionally necessary and can result in a marginal mandibular nerve injury. Fortunately, this usually resolves within 6 months, but it is definitely bothersome during recovery and quite often may be confused with an ischemic cerebral injury by ancillary staff. Removing the styloid process with a rongeur helps gain additional exposure of the distal ICA. If preoperative assessment suggests that distal exposure will be problematic, nasotracheal intubation should be used initially. Consultation with otolaryngology or oral and maxillofacial surgery preoperatively, for mandibular subluxation, should have already occurred, and those specialists should be available.

Systemic heparinization takes place after all the arteries are controlled and dissection is completed. The authors give a bolus of unfractionated heparin sulfate at 100 IU/kg and redoses every 2 h. The authors routinely check the activated clotting time after heparinization and then every hour thereafter. In cases of known heparin sensitivity, the authors' drug of choice is Argatroban. The authors also administer low-molecular-weight dextran 40 via a slow 50-cc intravenous bolus and then continue a maintenance drip at 10 cc/h overnight or until the patient can receive oral medications.

After clamping the ICA, CCA, and ECA, the artery is opened to a point above and below the recurrent disease. Shunting is at the surgeon's discretion. Performing an endarterectomy with patients awake is the most sensitive way for determining ischemia while clamped. The authors selectively shunt patients with (1) previous ipsilateral stroke, (2) contralateral carotid artery occlusion, (3) carotid stump pressures <50 mmHg, and (4) crescendo TIAs and/or a stroke in evolution. Other methods for determining whether a shunt is required include electroencephalography monitoring, somatosensory evoked potentials, transcranial Doppler monitoring. The criteria for determining whether or not a shunt should be used is not without controversy and should follow the surgeon's preference based upon his or her results. If regional anesthesia is used, communication with the patient during clamping determines the adequacy of cerebral perfusion. The authors use Sundt™ shunts (Integra® LifeSciences, Plainsboro, NJ, USA) and prefer clamps to hold them in place proximally and distally; Rummel tourniquets may also be used. The shunt is inserted distally first, de-aired, and then placed proximally and secured. The surgeon needs to be aware of possible proximal CCA disease when inserting the shunt proximally inorder to avoid embolization.

Recurrent CAD may be hyperplastic, atherosclerotic, or most frequently a combination of the two. The authors generally prefer "re-endarterectomy" and patching if technically possible. Occasionally, we will encounter a purely hyperplastic lesion that may be amenable to patch angioplasty alone. Otherwise, we attempt to remove the entire recurrent lesion, which is frequently quite tedious and without an easy end point, in contrast to primary CEA. Deep endarterectomy through both layers of media, however, is to be avoided because the authors feel this creates a very thrombogenic flow surface and weakens the arterial wall, making it susceptible to aneurysm formation. We recommend excision of the entire old patch including all suture material.

We do not routinely tack distal end points and we prefer "chasing" the plaque distally. The use of a Beaver® blade (Beaver-Visitec International, Inc., Waltham, MA, USA) is at times very helpful to establish a good distal end point. However, if there is any concern, the author recommends a running tacking suture between the intima and the endarterectomized arterial wall. Either a CV-8 Gore-Tex® (W.L. Gore & Associates, Inc., Flagstaff, AZ, USA) or an 8-0 polypropylene is the authors' suture of choice. A running suture eliminates scalloping of the transition area. Finally, when faced with loss of integrity of the arterial wall, or if the plaque appears to continue distally beyond an acceptable level, we do not hesitate to perform interposition bypass grafting and prefer autogenous grafts (with the saphenous vein or SFA) to prosthetic grafts. When SFA harvest is performed, it must be replaced with a polytetrafluoroethylene (PTFE) graft to avoid leg

ischemia. If the SFA is occluded, no bypass is required. Eversion endarterectomy of the occluded SFA segment is performed before sewing it into place as a carotid interposition graft.

The authors routinely patch all carotid artery closures unless the arteries are of extremely generous size and when patching would result in a patulous "aneurysmal" artery. Patch selection is up to the individual surgeon, with no study demonstrating superiority of one material over another. Bovine pericardium, PTFE, polyethylene terephthalate, and vein are all acceptable materials. Ankle saphenous vein, however, should be avoided based on a Cleveland Clinic study which noted an increased rupture rate when using veins from this location [14]. The author routinely uses a HEMASHIELD™ PLATINUM FINESSE knitted cardiovascular patch [Maquet, Rastatt, Germany]. Patch width should be tailored individually to prevent arterial narrowing while not making the artery diameter too large. The latter may result in mural thrombus formation in the patched area or low sheer stress predisposing to restenosis.

We routinely perform intraoperative completion angiography after all carotid operations. An 18-G angiocatheter is inserted through the ECA, aimed proximally, and contrast is gently injected under direct fluoroscopy. The authors visualize the entire operative site including the proximal carotid artery and portions of the intracranial circulation. More than one view may be required. We do not hesitate to reexplore the operative site if there is a problem noted on the arteriogram. Intraoperative completion duplex scanning may also be performed if the clinician is more comfortable with this modality, though duplex scanning cannot evaluate the intracranial circulation nor the aortic arch.

The authors routinely drain the wound with a 10-mm, fully perforated, flat, "Jackson-Pratt" drain placed through a separate stab incision and connected to a standard bulb suction. In our experience, drains are generally removed the morning after the operation. Drains do not prevent neck hematomas nor do they decrease return rates to the operating room for bleeding. However, we subjectively feel that postoperative neck edema is decreased when drains are used.

Postoperative Complications

Complications following RCEA are similar to those following primary CEA. The only difference is an increased incidence of cranial nerve injuries in redo operations. Based on our review of 219 RCEAs, 25 (13%) patients experienced nerve injuries of which four had prolonged recovery and one had a permanent injury. This is significant when compared to our nerve injury rate of 4% (44/1105) following primary CEA [5]. Operative mortality and neurologic morbidity were similar in both cohorts.

Postoperative carotid duplex scans are obtained within 1 month postoperatively, at 6 months, 12 months, and then yearly. Restenosis (>60%) occurred in three patients (1.5%) over an average of 2.1 years in our redo group compared to 0.4% (4/1105) over an average of 4.4 years in our primary CEA group.

Postoperative Management

Most patients may be discharged within 24 h of surgery. Patients are allowed to eat a standard meal the following morning, and ambulation is encouraged. The surgical drain is removed as soon as possible when drainage is minimal. Patients are placed on antiplatelet therapy, most commonly ASA 81 mg daily. They remain on their preoperative medications, and statins are prescribed if they are not part of their preoperative regimen. Patients are discharged with the 2-week office follow-up and are under surveillance with duplex imaging at intervals 1-month, 3-month, 6-months and yearly.

Case Example

A 63-year-old asymptomatic man with a history of bilateral CEA in 2002 was referred after a screening ultrasound (US) demonstrated left recurrent carotid stenosis in the 80–99% range. His first CEA was in 2002, and he was unaware of any problems with the artery until his US in 2009.

The patient underwent a left RCEA in February 2009 where the patch was completely removed and redo endarterectomy was performed removing diffuse, irregular plaque in the area of the patch. Postoperative scanning revealed a well-healed endarterectomy site without evidence of stenosis. Seven years later, the patient presented with left hemispheric TIAs and was found to have a new left recurrence in the 80–99% range. Risk factors included type II, insulin-dependent diabetes mellitus, and cigarette smoking. During repeat surgery, severe, diffuse plaque throughout the patch site with an area of "coral reef" plaque in the common carotid proximal to the patch was found (Fig. 13.1). Re-endarterectomy and patching were performed (Fig. 13.2). The patient went home within 24 h. Postoperative scanning has not revealed new problems <6 months out (Fig. 13.3). He is maintained on a statin, aspirin, and clopidogrel and has stopped smoking.

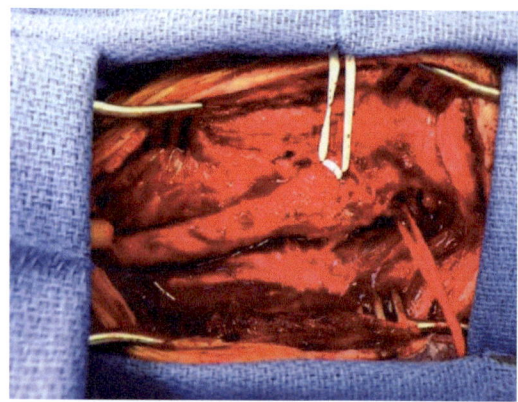

Fig. 13.1 Photograph of carotid artery bifurcation at completion of dissection for a redo procedure in 63-year-old asymptomatic man with a history of bilateral carotid endarterectomy (case example). When the artery was opened, severe and diffuse plaque throughout the patch site was found, with an area of "coral reef" plaque in the common carotid artery (CCA) proximal to the patch. The CCA is to the left, and the internal (ICA) and external (ECA) carotid arteries are to the right. White tape encircles the ECA, while pink tape encircles the ICA. From: Rubin J. Redo Carotid Endarterectomy. In: Hans SS, Shepard AD, Weaver MR, Bove P, Long GW. Endovascular and Open Vascular Reconstruction: A Practical Approach. Copyright © 2017, CRC Press, reproduced by permission of Taylor & Francis Books UK

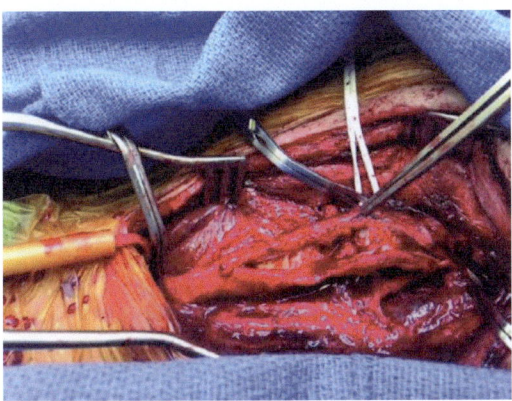

Fig. 13.2 Re-endarterectomy and patching of the 63-year-old patient. Operative photograph showing recurrent carotid stenosis after opening the artery. Orientation is the same as in Fig. 13.1. From: Rubin J. Redo Carotid Endarterectomy. In: Hans SS, Shepard AD, Weaver MR, Bove P, Long GW. Endovascular and Open Vascular Reconstruction: A Practical Approach. Copyright © 2017, CRC Press, reproduced by permission of Taylor & Francis Books UK

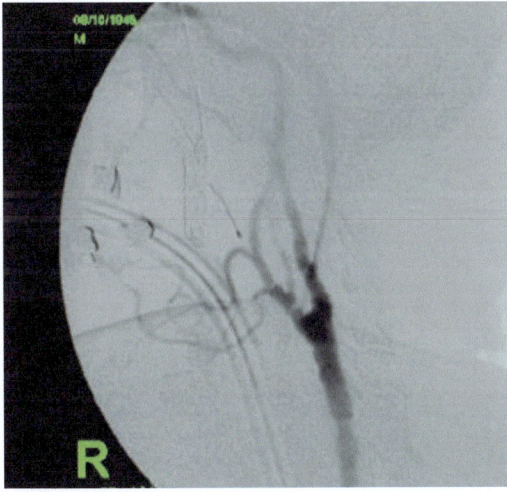

Fig. 13.3 Completion angiogram of the same patient following redo endarterectomy and patching. Postoperative scanning has not revealed new problems <6 months on. From: Rubin J. Redo Carotid Endarterectomy. In: Hans SS, Shepard AD, Weaver MR, Bove P, Long GW. Endovascular and Open Vascular Reconstruction: A Practical Approach. Copyright © 2017, CRC Press, reproduced by permission of Taylor & Francis Books UK

Review Questions

1. The incidence of carotid artery restenosis is:
   A. <4%
   B. 4–10%
   C. 11–20%
   D. >20%

   Answer: B

2. The incidence of cranial nerve injury during redo CEA is:
   A. Same as primary CEA.
   B. Greater than primary CEA.
   C. Cranial nerve injury almost never occurs during CEA.
   D. Permanent cranial nerve injuries are more common than temporary nerve palsy.

   Answer: B

3. Late (>5 years) restenosis following CEA is caused by:
   A. Technical problem at the initial operation
   B. Myointimal hyperplasia
   C. Recurrence of atherosclerotic disease
   D. Inflammatory response

   Answer: C

References

1. Hertzer NR, Martinez BD, Benjamin SP, et al. Recurrent stenosis after carotid endarterectomy. Surg Gynecol Obstet. 1979;149:360–4.
2. Moore WS, Kempczinski RF, Nelson JJ, et al. Recurrent carotid stenosis: results of this asymptomatic carotid atherosclerosis study. Stroke. 1998;29:2018–25.
3. Lal BK, Hobson RW 2nd, Goldstein J, et al. In-stent recurrent stenosis after carotid artery stenting: life table analysis and clinical relevance. J Vasc Surg. 2003;38:1162–8.

4. Attigah N, Külkens S, Deyle C, et al. Redo surgery or carotid stenting for restenosis after carotid endarterectomy: results of two different treatment strategies. Ann Vasc Surg. 2010;24:190–5.
5. Akingba AG, Bojalian M, Shen C, et al. Managing recurrent carotid artery disease with redo carotid endarterectomy: a 10-year retrospective case series. Ann Vasc Surg. 2014;28:908–16.
6. de Borst GJ, Zanen P, de Vries JP, et al. Durability of surgery for restenosis after carotid endarterectomy. J Vasc Surg. 2008;47:363–71.
7. Awad IA, Little JR. Patch angioplasty in carotid endarterectomy advantages, concerns, and controversies. Stroke. 1989;20:417–22.
8. Rerkasem K, Rothwell PM. Patch angioplasty versus primary closure for carotid endarterectomy. Cochrane Database Syst Rev. 2009;4:CD000160.
9. Wholey MH, Al-Mubarek N, Wholey MH. Updated review of the global carotid artery stent registry. Catheter Cardiovasc Interv. 2003;60:256–66.
10. CAVATAS Investigators. Endovascular versus surgical treatment in patients with carotid stenosis in the carotid and vertebral artery transluminal angioplasty study (CAVATAS): a randomized trial. Lancet. 2001;357:1729–37.
11. Levy EI, Hanel RA, Lau T, Koebbe CJ, et al. Frequency and management of recurrent stenosis after carotid artery stent implantation. J Neurosurg. 2005;102:29–37.
12. George J, Herz I, Goldstein E, et al. Number and adhesive properties of circulating endomedial progenitor cells in patients with in-stent restenosis. Arterioscler Thromb Vasc Biol. 2003;23:e57–60.
13. DePalma RG, Chidi CC, Sternfield WC, Koletsky S. Pathogenesis and prevention of trauma-provoked atheromas. Surgery. 1977;82:429–37.
14. O'Hara PJ, Hertzer NR, Krajewski LP, et al. Saphenous vein patch rupture after carotid endarterectomy. J Vasc Surg. 1992;15:504–9.

Carotid Interposition Grafting

14

Sachinder Singh Hans

As compared to carotid endarterectomy (CEA), carotid interposition grafting (CIG) is infrequently performed. Indications for CIG include:

- Locally advanced head and neck cancer involving the carotid artery
- Infected patch graft following CEA
- Failed endovascular therapy for restenosis following CEA or CAS
- Resection of extracranial carotid aneurysm when end-to-end anastomosis is not feasible
- Carotid artery trauma when local repair is not feasible
- Carotid stenosis secondary to neck irradiation

The conduit used for CIG includes straight or tapered PTFE graft (W.L. Gore. Newark, DE). In contaminated fields, autogenous reconstruction with the greater saphenous vein (GSV) or superficial femoral artery (SFA) can be used. The superficial femoral artery should be evaluated by duplex imaging and is preferred in patients undergoing resection of head and neck cancer invading the

carotid artery. For patients presenting with failed endovascular therapy for carotid restenosis following CAS, CIG is a satisfactory option. Failed CAS often occurs in patients with heavy calcified plaque burden or due to structural failure of the stent, removal of the stent with the distal CCA and proximal ICA followed by CIG. In patients with carotid stenosis following radiation to the neck for cancer, the author prefers resection of distal CCA and proximal ICA with CIG as CEA for radiation-induced lesions has higher incidence of recurrent stenosis than CEA for atherosclerotic occlusive disease.

Diagnostic Studies

Following evaluation by carotid duplex imaging, thin section computed axial tomography angiography should be performed to evaluate the distal of extension of the lesion (or distal end of the stent). If quality of CTA images is not satisfactory, catheter-based carotid/cerebral arteriography should be performed.

Patients with carotid in-stent stenosis following CAS should undergo carotid angioplasty with or without placement of additional stent if recurrent stenosis is greater than 80% or patient has focal neurological symptoms in the form of TIA or mild stroke. Carotid artery stenting is a satisfactory alternative to CEA for both symptomatic and asymptomatic carotid stenosis as demonstrated by the results of various trials (see Chapter 10 and Chapter

S. S. Hans
Medical Director of Vascular and Endovascular Services, Henry Ford Macomb Hospital, Clinton Township, MI, USA

Chief of Vascular Surgery, St. John Macomb Hospital, Warren, MI, USA

Department of Surgery, Wayne State University School of Medicine, Detroit, MI, USA

© The Editor(s) (if applicable) and The Author(s) 2018
S. S. Hans (ed.), *Extracranial Carotid and Vertebral Artery Disease*,
https://doi.org/10.1007/978-3-319-91533-3_14

16). The carotid revascularization endarterectomy versus stenting trial (CREST) showed equipoise between the results of CAS and CEA. However, the incidence of periprocedural stroke is higher with CAS but the incidence of myocardial infarction is higher following CEA. However, further subgroup analysis showed that the perioperative stroke and mortality were significantly lower among patients undergoing CEA for symptomatic patients and patients older than 80 years of age.

CIG for Failed Carotid Stenting

CIG for failed carotid stenting exposure of the distal end of the stent in the ICA is mandatory. This exposure may be difficult if upper end of the stent extends above the level of the body of second cervical vertebrae. The operative intervention should be performed under GA. It is important that any monitoring equipment does not obstruct the potential radiological imaging of the stent in the ICA in the event intraoperative imaging is necessary. The operative dissection is usually difficult because of the previous operations in patients with carotid restenosis as there is an inflammatory response due to the presence of the stent. Sharp dissection separating the CCA and ICA from surrounding structures is preferred.

Distal exposure of the ICA as outlined in Chap. 11 should be undertaken. The author prefers EEG monitoring to determine the need for the shunt in patients who do not tolerate carotid cross clamping if ischemic changes are observed by EEG and/or with median nerve somatosensory-evoked potential monitoring.

Interposition Graft Without Shunt

If the upper end of the stent extends above the cervical second vertebral body, intraoperative balloon occlusion is necessary to control retrograde bleeding through the ICA after systemic heparinization (100 units/kgm body wt), the CCA is punctured with a micropuncture needle, and using a microcatheter, 7 Fr sheath is inserted in the CCA just above the base of neck. 0.014 mm guidewire is advanced into the ICA toward the base of the skull, and over the wire #3 Fogarty catheter is inflated using 50% diluted contrast media solution. On the other hand, if the upper end of the stent is below the level of cervical second body, balloon occlusion is not necessary. Distal clamping of the ICA can be performed with careful mobilization after obtaining proximal control, and applying a vascular clamp, the ICA is divided transversely with a #15 blade scalpel a few millimeters below the upper end of the stent, which is then separated from the distal ICA with sharp dissection. The origin of the ECA is divided, its distal end is suture ligated, and the proximal end of the CCA is divided. Balloon occlusion catheter is deflated and removed, and a soft vascular clamp or a Yasargil clamp (Scanlan Int., St. Paul, MN) is applied. The distal anastomosis is performed first, blood is allowed to flow retrograde to remove any debris, a vascular clamp is applied (Fig. 14.1) proximal to the distal anastomosis, and proximal anastomosis is performed in an end-to-end fashion (Fig. 14.2). In some patients with discrepancy in the size of the CCA and graft, an end-to-side proximal anastomosis should be considered.

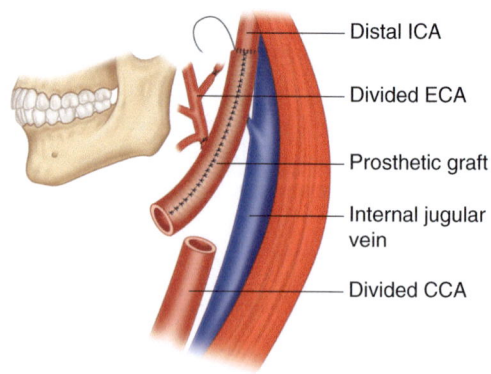

Fig. 14.1 Proximal anastomosis of CIG

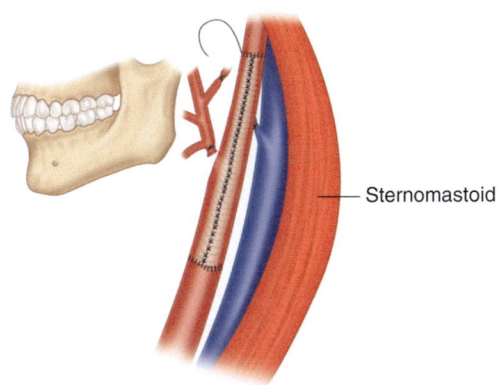

Sternomastoid

Fig. 14.2 Distal anastomosis of CIG

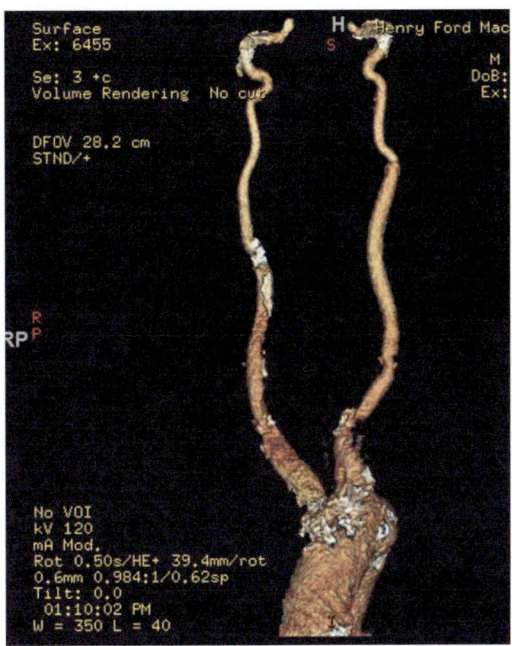

Fig. 14.3 Postoperative CTA of CIG on the left side with carotid atherosclerosis on the right

Shunt Placement

If the EEG and somatosensory median nerve somatosensory-evoked potentials indicated cerebral ischemia, or the SP is <40 mmHg, an indwelling shunt is required. The distal end of the shunt is first advanced into the divided ICA; after back-bleeding fills the shunt, the proximal end of the shunt is inserted into the CCA. The interposition graft is then passed over another shunt (second shunt). The first shunt is removed, and the second shunt with the interposition graft around it is inserted. Distal end-to-end anastomosis is performed first followed by proximal anastomosis to the divided CCA. Before proximal anastomosis is completed, the shunt is removed, and suturing is completed. If any technical difficulties are encountered, completion arteriogram is preferred by injecting the contract via a 5-F sheath inserted into the CCA, proximal to the CCA and graft anastomosis.

Author has performed four CIG for failed carotid stenting with tapered PTFE (7 mm × 5 mm) graft (Fig. 14.3). In one patient, nonreversed greater saphenous vein graft for infected carotid endarterectomy Dacron patch graft was performed. One patient had CIG (nonreversed greater saphenous vein) following resection of a malignant carotid body tumor with satisfactory late outcome. All PTFE grafts have remained patent for mean follow-up of 2 years. The saphenous vein interposition graft for infected Dacron patch graft following CEA developed stenosis due to myointimal hyperplasia, and patient subsequently underwent CAS. However, the stent occluded without any neurological symptoms, and the neck infection had resolved.

Complications

The majority of the complications of CIG are similar to those of CEA. The incidence of cranial nerve injury such as superior laryngeal and glossopharyngeal nerve is greater as cephalad exposure of the ICA in the neck is necessary.

Review Questions

1. Following CAS, patient develops a stent fracture and failure under which evaluation of stent extending to the level of C1 and C2. In order to remove the stent, the distal ICA is best controlled by:
   A. Usual atraumatic vascular clamp on the distal CEA.
   B. No control is necessary prior to removal of the stent.
   C. Distal intraluminal balloon occlusion.
   D. Clamp the origin of ICA including the stent with soft Fogarty jaw clamp.

   Answer: C

2. The best conduit for carotid interposition grafting (CIG) in a patient undergoing surgery for head and neck cancer with involvement of the ICA is:
   A. Autologous vein/superficial femoral artery
   B. Tapered PTFE graft
   C. Bovine xenograft
   D. External carotid artery

   Answer: A

3. Following carotid interposition grafting using synthetic graft, patient had increased drainage from sinus in the neck and CTA reveals infection surrounding the interposition graft. The best management option is:
   A. Antibiotics, removal of synthetic graft, and autologous vein/SFA graft and possible myocutaneous flap
   B. Debridement, antibiotics, and antibiotic-soaked synthetic graft
   C. Debridement, antibiotics, and removal of graft and ligation of proximal CCA
   D. Placement of a covered stent and antibiotics

   Answer: A

Suggested Reading

Berguer R. Function and surgery of the carotid and vertebral arteries. Philadelphia, PA: Lippincott Williams & Wilkins Health; 2014. p. 109.

Gonzalez A, Drummond MD, McCord S, et al. Carotid endarterectomy for treatment of in-stent stenosis. J Vasc Surg. 2011;54:1167–9.

Jacobs JR, Korkmaz H, Marks HC, Kline R, Buerger R. One stage carotid artery resection reconstruction in radiated head and neck carcinoma. Am J Otolaryngol. 2001;22:167–71.

Current Status of Carotid Endarterectomy and Carotid Stenting

Richard D. Fessler and Justin G. Thomas

Introduction

Atherosclerotic disease of the carotid artery is a major contributor to morbidity and mortality, accounting for 10–15% of patients diagnosed with stroke [1]. Surgical intervention of carotid artery disease with carotid endarterectomy (CEA) has been well studied and shown to reduce the risk of future ischemic stroke in patients with severe symptomatic carotid artery disease or in patients where maximal medical therapy has failed [2–4]. However, the role of carotid artery stenting (CAS) has not been as clear despite being a proposed treatment option for carotid artery disease since the 1990s [5, 6]. A significant contribution to the lack of clarity is partly due to the large number of clinical trials that have either confirmed or refuted the use of CAS to treat patients with carotid artery stenosis. The goal of this chapter is to provide the reader an overview of the clinical trials that have led to our current conclusions about stenting or endarterectomy in patients with carotid artery stenosis.

R. D. Fessler (✉)
Department of Surgery, St. John Hospital and Medical Centers, Detroit, MI, USA
e-mail: Richard.fessler2@ascension.org

J. G. Thomas
Section of Neurosurgery, Department of Surgery, Providence-Providence Park Hospital, Southfield, MI, USA

Overview of Clinical Trials

The following chapter will cover a significant majority of the landmark peer-reviewed publications and prospective research that has been published over the last 20 years regarding stenting or endarterectomy for carotid stenosis. A significant emphasis will be placed on identifying literature with randomized controlled trials (RCTs) or prospective studies, as this provided the highest quality evidence for treatment recommendations. Studies that had long-term follow-up data were also favored. An overview of these trials will be presented in a way to offer the reader a concise comprehensive summary of the literature that has led to our current practices today. However, it should be noted that there is a convoluted history surrounding many of the recommendations that have come from the literature on stenting versus endarterectomy; therefore, to help the reader better comprehend the time-relationship of the history behind carotid stenting versus endarterectomy (and avoid confusion that often stems from reading the literature), we will present each study in chronological order starting with the year of the initial patient randomization. This will help illustrate the extensive timeline for studying this disease while aiding the reader to consider the advances we have made since many of these clinical trials were published. Long-term data (when available) will also be discussed in each section. A summary of the trials can be seen in Table 15.1.

© The Editor(s) (if applicable) and The Author(s) 2018
S. S. Hans (ed.), *Extracranial Carotid and Vertebral Artery Disease*,
https://doi.org/10.1007/978-3-319-91533-3_15

Table 15.1 Summary of randomized controlled trials for carotid artery stenting versus endarterectomy in patients with extracranial carotid artery stenosis

Name	Trial name	Publication	Year of original publication or long-term follow-up study	Study design	Recruitment	Number of patients	Patient type	Follow-up	Distal embolization protection rate
CAVATAS	Carotid and vertebral artery transluminal angioplasty study	Endovascular versus surgical treatment in patients with carotid stenosis in the carotid and vertebral artery transluminal angioplasty study (CAVATAS): a randomized trial	2001	RCT	1992–1997	504	Stenosis of the common carotid artery, carotid bifurcation, or internal carotid artery that investigators believed needed treatment and was suitable for both carotid endarterectomy and endovascular treatment	1 year	0.0%
		Endovascular treatment with angioplasty or stenting versus endarterectomy in patients with carotid artery stenosis in the carotid and vertebral artery transluminal angioplasty study: long-term follow-up of a randomized trial	2009	Follow-up	–	413		4–5 years	–
EVA-3S	Endarterectomy versus angioplasty with symptomatic severe carotid stenosis	Endarterectomy versus stenting with symptomatic severe carotid stenosis trial	2006	RCT	2000–2005 trial was stopped early	527	Symptomatic hemispheric or retinal TIA or non-disabling stroke or retinal infarct within 120 days prior to enrollment *and* stenosis of 60–99% with NASCET criteria. Stenosis had to be confirmed with either catheter angiography *or* both U/S and MRA	6 months	92.0%
		Endarterectomy versus angioplasty with symptomatic severe carotid stenosis trial: results up to 4 years from a randomized, multicenter trial	2008	Follow-up	2005–2007	524		4 years	–
		Long-term follow-up study for endarterectomy versus angioplasty in patients with symptomatic severe carotid stenosis trial	2014	Retrospective, follow-up	2008–2012	493		7 years	–

SAPPHIRE	Stenting and angioplasty with protection in patients at high risk for endarterectomy	Protected carotid artery stenting versus endarterectomy in high-risk patients	2004	RCT	2000–2002	334	Symptomatic with >50% stenosis or asymptomatic with >80% and at least one high-risk criteria	3 years	95.6%
		Long-term results of carotid stenting versus endarterectomy in high-risk patients	2008	Follow-up	–	–	–	–	–
SPACE	Stent-protected angioplasty versus carotid endarterectomy	30-day results from the SPACE trial of stent-protected angioplasty versus carotid endarterectomy in symptomatic patients: a randomized non-inferiority trial	2006	RCT	2001–2006	1183	Symptomatic carotid artery stenosis with radiographic evidence of stenosis on imaging: at least 70% on duplex ultrasound or angiography according to ECST or 50% according to NASCET	30-days	27.0%
		Results of the stent-protected angioplasty versus carotid endarterectomy study to treat symptomatic stenosis at 2 years: a multinational, prospective, randomized trial	2008	Follow-up	–	1214	–	2 years	–

(continued)

Table 15.1 (continued)

Name	Trial name	Publication	Year of original publication or long-term follow-up study	Study design	Recruitment	Number of patients	Patient type	Follow-up	Distal embolization protection rate
ACST-2	Asymptomatic carotid surgery trial-2	Asymptomatic carotid surgery trial-2: rationale for a randomized clinical trial comparing carotid endarterectomy with carotid artery stenting in patients with asymptomatic carotid artery stenosis	2009	RCT	2008–2012	986	Asymptomatic carotid artery stenosis with low surgical risk and appropriately medical therapy	5 years	Not reported
		Status updated and interim results from the asymptomatic carotid surgery trial-2	2013	Follow-up	–	–	–	–	–
CREST	Carotid revascularization endarterectomy versus stenting trial	Stenting versus endarterectomy for treatment of carotid artery stenosis	2010	RCT	2005–2008	2502	Please see below table on "Radiographic Criteria Used for Randomization in CREST"	4 years	96.1%
		Long-term results of stenting versus endarterectomy for carotid artery stenosis	2016	Follow-up	–	1607	–	10 years	–

ICSS	International carotid stenting study	Carotid artery stenting compared with endarterectomy in patients with symptomatic carotid stenosis: an interim analysis of a randomized controlled trial	2010	RCT	2004 to not reported	1713	Symptomatic carotid artery stenosis (within 365 days of TIA or non-disabling stroke) and stenosis of at least 50% diagnosed with NASCET criteria. Patients had to be deemed suitable for surgery and low surgical risk prior to intervention	120 days	72%
		Long-term outcomes after stenting versus endarterectomy for treatment of symptomatic carotid stenosis: the international carotid stenting study randomized trial	2015	Follow-up	–	–		Up to 10 years	–
ACT-1	Asymptomatic carotid trial-1	Randomized trial of stent versus surgery for asymptomatic carotid stenosis	2016	RCT	2005–2013	1453 (with 3:1 randomization)	<80 years old, asymptomatic with 70–99% stenosis, and not high surgical risk	5 years	97.6%

General Considerations

There are many different end points and definitions used by the authors of the following papers. For clarity, we will define the following generalizations and make note of any differences made by investigators as they present:

Stroke is generally defined as an ischemic neurological deficit that persisted for more than 24 h. A *non-disabling stroke* is generally considered patients with a modified Rankin Scale (mRS) score of 0–2, with disabling strokes being scores of 3–5 (higher the score indicates a worse stroke). *Myocardial infarction* was not always clearly defined in each study but for our generalization is defined as an elevation of creatinine kinase higher than two times the upper limit of normal with positive serum MB fractions. *Composite cardiovascular events* are defined as stroke, myocardial infarction, or death.

Criteria for measuring stenosis were performed either by using techniques from the NASCET trial [2] or ECST trial [3]. Degrees of stenosis with ultrasound measurements were assigned with standard ultrasound criteria: mild (<50%), moderate (50–69%), severe (70–99%), and occluded (100%) [7].

1992: Carotid and Vertebral Artery Transluminal Angioplasty Study (CAVATAS)

This study [8], along with the long-term follow-up [1], was a multicenter RCT that compared a rather generalized patient population with carotid artery stenosis to endovascular treatment (with either angioplasty and/or stenting) to endarterectomy. A total of 504 patients from 1992 to 1997 were randomized. Prior to 1994, patients randomized in the study to receive endovascular treatment underwent percutaneous transluminal angioplasty with balloon catheters. Carotid stents were being developed prior to this time and when they became available they were used from 1994 onward when the radiologists believed there was a treatment benefit. Stents were allowed as either a secondary procedure after unsatisfactory balloon dilation *or* stenting alone without attempting balloon dilation first. Among other exclusion criteria, patients were specifically excluded from the study if they had "unsuitable" surgical risk factors defined as recent myocardial infarction, poorly controlled hypertension or diabetes mellitus, renal disease, respiratory failure, inaccessible carotid stenosis, or severe cervical spondylosis. Contralateral carotid artery occlusion was not an exclusion criterion. Patients also did not have pretreatment-defined criteria for randomization based on their degree of stenosis and investigators "used their own protocol to establish the presence of clinically important carotid stenosis before treatment." Only 3% of patients were asymptomatic from their carotid artery stenosis.

Based on these criteria, 251 patients were randomized to endovascular treatment and 253 to CEA. The degree of ipsilateral carotid artery stenosis was 86.4% in the endovascular group and 85.1% in the surgical group. In addition to their stenosis, 24 patients (10%) in the endovascular arm and 20 patients (8%) in the surgical arm were diagnosed with a contralateral carotid occlusion prior to ipsilateral carotid artery intervention.

The rates of major outcomes within the first 30 days did not differ significantly between endovascular and surgical intervention: 6.4% versus 5.9% for 30-day disabling stroke or death and 10.0% and 9.9% for any stroke lasting for more than 7 days or death. The rate of periprocedural cranial neuropathy was higher in the surgical group (8.7%) compared to none in the endovascular group. Major groin or neck hematomas also occurred less frequently in the endovascular group than after surgery (1.2% versus 6.7%).

At 1 year of follow-up, severe ipsilateral carotid stenosis was seen more often after endovascular treatment (14% versus 4%). At long-term follow-up of endovascular treatment (mean 5 years) and surgical treatment (mean 4 years), severe carotid restenosis of at least 70% occurred more often in the endovascular group than the surgical group. The adjusted 5-year incidence of restenosis was 30.7% in the endovascular treatment compared to 10.5% in the surgical group. The long-term general conclusion was that restenosis was more likely, approximately three times, after endovascular treatment than endarterectomy and that endovascular treatment was associated with recurrent ipsilateral cerebrovascular symptoms.

The CAVATAS study and its long-term follow-up reported some interesting findings but drew criticism. First, there was no clear indication for treatment: patients were left at the operator's discretion of their own protocol if an individual, regardless of symptoms, had carotid artery disease that warranted intervention. There was no specific mention about what protocols, if any, were used for operators to decide on whether a patient required therapy. Second, there was a lack of protection against distal emboli, which the lack of doing so has largely been abandoned as it has been shown to significantly increase the risk of stroke [9]. Third, endovascular treatment consisted of balloon angioplasty in almost three quarters of patients with only 55 of the 213 patients (26%) receiving a stent. Finally, this population is rather limited when compared to the generalized population with carotid stenosis, as most patients have significant comorbidities that were excluded from this study or are asymptomatic and CAVATAS included only 3% of patients with asymptomatic disease. Therefore, the conclusions do not necessarily apply to many, if not most, patients with carotid artery disease and follow-up studies from CAVATAS would illustrate many of these points.

2000: Endarterectomy Versus Angioplasty with Symptomatic Severe Carotid Stenosis (EVA-3S)

The EVA-3S clinical trial and its two long-term follow-up publications [10–12] reported an extensive series on patients with severe symptomatic carotid stenosis treated with carotid endarterectomy or stenting. In the first study, a total of 527 symptomatic patients were randomized to stenting (with distal emboli protection used in 92% of patients) or endarterectomy. Patients with symptomatic hemispheric or retinal TIA *or* non-disabling stroke or retinal infarct within 120 days prior to enrollment were enrolled if

they had carotid stenosis of 60–99% confirmed with either catheter angiography or both duplex ultrasound and magnetic resonance angiography of the carotid vessels. Initially patients were only treated if they had 70% carotid stenosis, but the study protocol was modified to include patients up to 60% after there was a potential benefit to surgically treat patients with 50–69% stenosis [4]. Patients in the initial study were followed for the perioperative 30-day period along with follow-up at 3 and 6 months post-intervention.

The first study was stopped early because of "safety and futility" at the recommendations of the trials safety committee. Patients with stenting had higher rates of 30- and 60-day stroke or death. Patients with stenting also had higher relative risks of nonfatal stroke or death within this period. There were also more local complications with stenting, mainly from injuries related to the puncture site (femoral pseudoaneurysm, arteriovenous fistula formation, lower limb arterial occlusion, or thrombosis), but these results were not statistically significant. Patients with endarterectomy had more systemic complications, mainly from pulmonary issues, but again were not statistically significant. There were significantly more cranial nerve injuries with surgery (7.7% versus 1.1%, $P < 0.001$), and shorter hospital stays with stenting (3 versus 4 days, $P = 0.01$); however, there was no statistically significant difference in myocardial infarction ($P = 0.62$). The overall conclusion at the early termination of this trial was that patients with symptomatic carotid stenosis of at least 60% had lower rates of stroke or death at 30 days and 6 months with endarterectomy when compared to stenting.

However, there were some limitations to the first publication. The most significant limitation of the first study (identified by both the primary investigators and investigators of other clinical trials) was that the stents could be placed by physicians with various degrees of experience. Interventionalists could be included if they had performed as few as five previous carotid stent procedures *or* while working under the supervision of a qualified tutor if they had no previous experience. Another limitation was that high surgical risk patients were excluded, limiting the generalizing conclusions that were made. Finally, the consideration of patients with contralateral carotid disease was not considered during the inclusion or exclusion of criterial in this trial.

Two follow-up studies at both 4- and 7-year follow-up were published after the initial trial was completed [10, 12]. The first publication had an overall retention rate of 99% with only three patients lost to follow-up, the second having a 94% retention with only 88 patients lost. Long-term conclusions were largely influenced by the initial study with high perioperative rate of 30-day stroke or death within the stenting group. The composite incidence of periprocedural stroke or death *or* any non-procedural ipsilateral stroke was significantly higher for stented patients at 4 years (11.1% versus 6.2%, $P = 0.03$) and 7 years (11.0% versus 6.0%, $P = 0.04$). However, after the periprocedural period was over both follow-up studies concluded the long-term risk of stroke or death was low and not significant in either both treatment groups, with both treatment arms having similar hazard ratios. Furthermore, the 2014 data suggested there was no difference in restenosis, occlusion, myocardial infarction, or need for revascularization at long-term in both intention-to-treat and per-protocol analyses.

Overall it was concluded that the perioperative safety of carotid stenting had to improve before more patients were subjected to this treatment modality, and operator experience interestingly was not a determining factor in the 30-day risk of stroke or death in this study.

2000: Stenting and Angioplasty with Protection in Patients at High Risk for Endarterectomy (SAPPHIRE)

The SAPPHIRE trial included data published from *Protected Carotid-Artery Stenting versus Endarterectomy in High-Risk Patients* [13], and its subsequent long-term follow-up publication [14] was an RCT that compared stenting *with* distal embolic protection to endarterectomy alone in patients specifically with identified "high-risk"

surgical features that increased the risk of both short- and long-term complications. A total number of 334 patients were randomized in a 1:1 ratio from 2000 to 2002 and followed for a mean of 3 years post-procedure. Patients were included if they had at least one high-risk criteria and *either* symptomatic carotid stenosis >50% *or* asymptomatic stenosis >80%. Distal embolization protection was used in 96% of the stented patients.

Criteria for High Risk in SAPPHIRE
At least one factor was required for treatment in this study [14].

- Clinically significant cardiac disease
  - Congestive heart failure, abnormal stress test, or need for open-heart surgery
- Severe pulmonary disease
- Contralateral carotid occlusion
- Contralateral laryngeal nerve palsy
- Previous radical neck surgery or radiation therapy to the neck
- Recurrent stenosis after endarterectomy
- Age >80 years of age

Composite cardiovascular events at one year did not show a significant difference in outcome between stenting and endarterectomy in patients with both severe carotid artery stenosis *and* classified as an increased surgical risk. Stenting patients experienced a 12.2% composite cardiovascular event rate, whereas surgical patients had a 20.1% event rate ($P = 0.004$ for non-inferiority). Carotid revascularization rates were also lower at one year post-procedure in patients who had received a stent (0.6%) compared to the surgical group (4.3%, $P = 0.04$). Patients in the stenting group had a lower rate of cranial nerve palsies (0% versus 4.9%, $P = 0.004$) and shorter inpatient length of stay (1.84 ± 1.75 days versus 2.85 ± 3.67 days, $P = 0.002$).

Long-term data published four years later further supported the primary outcomes of the initial study, albeit with only a 77.8% overall follow-up rate. Kaplan-Meier for estimating cumulative incidence of the primary outcome was the method used to partially correct for the loss of follow-up. Composite cardiovascular events at one year plus death or ipsilateral stroke between 1 and 3 years were 24.6% for the stenting group and 26.9% for the endarterectomy group ($P = 0.71$) and 26.2% and 26.9%, respectively, with the Kaplan-Meier method. There was an overall high incidence of death in the 1–3-year period follow-up study, with 18.6% of stented patients and 21.0% of surgical patients experiencing mortality (20.0% and 24.2%, respectively, with the Kaplan-Meier method). However, the majority of deaths were contributed to non-neurological causes of death. Cardiac-related death was a contributor in both treatment groups, with 15 cardiac deaths occurring in both the stenting and surgical groups; however, there was no statistical difference when comparing the two groups ($P = 0.99$). Furthermore, it was noted the cumulative incidence of death in this study was likely related to "high-risk" patients themselves, with every patient having at least one identified high-risk factor and approximately 20% of the patients being over 80 years of age.

This study highlights that stenting is non-inferior to endarterectomy in patients with severe carotid stenosis *and* with a high surgical risk. Furthermore, there are fewer perioperative cranial nerve injury associated with stenting these patients along with a shorter length of stay. However, it should be noted that this study illustrates only a specific patient population (severe stenosis, high surgical risk) and does not provide any insight into patients with low or moderate surgical risk. This study differed from SPACE and EVA-3S (where they reported worse outcomes with stenting compared to endarterectomy) and that they did not include high surgical risk patients or asymptomatic patients. Furthermore, distal emboli protection devices, which by now were expected to be used when feasible in carotid stenting procedures, were only used in 92% of patients in the EVA-3S trial and 27% of patients in the SPACE trial.

2001: Stent-Protected Angioplasty Versus Carotid Endarterectomy (SPACE)

The SPACE trial [15] and its 2-year follow-up [16] compared carotid stenting to endarterectomy in patients with severe symptomatic carotid artery stenosis. In an RCT from 2001 to 2006, a total of 1183 patients with symptomatic carotid artery stenosis and radiographic evidence of stenosis on imaging (at least 70% on duplex ultrasound or angiography according to ECST or 50% according to NASCET) were randomized to treatment and followed for 30 days and then two years.

Patients had similar rates of death or ipsilateral ischemic stroke from either carotid artery stenting or endarterectomy at both short- (6.8% versus 6.3%, respectively, $P = 0.09$ for noninferiority) and long-term intervals (9.5% versus 8.8%, respectively, $P = 0.62$). At long term, patients appeared to have a statistically significantly higher rate of recurrent stenosis of at least 70% in the stenting group in both intention-to-treat and per-protocol analyses (10.7% versus 4.6%, $P < 0.01$, and 11.1% versus 4.6%, $P < 0.01$, respectively). However, the overall mortality rate along with the rate of disabling stroke at both short- and long-term intervals was not inferior with stenting compared to endarterectomy.

In a subgroup analysis on the patients from SPACE [17], potential risk factors were examined including age, sex, type of qualifying event, side of intervention, degree of stenosis, and presence of high-grade contralateral stenosis or occlusion. Overall age was determined to give the greatest separation between high- and low-risk patients, particularly in the stenting population. There was an overall statistical significance of ipsilateral stroke or death within the first 30 days with increased age in the stenting population ($P = 0.001$) but not in the surgical group ($P = 0.534$). In patients under the age of 68 years old, there was a lower periprocedural risk of stroke or death with CAS than CEA ($P = 0.001$); however, the opposite trend was seen in patients over the age of 68, with patients having a lower risk of stroke or death at 30 days with surgery compared to stenting ($P = 0.026$). All the other aforementioned risk factors examined in the subgroup analysis did not have a statistically different prediction of ipsilateral stroke or death at 30 days, including sex, degree of stenosis, or degree of pathology in the contralateral carotid artery.

An important limitation of the SPACE study was the low use of distal embolic protection in the stenting population. The SPACE collaborators suggested there was a "tendency towards better results in the carotid endarterectomy group within 30 days, apart from death and hemorrhagic stroke"; however, only 27% of patients received some form of distal embolic protection during the stenting procedure, which may have influenced the outcome. The results may have favored stenting if the use of distal embolic protection been more universal in this study. High surgical risk patients also were not included, and the SPACE conclusions cannot necessarily be generalized toward this patient population.

2004: International Carotid Stenting Study (ICSS)

The ICSS was an RCT enrolling 1713 patients starting in 2004 with the primary goal to establish safety and efficacy. The ICSS addressed some of the concerns and limitations in previous trials, namely, by expanding some of the safety parameters and requirements needed for physicians to enroll in the study. Centers had to have providers that had performed at least 50 carotid operations (10 or more cases per year), and a physician had to have done a minimum of 50 stenting procedures, 10 of which had to be in the carotid artery. This requirement was more rigorous than other previous studies, namely, the EVA-3S trial. Patients enrolled in the study had to have symptomatic carotid stenosis of >50% measured by NASCET criteria (or another noninvasive equivalent), and symptoms had to occur within 12 months prior to the patient's enrollment. Distal embolic protection was used in only 72% of patients.

The primary outcome measured in the first ICSS publication was a 3-year rate of fatal or disabling

stroke in any vascular territory [18]. Between the time of randomization and 120-day post-intervention, the event rate for disabling stroke or death was 4.0% in the stenting group and 3.2% in the surgical group. The composite cardiovascular risk (stroke, myocardial infarction, or death) was 8.5% in patients who received a stent compared to 5.2% in the endarterectomy group ($P = 0.006$). Risks of stroke and overall all-cause death within the stenting group were also higher compared to the endarterectomy group. Cranial nerve palsies were significantly higher in the surgical group, and there were fewer hematomas in the stented patients. Overall, the initial data from ICSS suggested that carotid endarterectomy is a safer treatment option for patients with symptomatic carotid stenosis. At the time of their initial publications, the data from SPACE, EVA-3S, and ICSS all appeared to favor carotid endarterectomy over stenting, specifically because of the high perioperative risk associated with stenting. At the time of the ICSS publication, it was also recommended that endarterectomy remain treatment of choice given the more inferior outcomes linked to stenting.

The long-term data from ICSS [19] was consistent with most other long-term studies: in this study the number of fatal or disabling strokes and the overall 5-year cumulative risk of adverse outcome did not differ between stenting and endarterectomy. However, the ICSS did suggest that *any* stroke (including non-disabling strokes) was more frequent in the stenting population. Restenosis of at least 70% was not significantly different between the two groups. Subgroup analysis was performed in ICSS but not discussed at length because the study lacked the statistical power to draw appropriate conclusions.

2005: Carotid Revascularization Endarterectomy Versus Stenting Trial (CREST)

The CREST trial is one of the most widely cited and discussed trials on intervention for carotid artery stenosis in recent years. This RCT, which began randomization in 2005 and completed enrollment in 2008, included 2502 patients with either symptomatic or asymptomatic stenosis of varying degrees depending on the modality used to detect. Distal embolic protection was used in 96.1% of patients who underwent stenting. Initial results were published in 2010 [20], and a 10-year follow-up was reported in 2016 [21].

The initial study reported no significant dif-

Radiographic Criteria Used for Randomization in CREST

At least one was required for enrollment [20].

- Symptomatic stenosis of at least 50% on angiography
- Symptomatic stenosis of 70% or more on ultrasonography
- Symptomatic stenosis of 70% or more on computed tomographic angiography or magnetic resonance angiography if the stenosis on ultrasound was 50–69%
- Asymptomatic stenosis of at least 60% on angiography
- Asymptomatic stenosis of at least 70% on ultrasonography
- Asymptomatic stenosis of at least 80% on computed tomographic angiography or magnetic resonance angiography if the stenosis on ultrasound was 50–69%

ference in primary composite cardiovascular end point (stroke, myocardial infarction, or death) within the immediate periprocedural period or during the first 4-year postoperative period. There was a higher rate of stroke or death within 4 years of randomization among combined symptomatic and asymptomatic patients with carotid stenosis treated with stenting compared to endarterectomy (6.4% versus 4.7%, $P = 0.03$) with a difference only observed in the asymptomatic population but *not* when patients with symptomatic disease were separately examined (8.0% versus 6.4%, $P = 0.14$). Rates of myocardial infarction were higher in patients treated with endarterectomy (2.3% versus 1.1%, $P = 0.03$). While there was also no significant difference when comparing all symptomatic statuses ($P = 0.84$) or sex ($P = 0.34$)

collectively, there were differences in subgroup analysis. A crossover age of 70 years was noted for patients undergoing stenting or endarterectomy, with patients younger than 70 years of age doing better with stenting and older patients doing better with endarterectomy. Patients with stenting also had far fewer rates of cranial nerve palsies compared to endarterectomy (0.3% versus 4.7%).

In the CREST long-term follow-up study, where the median follow-up was 7.4 years but up to 10 years, there was no significant difference in primary composite end points (stroke, myocardial infarction, or death) between the stenting and endarterectomy groups. When symptomatic patients were separately analyzed from asymptomatic patients, there was no statistical difference at outcomes up to 10 years. Other end points that were of importance were the lack of statistical significance in restenosis, as there was no difference observed in restenosis between the two patient populations. One of the major limitations, however, was the high number of patients lost to follow-up and was not included in this study (36% of patients initially randomized from the 2010 publication). The high loss was mainly from patients who did not consent to long-term follow-up, withdrew from the study, or expired.

The CREST trial and its long-term follow-up, however, illustrated some key findings. The study suggested that "symptomatic status is of relevance in the context of periprocedural risk but ceases to be of useful characterization of patients at 5 and 10 years after revascularization" highlighting the importance of correctly identifying the perioperative risk factors that may contribute to a poor outcome after treatment [21]. The CREST trial also illustrated the importance in applying appropriate patient selection to individual treatments.

2005: Asymptomatic Carotid Trial-1 (ACT-1)

The ACT-1 trial [22] was an RCT comparing CAS *with* distal embolic protection to CEA in patients <80 years of age with severe carotid artery stenosis. A total number of 1453 patients were randomized in a 3:1 stent to surgery ratio from 2005 to 2013 and followed for a mean of 5 years post-procedure. Patients were included if they were <80 years of age with asymptomatic carotid stenosis and specifically *not* a high-risk patient. Patients were considered asymptomatic if they never had a stroke, TIA, or amaurosis fugax within the 180 days prior to enrollment.

All the patients had stenosis of the carotid bifurcation of 70–99% based on ultrasound or angiography *without* contralateral carotid stenosis (>60%). Distal embolization protection was used during the CAS in 97.6% of the patients. The primary outcome was assessed by either (1) a composite cardiovascular event of death, a major or minor stroke (either ipsilateral or contralateral), or a myocardial infarction during the first 30 days after the procedure *or* (2) an ipsilateral stroke during the first 365 days after the procedure.

Comparing the two treatment groups of asymptomatic patients with (1) significant carotid stenosis, (2) <80 years of age, and (3) not at high surgical risk, there was no difference in primary outcome at both 30 days and 1 year when comparing CAS with CEA (3.8% and 3.4%, respectively, $P = 0.01$ for non-inferiority). However, there was a greater number of cranial nerve injury during the periprocedural period in patients treated with endarterectomy (1.1% versus 0.1%, $P = 0.02$).

In a long-term follow-up, there was also no difference in rates of ipsilateral stroke from 30 days to 5 years between the two treatment groups. Five-year overall survival rates were also non-inferior in CAS (93.1%) compared to CEA (94.7%, $P = 0.44$); however, there was a higher rate of restenosis in patients treated with endarterectomy after 1 year post-procedure.

A few of the significant limitations identified by the authors of this chapter were a slightly high rate of patients lost to follow-up (over 10%) and a long period of study enrollment to complete the study (8 years); however, overall, this study highlighted some key points: in the younger and asymptomatic patient population, stenting was non-inferior to endarterectomy, as previously suggested by some of the findings from the trials above. This is likely due to the rather selective patient population that underwent stenting versus endarterectomy, a reflection of good practice in a randomized trial. Furthermore, there was a higher perioperative risk of cranial nerve injury in the surgical arm compared to the endovascular arm. There was also a higher rate of revascularization in the stenting group at 1 year (99.4%) compared to the surgical group (97.4%, $P = 0.005$).

2008: Asymptomatic Carotid Surgery Trial-2 (ACST-2)

The ACST-2 clinical trial is currently an ongoing study to assess asymptomatic patients with high-grade carotid artery stenosis randomized to either carotid artery stenting or endarterectomy. Randomization for the study began in 2008 [23] and has recently had interim results published for patients enrolled up to 2012. A total of 986 patients with asymptomatic stenosis (no ipsilateral carotid territory neurological symptoms for at least 6 months and no previous ipsilateral carotid procedure) with low surgical risk (appropriately medically managed up to the point of randomization with adequate time for recovery from any recent procedures or events and with an expected life-span of at least 5 years) were enrolled. Baseline characteristics and 30-day results were recently reported [24].

The study had a majority of patients with baseline ipsilateral carotid stenosis >70% (96% of patients) and no significant contralateral carotid disease in 63% (a carotid occlusion was present in 8% of patients). Initial 30-day results revealed that both patients who undergo stenting and endarterectomy have a 1.0% risk of major disabling stroke, fatal myocardial infarction, or death with a 2.9% risk for a non-disabling stroke.

The trial plans to report long-term results of this study after all patients randomized undergo a follow-up of 5 years.

Authors' Recommendations

When a physician considers treating carotid artery stenosis, a decision to intervene with either stenting or endarterectomy should be based on the current clinical evidence along with provider experience. However, as seen above, the timeline and extensive history of these clinical trials can make decisions quite difficult and confusing, given the convoluted and extensive literature that currently exists. This summary is intended to weave together the past 20+ years of clinical evidence with modern medical practice.

Some general considerations need to be addressed about the abovementioned trials. None of the randomized trials published to date have examined the role of intense medical therapy compared to revascularization *with* intense medical therapy. However, the CREST-2 trial is currently underway to examine the role of intense medical therapy versus revascularization with modern techniques (i.e., endarterectomy or stenting with distal embolic protection). This study is currently ongoing and its protocol was recently published [25].

All of the trials illustrated the importance of identifying perioperative risk to individual patients. The CREST trial highlighted the importance of age as a consideration for intervention: older patients (above 70 years of age) did better with endarterectomy, whereas younger patients did better with stenting [20]. However, this information should be weighed with a patient's perioperative risk factors, as patients undergoing endarterectomy had a higher risk of myocardial infarction, whereas patients undergoing stenting had a higher risk of stroke. These potential perioperative complications should also be delicately weighed in patients with an extensive cardiac history or vasculopathy. The rates of stroke or death among patients after stenting and endarterectomy were lower when compared to the SPACE, EVA-3S, and ICSS trials. However, it is important to note the advancements that were being made in patient safety, selection, and physician training for the procedure during the time of these trials. "High surgical risk" itself should not preclude a patient from stenting. Yadav et al., in the SAPPHIRE trial, noted some of the highest-risk candidates for stenting "resulted in rates of complications for all major adverse events (death, stroke or myocardial infarction) that were statistically equivalent to or lower than those among patients who underwent endarterectomy both in the overall study population and in the subgroups" [13]. Patients with stenting also had lower cranial nerve palsy rates and higher target vessel revascularization compared to endarterectomy. Finally, both SPACE and ICSS had a rather low use of distal embolic protection during stenting, thereby certainly potentially increasing the risk of ischemic stroke following vessel manipulation during endovascular treatment.

Given the information from clinical trials (particularly later investigatons) combined with clinical experience, it is the suggestion of the authors for the following:

Appropriate choices for CEA:

1. Anatomically difficult to access, i.e., C2 vertebral body level or higher
2. Contralateral carotid occlusion
3. Isolated hemispheres, i.e., an absence of collateral circulation from the contralateral or posterior cerebral circulation
4. Contralateral cranial nerve palsy
5. Ipsilateral restenosis, previous irradiation, or major surgery
6. Age <70

Appropriate choices for CAS:

1. Anatomically accessible lesions
2. Type III arch, severe atherosclerotic disease aortic arch
3. Age 70–80

Consideration About Clinical Equipoise

Consideration of the patient, their age, medical comorbidity, and the natural history of atherosclerotic disease and stroke is important. Patients over the age of 80 with incidental asymptomatic carotid artery disease may not benefit from intervention whether it is CEA or CAS. The 5-year nontarget vessel rate versus the risk of CEA or CAS in this cohort is essentially the same and approaches 20%. Thus, a strong argument can be made to only treat *symptomatic* target vessels which have failed best medical therapy. We are sworn to "do no harm," and subjecting patients with asymptomatic disease to significant periprocedural morbidity in the absence of compelling data to suggest significant benefit should be avoided.

Review Questions

1. Which of the following are false: the Carotid and Vertebral Artery Transluminal Angioplasty Study (CAVATAS) trial:
   A. Was a multicenter randomized control trial with a generalized patient population
   B. Was initiated at a time when carotid stents were commercially available
   C. Included both symptomatic and asymptomatic patients with carotid artery stenosis
   D. Used stenting as second-line treatment for patients randomized to endovascular therapy, only after they failed attempted treatment with balloon angioplasty
   E. Did not exclude patients with contralateral carotid artery occlusions

   Answer: B: Experimental carotid stents were only in development in 1992 when the trial initiated. The first FDA-approved carotid stent was not released for commercial use until 1994.

2. The International Carotid Stenting Study (ICSS) addressed limitations and safety concerns by:
   A. Certifying that centers enrolled in the study had surgeons who performed at least 50 carotid operations (10 or more cases per year).

   B. Requiring that interventionalists had performed a minimum or 50 stenting procedures, 10 of which had to be in the carotid artery.
   C. Patients had to have symptomatic carotid stenosis >50% measured by NASCET criteria or another noninvasive equivalent.
   D. All of the above are true.

   Answer: D

3. The Carotid Revascularization Endarterectomy versus Stenting Trial (CREST):
   A. Included both symptomatic and asymptomatic patients with distal embolic protection in over 95% of patients randomized to endovascular treatment.
   B. Demonstrated a higher rate of myocardial infarction in patients treated with endarterectomy during the periprocedural period.
   C. Revealed patients had fewer cranial nerve palsies with endovascular treatment compared to endarterectomy.
   D. Demonstrated there was no significant difference in stroke, myocardial infarction, or death between stenting and endarterectomy at a 10-year follow-up.
   E. All of the above are true.

   Answer: D

References

1. Bonati LH, Ederle J, McCabe DJ, Dobson J, CAVATAS Investigators, et al. Long-term risk of carotid restenosis in patients randomly assigned to endovascular treatment or endarterectomy in the carotid and vertebral artery transluminal angioplasty study: long-term follow-up of a randomised trial. Lancet Neurol. 2009;8(10):908–17.
2. North American Symptomatic Carotid Endarterectomy Trial Collaborators, Barnett HJM, Taylor DW, Haynes

RB, et al. Beneficial effect of carotid endarterectomy in symptomatic patients with high-grade carotid stenosis. N Engl J Med. 1991;325(7):445–53.

3. Randomised trial of endarterectomy for recently symptomatic carotid stenosis: final results of the MRC European carotid surgery trial (ECST). Lancet. 1998;351(9113):1379–87.

4. Rothwell PM, Eliasziw M, Gutnikov SA, Fox AJ, Carotid Endarterectomy Trialists' Collaboration, et al. Analysis of pooled data from the randomised controlled trials of endarterectomy for symptomatic carotid stenosis. Lancet. 2003;361(9352):107–16.

5. Yadav JS, Roubin GS, Iyer S, Vitek J, King P, Jordan WD, Fisher WS. Elective stenting of the extracranial carotid arteries. Circulation. 1997;95(2):376–81.

6. Salzler GG, Farber A, Rybin DV, Doros G, Siracuse JJ, Eslami MH. The association of carotid revascularization endarterectomy versus stent trial (CREST) and centers for medicare and medicaid services carotid guideline publication on utilization and outcomes of carotid stenting among "high-risk" patients. J Vasc Surg. 2017;66(1):104–111.e1.

7. Sidhu PS, Allan PL. Ultrasound assessment of internal carotid artery stenosis. Clin Radiol. 1997;52(9):654–8.

8. Endovascular versus surgical treatment in patients with carotid stenosis in the carotid and vertebral artery transluminal angioplasty study (CAVATAS): a randomised trial. Lancet. 2001;357(9270):1729–37.

9. Mas JL, Chatellier G, Beyssen B, EVA-3S Investigators. Carotid angioplasty and stenting with and without cerebral protection: clinical alert from the endarterectomy versus angioplasty in patients with symptomatic severe carotid stenosis (EVA-3S) trial. Stroke. 2004;35(1):e18–20

10. Mas JL, Arquizan C, Calvet D, Viguier A, EVA-3S Investigators, et al. Long-term follow-up study of endarterectomy versus angioplasty in patients with symptomatic severe carotid stenosis trial. Stroke. 2014;45(9):2750–6.

11. Mas JL, Chatellier G, Beyssen B, Branchereau A, EVA-3S Investigators, et al. Endarterectomy versus stenting in patients with symptomatic severe carotid stenosis. N Engl J Med. 2006;355(16):1660–71.

12. Mas JL, Trinquart L, Leys D, Albucher JF, EVA-3S investigators, et al. Endarterectomy versus angioplasty in patients with symptomatic severe carotid stenosis (EVA-3S) trial: results up to 4 years from a randomised, multicentre trial. Lancet Neurol. 2008;7(10):885–92.

13. Yadav JS, Wholey MH, Kuntz RE, Fayad P, Stenting and Angioplasty with Protection in Patients at High Risk for Endarterectomy Investigators, et al. Protected carotid-artery stenting versus endarterectomy in high-risk patients. N Engl J Med. 2004;351(15):1493–501.

14. Gurm HS, Yadav JS, Fayad P, Katzen BT, SAPPHIRE Investigators, et al. Long-term results of carotid stenting versus endarterectomy in high-risk patients. N Engl J Med. 2008;358(15):1572–9.

15. SPACE Collaborative Group, Ringleb PA, Allenberg J, Brückmann H, et al. 30 day results from the SPACE trial of stent-protected angioplasty versus carotid endarterectomy in symptomatic patients: a randomised non-inferiority trial. Lancet. 2006;368(9543):1239–47.

16. Eckstein HH, Ringleb P, Allenberg JR, Berger J, et al. Results of the stent-protected angioplasty versus carotid endarterectomy (SPACE) study to treat symptomatic stenoses at 2 years: a multinational, prospective, randomised trial. Lancet Neurol. 2008;7(10):893–902.

17. Stingele R, Berger J, Alfke K, Eckstein HH, et al. Clinical and angiographic risk factors for stroke and death within 30 days after carotid endarterectomy and stent-protected angioplasty: a subanalysis of the SPACE study. Lancet Neurol. 2008;7(3):216–22.

18. International Carotid Stenting Study investigators, Ederle J, Dobson J, Featherstone RL, et al. Carotid artery stenting compared with endarterectomy in patients with symptomatic carotid stenosis (international carotid stenting study): an interim analysis of a randomised controlled trial. Lancet. 2010;375(9719):985–97.

19. Bonati LH, Dobson J, Featherstone RL, Ederle J, et al. Long-term outcomes after stenting versus endarterectomy for treatment of symptomatic carotid stenosis: the international carotid stenting study (ICSS) randomised trial. Lancet. 2015;385(9967):529–38.

20. Brott TG, Hobson RW, Howard G, Roubin GS, CREST Investigators. Stenting versus endarterectomy for treatment of carotid-artery stenosis. N Engl J Med. 2010;363(1):11–23.

21. Brott TG, Howard G, Roubin GS, Meschia JF, CREST Investigators, et al. Long-term results of stenting versus endarterectomy for carotid-artery stenosis. N Engl J Med. 2016;374(11):1021–31.

22. Rosenfield K, Matsumura JS, Chaturvedi S, Riles T, ACT I Investigators, et al. Randomized trial of stent versus surgery for asymptomatic carotid stenosis. N Engl J Med. 2016;374(11):1011–20.

23. Rudarakanchana N, Dialynas M, Halliday A. Asymptomatic carotid surgery trial-2 (ACST-2): rationale for a randomised clinical trial comparing carotid endarterectomy with carotid artery stenting in patients with asymptomatic carotid artery stenosis. Eur J Vasc Endovasc Surg. 2009;38(2):239–42.

24. ACST-2 Collaborative Group, Halliday A, Bulbulia R, Gray W, et al. Status update and interim results from the asymptomatic carotid surgery trial-2 (ACST-2). Eur J Vasc Endovasc Surg. 2013;46(5):510–8.

25. Howard VJ, Meschia JF, Lal BK, Turan TN, CREST-2 Study Investigators, et al. Carotid revascularization and medical management for asymptomatic carotid stenosis: protocol of the CREST-2 clinical trials. Int J Stroke. 2017;12(7):770–8.

Technical Aspects of Carotid Artery Stenting

16

Robert G. Molnar and Nitin G. Malhotra

Indications

Previous chapters have outlined the results of CAS and CEA trials. The current indications for carotid artery stenting (CAS) include symptomatic patients with carotid stenosis greater than 70% who are determined to be high risk for surgery following appropriate surgical consultation [1, 2]. Patients can also undergo CAS when enrolled in clinical trials under the auspices of the FDA.

Procedure Planning

One of the critical aspects of safe endovascular carotid intervention is to ensure that the anatomy present does not confer a higher risk from intervention to the patient. Computed tomography angiography (CTA) allows an assessment of the arch, great vessels, and carotid anatomy with specific attention to the angulations and degree of calcifications. Both a magnetic resonance angiography (MRA) or a diagnostic arch and carotid angiogram can also be obtained, but the first limits a good assessment of the calcification burden, while the second is invasive and thus carries the risks associated with carotid endovascular intervention, the major being stroke. By assessing the anatomy and calcification pre-procedurally, one can assess whether carotid cannulation can be safely and effectively performed. Excessive calcification, tortuosity, and severe angulations to the great vessels should be avoided and in some cases would be absolute contraindications and surgical endarterectomy performed. It is very important to note that a meticulous approach to any carotid intervention is mandatory, as the consequences of embolization or thrombosis are much more devastating than in other vascular beds treated via endovascular means. Patients can also be approached with an arch and carotid arteriogram with intent to treat, recognizing that unfavorable arch anatomy, excessive calcification, or unfavorable carotid anatomy might lead to a diagnostic study only based upon the procedural findings. A thorough discussion with the patient and their family is important so that their expectations are realistic and that often decisions on treatment have to be made real-time during the procedure.

Prior to the procedure, all patients should be counseled on expectations during the procedure and a detailed neurologic exam completed to document their baseline status. If not already on dual antiplatelet therapy, they should receive 300 mg of Plavix and should also be on aspirin

R. G. Molnar (✉) · N. G. Malhotra
Division of Vascular Surgery, Michigan Vascular Center, McLaren Regional Medical Center, Michigan State University, Flint, MI, USA

© The Editor(s) (if applicable) and The Author(s) 2018
S. S. Hans (ed.), *Extracranial Carotid and Vertebral Artery Disease*,
https://doi.org/10.1007/978-3-319-91533-3_16

therapy. The conduct of the procedure should be reviewed with the patient so they are comfortable with instructions of breathing and head positioning. The importance of not moving during image acquisition should be stressed, and it is often helpful to review the instructions that will be used during the procedure. CAS can be performed via the transfemoral route or a transcervical route requiring surgical cutdown. The procedural steps are outlined below with attention to best practice steps to avoid complications.

Transfemoral Procedural Details

Patients are placed in standard supine position with blood pressure, electrocardiogram tracing, and pulse oximetry monitored. Supplemental oxygen should be used routinely with any conscious sedation, and both groin regions are prepped to allow access to the best femoral artery for safe access. Standard angiographic equipment is utilized, and strict attention to avoiding air embolization is critical.

Once safe femoral access is obtained, the patient is anticoagulated with weight-based heparin, argatroban, or anticoagulant of choice with activated clotting time (ACT) levels documented between 250 and 300. A pigtail catheter is advanced into the ascending aortic arch and the image intensifier is then rotated until the catheter is visualized in its widest plane. Most textbooks report using a standard 30° left anterior oblique view; however, occasionally the best angle may be up to 50°. This becomes very important as some with an aortic arch that appears to be very angulated at 30° may actually appear more normal using a steeper image intensifier angle (e.g., >30°) due to the elongation of the aortic arch in some patients.

After confirming that the anatomy is acceptable for safe carotid cannulation, the anticoagulation level is confirmed by ACT. It is better to selectively cannulate the contralateral carotid first as this will allow evidence of any cross-hemispheric flow with the contralateral carotid injection. The catheter to be used for cannulation is at the discretion of the interventionist.

For a standard type I arch and many mild type II arches, a JB1 or Berenstein catheter is usually an excellent choice, but many catheters have a similar shape and profile and can be used for selective vessel catheterization. For a type II arch or severely angulated origins of the great vessels, use a Simmons 1 or Vitek catheter for safe cannulation. It is best to have a few catheters that are used routinely, as this familiarity with the catheters allows you to develop a significant "feel" for the catheter and how it will react with tortuosity and resistance and how it will react to your manipulations. In summary, the catheters routinely used are the pigtail for a flush arch aortogram, a JB1 for cannulation of most type I arches, and a Simmons 1 for type II or bovine arch configurations (Fig. 16.1). While there are many brands and shapes available for selective catheterization of the great vessels, it is most important that you identify a few as your catheters of choice to allow for a reliable response during manipulation and to avoid excessive "attempts" which increases the risk of embolization.

The selective catheter should be advanced to the mid-common carotid artery (assuming the disease is distal to this segment), and anterior-posterior (AP), lateral, and oblique images should be obtained, including intracerebral runoff to assess for cross fill from one hemisphere to the other. Once the contralateral artery is assessed,

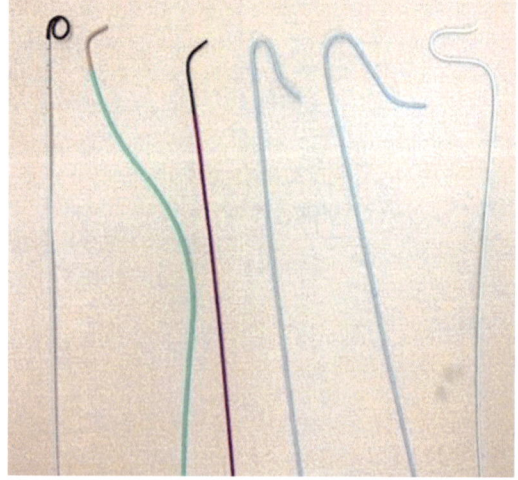

Fig. 16.1 Catheters—from L to R: Pigtail, JB1, Berenstein, Simmons 1, Simmons 2, Vitek

the ipsilateral or treatment side is selected. Again, baseline AP, lateral, and oblique images are obtained to quantify and measure the degree of stenosis. Visualizing bony landmarks as to the distal extent of the lesion will assist with stent positioning and deployment.

Vessel reference measurements are made and include the diameter of the mid to distal ICA where filter placement would be anticipated. The CCA just proximal to the bifurcation will determine the size of the stent used. The stent size is chosen to be a minimum of 1 mm wider than the CCA measurement. The distal filter size is slightly larger than the diameter of the distal ICA to ensure complete filter apposition to the vessel wall. If the lesion is severely stenosed, it is recommended that pre-dilatation with a 3.5 or 4 mm balloon be used. This will allow safe passage of the stent delivery catheter and, more importantly, limit the chance that the "olive tip" of the delivery system does not get caught in the stent cells upon attempted removal. If post-dilatation is anticipated, a 0.014 angioplasty balloon is used that is of equal size to the distal ICA reference vessel diameter. Once all the equipment is prepared/flushed and ready for use, a short floppy tip Amplatz wire (1 cm floppy tip) is slowly advanced through the selective catheter, and the wire tip is placed to the distal CCA. If needed, the wire can be advanced and selectively placed in the external carotid artery for additional wire support, but it is rarely needed. By not crossing the bifurcation (which is usually a diseased segment) with the wire or a selective catheter to assist with ECA selection, there is less chance of manipulation of the diseased segment and embolization without distal protection in place. However, for extreme tortuosity or type II arches, selection of the external carotid artery will help with safe sheath positioning. While maintaining fluoroscopic monitoring of the wire tip, the short femoral sheath is removed, and a 90 cm sheath is slowly advanced over the Amplatz wire. It is recommended that a Tuohy-Borst connector be used rather than a Check-Flo® valve as air will less likely be introduced with the back-bleeding that occurs with the Tuohy-Borst use. As the sheath is slowly advanced while the wire tip is monitored,

the sheath is placed into the CCA, and the dilator is held in place as the sheath is advanced to the distal CCA. It is very important to note that the dilator for the sheath can extend beyond the sheath tip by 3–6 cm and is difficult to visualize by fluoroscopy. This can lead to inadvertent dilator passage beyond the 0.035 wire without recognition and can lead to intimal damage or dissection. For this reason, once the radiopaque sheath tip is seen in the proximal CCA, the dilator and wire are pinned, and the sheath is slowly advanced over the wire to the distal CCA or 2 cm proximal to a lesion in the CCA.

With the sheath in place, the wire and dilator are slowly removed, and the sheath is thoroughly aspirated/debubbled. The sheath is then connected to a power injector, and the line is prepped and debubbled using the three-way stopcock. A manifold system may also be used, but it is imperative that strict adherence to avoiding air embolization is maintained. An additional magnified angiogram is obtained with attention to centering the lesion on the viewing monitor. This allows for the proximal CCA to the distal ICA to be imaged. A pre-assessment neurological check is made by having the patient follow motor commands of the contralateral extremities with assessment by cath lab staff. Under fluoroscopic guidance, the distal protection device is advanced past the lesion and positioned in the distal ICA, preferably in a straight segment. Should there be significant tortuosity in the ICA, it may be safer to approach the lesion with retrograde flow protection using the MOMA device which provides CCA and ECA occlusion and retrograde flow through the ICA for distal cerebral protection. After the filter is deployed, a small amount of contrast is delivered to ensure antegrade flow through the filter and to ensure the lesion location has not moved from the bony landmarks established with the placement of the filter. The stent is advanced over the wire and past the lesion then slowly brought back to the target lesion based upon the bony landmarks to remove any redundancy in the system and to help prevent the stent from jumping during deployment. A small puff of contrast is administered to ensure positioning prior to stent deployment. If the stent delivery system occludes the antegrade flow, the stent can still be deployed using the bony landmarks established prior to loss of antegrade flow.

After stent deployment, another small puff of contrast is administered to check for antegrade flow, and a neurological test is performed. If the stent has a 30% or less residual stenosis, it is left as is. If greater than 30%, angioplasty is performed based upon reference vessel diameter of the ICA. If angioplasty is performed, the patient can be given atropine for possible bradycardia at the interventionist's discretion. After two orthogonal views are obtained to ensure no additional intervention is required, the filter is recaptured and another neurological test completed. AP and lateral views including intracranial views are obtained to document post-procedure flow. The sheath is then withdrawn over a J wire and exchanged for a short sheath. There is no need to reselect the contralateral carotid artery for completion arteriogram. A femoral closure device is used at the discretion of the interventionalist.

Trans-carotid Artery Revascularization (TCAR)

In patients with steep aortic arches, significant proximal vessel or ICA tortuosity, or excessive proximal calcification, the ENROUTE® TCAR approach can be utilized. This method requires 5 cm of normal CCA proximal to the bifurcation as measured from the clavicle. This measurement is easily obtained on pre-procedural carotid duplex examination. It is also advised that the CCA be relatively disease-free at the proposed access site. Patients can be approached either under general anesthesia or under regional block. The patient is positioned as for a standard carotid endarterectomy with a shoulder roll in place and the neck rotated to allow for dissection of the proximal carotid artery. Either a transverse or small vertical incision is created just above the clavicle to dissect to the CCA. Approximately 2 cm of the artery is circumferentially exposed with care to avoid nerve or lymphatic injury. After exposure,

the proximal artery is encircled with a Rummel tourniquet (umbilical tape with short red rubber segment to allow for proximal occlusion) or vessel loop control. A 0.018 microcatheter is placed ensuring that the wire advancement is not beyond the bifurcation during placement. If the CCA is located in a deep location in the neck, the microcatheter may be tunneled through a counterincision to aid in appropriate angulation for safe arterial access in order to prevent dissection. An arteriogram is performed confirming adequate anatomy to proceed with safe sheath placement and stenting.

An 8 French femoral venous sheath supplied with the ENROUTE® system is placed in the contralateral femoral vein under ultrasound guidance, and the sheath is flushed and suture secured to the thigh. The micropuncture sheath is exchanged out for the ENROUTE® 6 French carotid sheath under fluoroscopic guidance to ensure the system wire does not cross the bifurcation/lesion. The sheath is flushed and the retrograde filter flow system is connected first to the carotid sheath and then to the venous sheath, and passive retrograde flow is established without CCA occlusion. Retrograde flow is confirmed as is the patient's hemodynamic status (SBP should be maintained between 140 and 160 mmHg) and anticoagulation status. As with the transfemoral approach, all intervention equipment should be prepped and flushed ready for use. The Rummel or vessel loop on the CCA is then actuated to occlude the vessel, and retrograde flow is again confirmed. A 0.014 wire is advanced fluoroscopically into the distal ICA, the stent is positioned, and a small amount of contrast is administered with cessation of retrograde flow to confirm stent position. The stent is deployed, the stent is post-dilated if needed, and two orthogonal images are attained with brief retrograde flow cessation prior to removing the 0.014 wire. The CCA is then opened by releasing the Rummel or vessel loop to again establish passive retrograde flow, and finally the system is disengaged to allow normal antegrade flow. The ENROUTE® filter system is drained into the femoral sheath, and the filter can be checked for debris. Completion angiograms are obtained, and the 6 Fr sheath is removed with suture repair of the CCA. The wound is closed and the femoral sheath removed.

Complications and Salvage Techniques

The most dreaded complication of CAS is stroke, and this can occur due to thrombosis or embolization. Thrombosis should be a rare occurrence if patients are being treated with dual antiplatelet agents and are adequately anticoagulated during the procedure. During transfemoral CAS, should there be a change in the neurological status of the patient, a brisk aspiration of the sheath should be done to eliminate thrombotic, embolic, or inadvertent air embolus within the carotid system. Simultaneously, the vitals should be checked with blood pressure, heart rate, and oxygen saturation confirmed. A small amount of contrast can be administered to evaluate for antegrade flow through the filter system. Should there be occlusion of the ICA flow, quickly evaluate the stent for deformity or irregularity. An export catheter can be advanced up to the level of the filter and aspirated; however embolic or thrombotic material of larger size will be more easily aspirated with the 6 Fr sheath. The sheath can be slowly advanced through the stent up to the filter and a number of aspirations can be performed which will usually remove any debris. Any spasm related to manipulation of the ICA can be relieved with intra-arterial injection of nitroglycerin. If there is suspicion of thrombus, 1–2 mg of alteplase can be administered directly into the ICA. The filter retrieval system can then be used to partially collapse the filter (to avoid spillage around the filter should there be significant embolic load) and bring it directly into the sheath. Aspirations should again be made to ensure no residual material remains and arteriograms can be obtained to assess the intracranial flow, comparing them to the pre-intervention images. Intracranial defects should be documented, but there should be no attempt

at retrieval unless the interventionist is skilled in intracerebral interventions. Consultation with a neuro-interventionist should be made and the patient's clinical status supported.

Occasionally, angioplasty and stenting of the carotid bulb will result in activation of the associated baroreceptor, and the patient will experience bradycardia or even cardiac pause. This can be pretreated in patients with relative bradycardia by administering 1 mg atropine prior to stenting and angioplasty. Should the heart rate fall during angioplasty, it is imperative to immediately deflate the balloon and reassess the heart rate. Asking the patient to cough can often help elevate the HR. Should there be persistent bradycardia with hypotension, temporary pacing may be necessary.

TCAR has proven to have the lowest stroke rate in any reported prospective, multicenter trials [3]. While it appears there is less risk of embolization given the initiation of retrograde flow, the fact that embolic material can be significant underscores the need to be diligent in the treatment of carotid lesions (Fig. 16.2). Just as for transfemoral CAS, similar principles would govern any change in the patient's neurologic status undergoing a TCAR procedure. An immediate aspiration of the sheath should be performed in an attempt to remove any thrombotic, embolic, or air embolus complication. Ensuring safe sheath placement to avoid any dissection of the CCA is also important, and should any evidence of dissection be found, angiographic evaluation should be made with possible open repair or stenting of the dissection if amenable. In patients undergoing TCAR with sedation and regional block, should there be evidence that retrograde flow is not tolerated, the procedure should be stopped, and there should be a consideration of standard endarterectomy with shunting or transitioning to a CAS with filter protection to allow antegrade flow during the procedure.

Other complications from arterial access can occur as with any endovascular intervention; however the critical importance of meticulous technique when intervening on the carotid arteries cannot be overemphasized. There is very

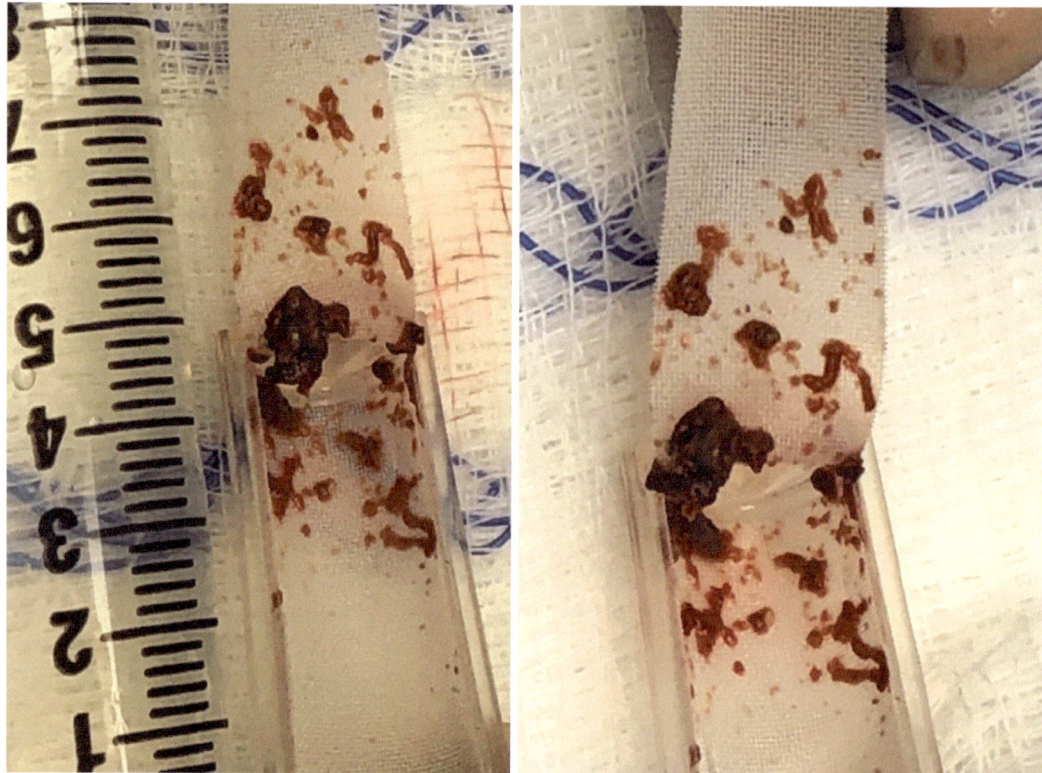

Fig. 16.2 Embolic debris captured in a TCAR procedure using retrograde flow

minimal room for error, and any complication can have devastating consequences. Strict attention to sheath management, to anticoagulation status, and to establishing a team with knowledge of the procedure is paramount to safe and effective CAS. In addition, efficiency of time is important as any delays encountered during the intervention can lead to potential complications. All members of the team should be focused on the procedure and potential distractions minimalized.

Post-procedural Care

Patients are admitted for 23-h observation to include blood pressure monitoring, access site evaluation, and neurological assessments. Any hypotension or hypertension should be appropriately treated and change in neurologic exam immediately assessed. Peri-procedural strokes can occur due to late embolization through the stent struts or due to thrombus formation. Patients should be

continued on dual antiplatelet medication as well as a cholesterol-lowering or cholesterol-stabilizing agent. Carotid duplex exams should be performed at 1, 6, and 12 months followed by yearly examinations to assess for restenosis.

Contraindications/Pitfalls to Avoid

The arch anatomy is one detail that cannot be overlooked nor its importance disregarded. Steep arches in which the origins of the great vessels have shifted to a right inferior orientation to the apex of the arch make cannulation and safe delivery of the stent delivery catheter difficult and can lead to inadvertent embolization from the aortic arch itself. The standard classification of arch anatomy as it pertains to safe cannulation of the great vessel rates the complexity of the arch as type I, II, or III. In general, as the great vessels come off more proximally on the ascending aorta, the ability to traverse up

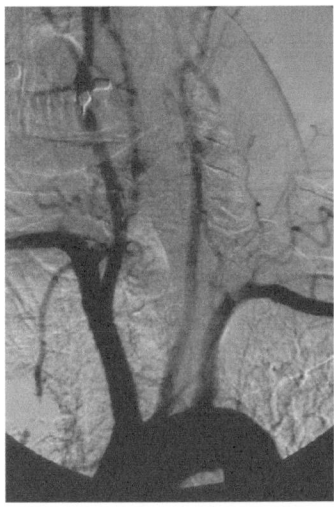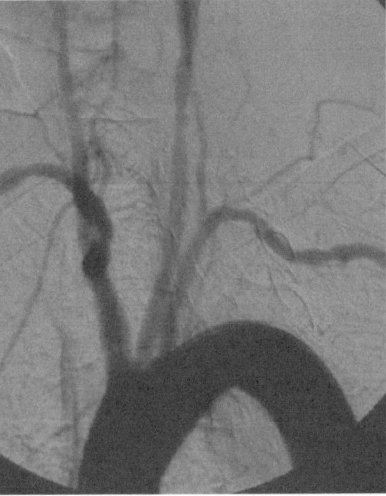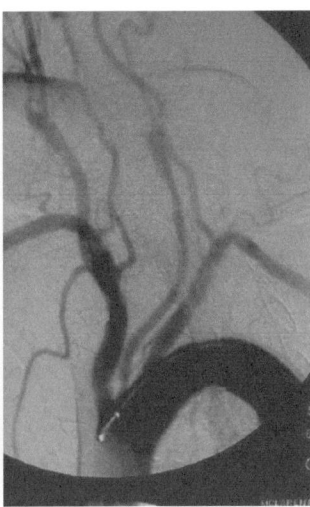

Fig. 16.3 Proximal progression of the origins of the great vessels for a type I (left), type II (middle), and type III (right) arch. From: Molnar RG, Zuhaili B. Carotid angioplasty and stenting. In: Hans SS, Shepard AD, Weaver MR, Bove P, Long GW. Endovascular and open vascular reconstruction: a practical approach. Copyright © 2017, CRC Press, reproduced by permission of Taylor & Francis Books UK

Fig. 16.4 Complex lesions prone to embolization with intervention. From: Molnar RG, Zuhaili B. Carotid angioplasty and stenting. In: Hans SS, Shepard AD, Weaver MR, Bove P, Long GW. Endovascular and open vascular reconstruction: a practical approach. Copyright © 2017, CRC Press, reproduced by permission of Taylor & Francis Books UK

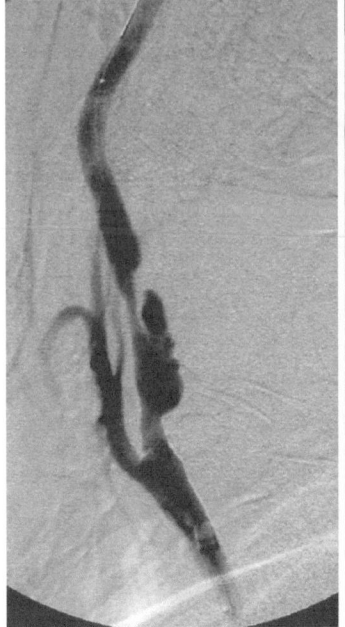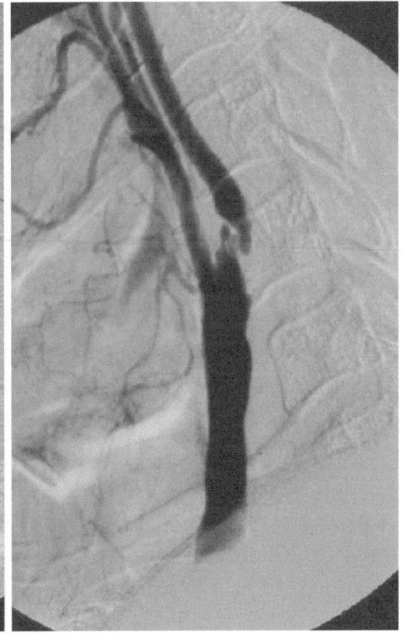

the descending aorta, over a peaked aortic arch, inferiorly into the ascending aorta followed by acute angulations to the origins of the great vessels becomes more difficult. This results in additional manipulation of catheters in a potentially diseased aortic arch. While some cannulations will be nearly impossible, others can be performed with excellent endovascular skills; yet this may confer accepting a significant additional embolization risk. Figure 16.3 provides angiographic depictions of three examples of aortic arch anatomy.

Concentric calcification or severe complexity of the lesion itself (Fig. 16.4), thrombus/near

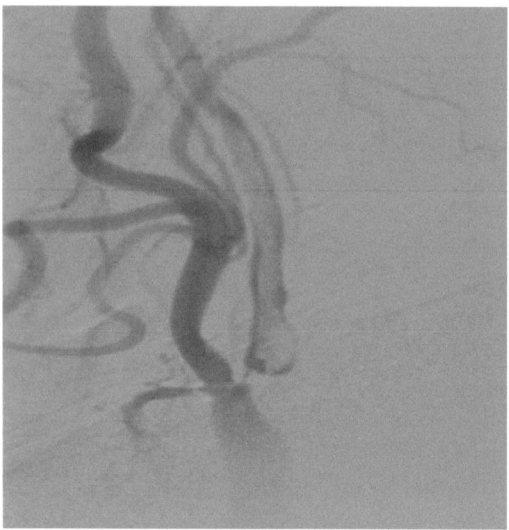 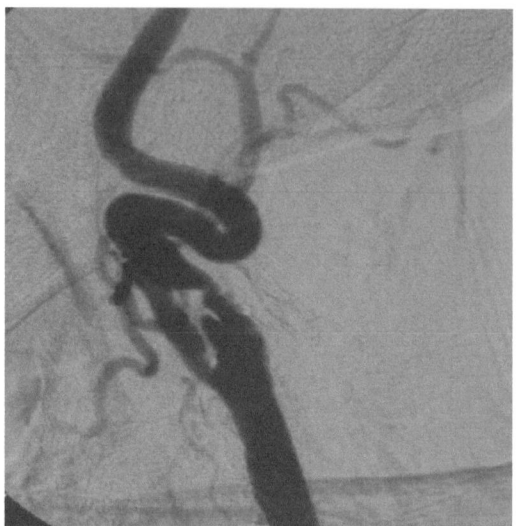

Fig. 16.5 Severe carotid stenosis with thrombus. From: Molnar RG, Zuhaili B. Carotid angioplasty and stenting. In: Hans SS, Shepard AD, Weaver MR, Bove P, Long GW. Endovascular and open vascular reconstruction: a practical approach. Copyright © 2017, CRC Press, reproduced by permission of Taylor & Francis Books UK

Fig. 16.6 Excessive ICA tortuosity making filter placement contraindicated. From: Molnar RG, Zuhaili B. Carotid angioplasty and stenting. In: Hans SS, Shepard AD, Weaver MR, Bove P, Long GW. Endovascular and open vascular reconstruction: a practical approach. Copyright © 2017, CRC Press, reproduced by permission of Taylor & Francis Books UK

occlusion (Fig. 16.5), and excessive tortuosity of the distal internal carotid artery if distal filter protection is to be used (Fig. 16.6) are all relative and, depending on severity, can be definitive contraindications to CAS.

Conclusions

Carotid artery stenting (CAS) has been proven to be safe and effective in certain patient populations. While some patients are deemed to be high risk for carotid endarterectomy, other patients are certainly high risk for CAS as outlined above. In addition, our recent work has identified stent fractures in patient's having received CAS, and the long-term durability remains to be studied. Patients at high risk for CAS include those with type II and III arches, those with arch and circumferential carotid calcification, and those with severe ICA tortuosity, especially adjacent to the area of dis-

ease. New technologies and approaches, such as TCAR, do eliminate some of the risks, but patient selection will always require a complete understanding of potential complications and steps taken to eliminate risks as possible. In the case of a procedural complication, steps reviewed in the above chapter can help facilitate an acceptable outcome; however proper selection of patients will allow for these risks to occur in very limited circumstances. It will be important to continue a critical assessment of carotid stent technology to finely focus on those characteristics that create a higher risk for patients undergoing CAS and to better define who will be best suited for CAS versus CEA. While this clarity is being defined, it is of critical importance that interventionists who either perform or wish to perform carotid interventions pay close attention to a meticulous approach to patient selection as well as procedural technique.

Review Questions

1. Relevant contraindications for transfemoral carotid artery stenting include all of the following, except:
   A. Circumferential calcification
   B. A type I arch
   C. Thrombus
   D. Internal carotid artery tortuosity

   Answer: B

2. During transfemoral carotid stenting with filter protection, there is loss of antegrade flow, and the patient exhibits neurological changes. Bailout procedures include all of the following, except:
   A. Flushing the sheath
   B. Using an export catheter
   C. Administering alteplase
   D. Aspirating the sheath

   Answer: A

3. TCAR (trans-carotid artery revascularization) might be a better approach to carotid stenting in which of the following circumstances?
   A. Disease in the common carotid artery 4 cm above the clavicle
   B. Patients with a type III aortic arch
   C. Patients with a contralateral recurrent laryngeal nerve injury
   D. Patients with bilateral common femoral venous thrombosis

   Answer: B

4. Which of the following regarding the procedure of carotid artery stenting is true?
   A. Patients should be on antiplatelet therapy, but anticoagulation is not needed.
   B. TCAR should be performed with the SBP < 110.
   C. Strokes will not occur if a distal protection filter is used.
   D. A meticulous attention to detail is needed for those performing CAS.

   Answer: D

References

1. Brott TG, Hobson RW II, Howard G, Roubin GS, et al. Stenting versus endarterectomy for treatment of carotid-artery stenosis. N Engl J Med. 2010;363:11–23.
2. Hobson RW, Howard VJ, Roubin GS, et al. Carotid artery stenting is associated with increased complications in octogenarians: 30-day stroke and death rates in CREST lead-in phase. J Vasc Surg. 2004;40(6):1106–11.
3. Kowlek CJ, Jaff MR, Leal JI, Hopkins LN, Shah RM, Hanover TM, Macdonald S, Canbria RP. Results of the ROADSTER multicenter trial of transcarotid stenting with dynamic flow reversal. J Vasc Surg. 2015;62:1227–35.

Mitchell R. Weaver

Introduction

Arterial occlusive disease of the supra-aortic trunk vessels, namely, the brachiocephalic artery (BCA), proximal left common carotid artery (LCCA), and proximal left subclavian artery (LSCA), which is symptomatic and requires intervention, is not frequently encountered [1, 2]. Symptoms may manifest as neurologic events such as stroke, transient ischemic attack, or vertebrobasilar insufficiency when the cerebral hemispheres are involved or tissue loss or effort fatigue when affecting the upper extremities. Treatment options in these cases include both extra and transthoracic open arterial reconstructions and endoluminal arterial reconstructions. The location and extent of the disease as well as patient's overall physical condition are factors in the choice of repair.

Atherosclerosis is the primary pathologic process leading to supra-aortic trunk vessel occlusive disease; however other etiologies exist including arteritis, congenital malformations, and mechanical or radiation-induced trauma. Each of these processes may lead to symptoms and the need for intervention [3–6]. The pathophysiologic mechanism by which these lesions produce symptoms is the result of tissue ischemia secondary to low flow or atheroembolization.

Clinical presentation to the vascular surgeon may include the asymptomatic finding of unequal blood pressures between the arms or an abnormal pulse exam, neurologic symptoms, or upper extremity symptoms. Neurologic symptoms include focal hemispheric symptoms, such as stroke, TIA, or amaurosis fugax, or more global bilateral hemispheric or vertebrobasilar symptoms. Upper extremity symptoms include complaint of arm fatigue with activity which may also be associated with vertebrobasilar symptoms (subclavian steal syndrome) or evidence of atheroembolization in the distal upper extremity. Patients with prior coronary artery bypass via an internal mammary artery may present with symptoms coronary insufficiency.

As atherosclerosis is the most common etiology of supra-aortic trunk arterial occlusive disease, these patients should be thoroughly evaluated for associated risk factors including tobacco abuse, dyslipidemia, hypertension, diabetes mellitus, renal insufficiency, and family history of atherosclerosis. Identified risk factors should be aggressively medically optimized. Symptoms or history of arterial occlusive disease in other vascular beds including the coronary arteries and lower extremities (claudication) should be sought.

The physical exam includes measurement of blood pressure in both upper extremities. A complete pulse examination of the neck and upper and lower extremities is essential. A decreased

M. R. Weaver
Wayne State University College of Medicine,
Vascular Surgery, Henry Ford Hospital,
Detroit, MI, USA
e-mail: mweaver1@hfhs.org

© The Editor(s) (if applicable) and The Author(s) 2018
S. S. Hans (ed.), *Extracranial Carotid and Vertebral Artery Disease*,
https://doi.org/10.1007/978-3-319-91533-3_17

or absent pulse indicates a proximal high-grade stenosis or occlusion; however the presence of a pulse does not completely exclude proximal disease, particularly in the setting of a chronic occlusion, given the rich collateral pathways present in the upper extremity. An irregular pulse should prompt for a more detailed cardiac examination to identify atrial fibrillation or other arrhythmias that may predispose to cardioembolism. Auscultation for bruits over all major arteries should be per-formed. The skin envelope of the digits is examined for signs of color or temperature differences, tissue loss, or trophic changes.

Diagnostic Studies

Patients with upper extremity (UE) ischemic symptoms should undergo bilateral UE arterial segmental pressure testing (Fig. 17.1). This

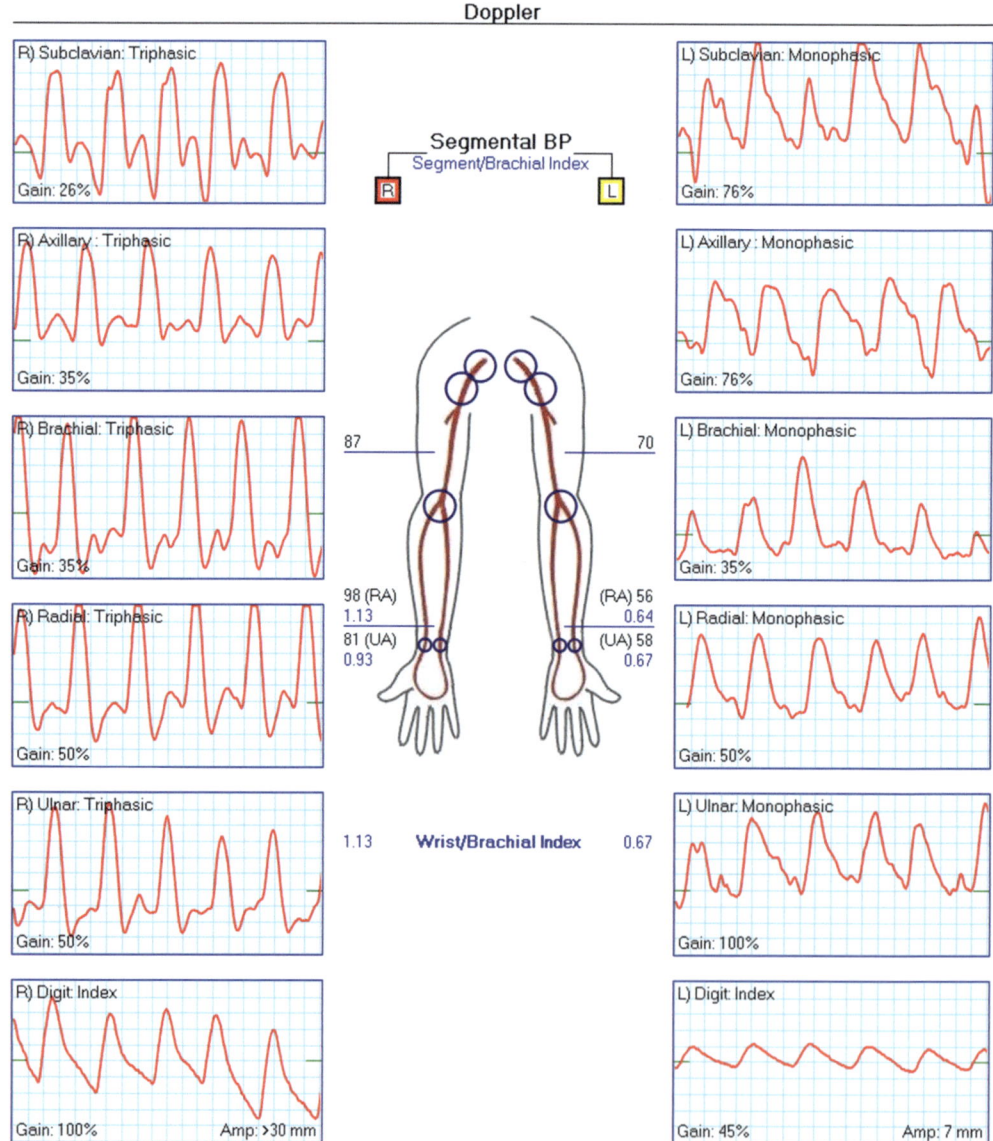

Fig. 17.1 Bilateral upper extremity segmental pressure study in patient with proximal left subclavian artery occlusion. Note significant pressure differential between right upper extremity and left upper extremity. Triphasic Doppler waveforms are noted in the normal right upper extremity, while abnormal monophasic Doppler waveforms are noted in the left upper extremity

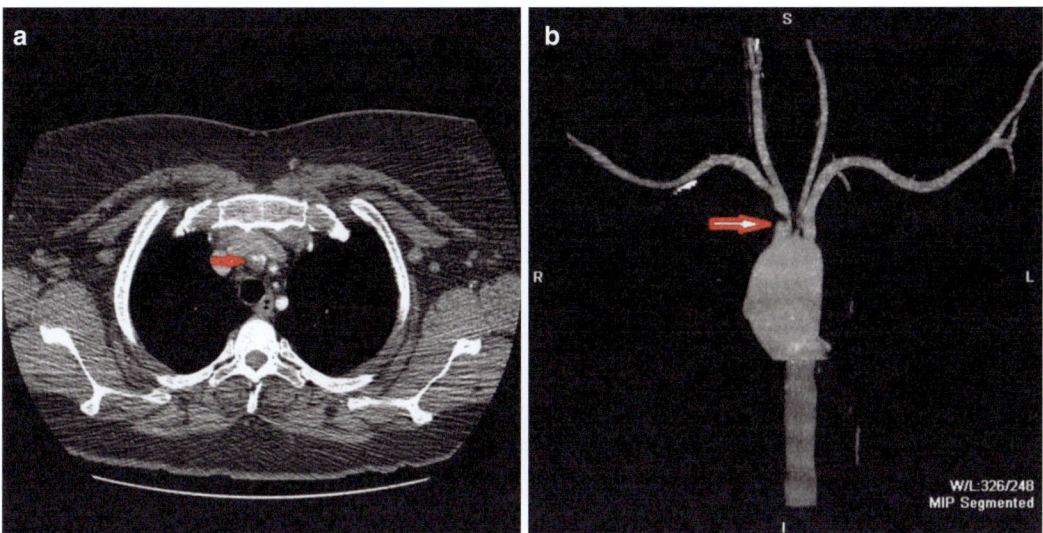

Fig. 17.2 (**a**) Cross-sectional computed tomography imaging demonstrating severe BCA stenosis (arrow); (**b**) A 3-D reconstruction computed tomography image demonstrating severe BCA stenosis (arrow)

testing provides objective and reproducible data which may identify fixed obstructions as well as inducible vasospasm, while also quantifying the degree of arterial insufficiency. Serial examinations allow for objective assessment of disease status and evaluation of the effectiveness of therapeutic interventions. Bilateral brachial, upper forearm, and wrist systolic pressures are obtained along with associated Doppler waveforms. The normal pressure differential between arms should not exceed 15 mmHg, and a pressure drop of 20 mmHg or more between levels indicates an intervening hemodynamically significant lesion. Reduced brachial pressures bilaterally, particularly when associated with blunted or monophasic Doppler waveforms, should prompt high thigh pressure measurements to exclude the possibility of bilateral proximal UE arterial disease.

Duplex ultrasound is useful for imaging the cervical carotid arteries and the more distal subclavian arteries; however due to the intrathoracic location, the supra-aortic vessels and specifically their origins are not satisfactorily visualized with this modality. However, decreased flow velocities or damped waveforms within the common carotid arteries or reversal of flow in the vertebral arteries may suggest supra-aortic trunk vessel stenosis or occlusion.

Cross-sectional imaging with computed tomography angiography (CTA) (Fig. 17.2) and magnetic resonance angiography (MRA) are the studies of choice for confirming diagnosis and planning operative intervention. Complete imaging of not only the aortic arch but also the outflow including the entire cervical and intracranial vasculature and/or upper extremities is important. Assessment for carotid bifurcation occlusive disease is made to determine need for concomitant carotid endarterectomy. Imaging is reviewed to determine feasibility of both open and endovascular options for arterial reconstruction. In the case of transthoracic approaches, evaluation should be made to determine appropriate disease-free clamping sites for the proximal ascending aortic anastomosis as well as distal targets for the bypass (i.e., distal BCA verse right subclavian artery or carotid arteries). Open extra-thoracic arterial reconstructions require identification of a disease-free donor vessel.

There are several factors to consider on preoperative imaging in order to execute a successful endovascular intervention. First is determining the site of access in order to be prepared with the appropriate endovascular equipment. If transfemoral access is planned, one must ensure that the femoral-iliac-aortic system is patent giving

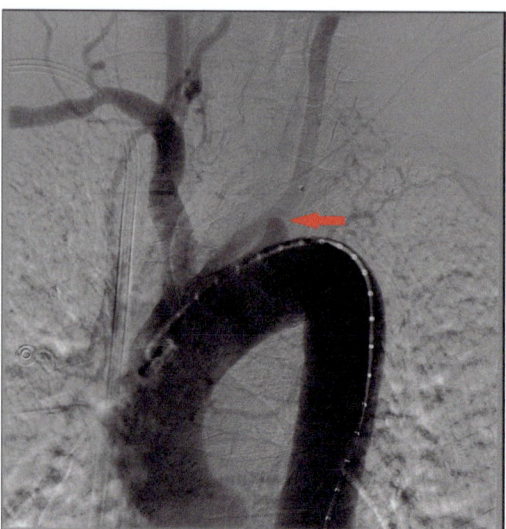

Fig. 17.3 Image demonstrates digital subtraction catheter-directed angiography of the aortic arch performed in a steep left anterior oblique projection to "open up" the arch. Noting equidistance of the markers on the pigtail catheter helps to confirm ideal c-arm angulation. Occlusion of the LSCA is noted (arrow)

access to the aortic arch. A review of the aortic arch anatomy is important including the origins of the great vessels. Great vessel origins that originate at the apex of the aortic arch tend to be easier to access than those arising below the apex. The relationship of the origins of the vessels also needs to be assessed, as the treatment of the origin of one vessel may affect the origin of another. This includes the presence of a common origin of the BCA and LCCA or if they share a true common trunk. In such cases if an endovascular procedure is planned, the non-diseased vessel may need to be protected with a second stent. A flush occlusion with the aorta may also prohibit femoral access, and retrograde brachial or carotid access will need to be considered. The distal extent of the disease to be treated should be determined and how this may affect branch vessels such as the origins of the right subclavian and carotid arteries in the treatment of BCA disease and the vertebral artery origin in the treatment of LSCA disease. In general short, non-calcified, stenotic lesions appear to be most ideal for endovascular therapy, whereas those lesions that are longer and have heavy calcification or a total occlusion have

a greater chance of failure with endovascular techniques [7–9]. Catheter-directed angiography (Fig. 17.3) as a diagnostic tool alone may also be of value in assessing aortic arch branch vessel disease especially when heavily calcified vessel makes it difficult to truly determine the degree of stenosis on other cross-sectional imaging.

Indications

The most common indications for intervention on the supra-aortic trunk vessels are neurologic symptoms such as stoke and vertebral basilar insufficiency, severe lifestyle-limiting upper extremity effort fatigue, or evidence of upper extremity atheroembolism. An additional indication for treatment of proximal left subclavian artery occlusive disease includes providing adequate arterial inflow into a left internal mammary artery (LIMA) being used to bypass to a coronary artery. Patients with hemodynamically significant bilateral upper extremity arterial occlusive disease who are otherwise asymptomatic but have no accurate way to monitor blood pressure may be considered for intervention to facilitate management of their hypertension. Some authors have also used severe but asymptomatic stenosis of the BCA or LCCA as an indication for intervention [4, 7]. It should be emphasized that the majority of patients with asymptomatic proximal subclavian artery stenosis or occlusion do not require invasive intervention for this but the patients should be informed that their blood pressure should be measured from the contralateral arm.

Endovascular Therapy

Endovascular techniques have become the first-line therapy for the treatment of short-segment occlusive lesions of the supra-aortic trunk vessels with the LSCA being the most commonly treated vessel in most series [3, 5, 10–13]. Standard endovascular techniques are utilized in the treatment of supra-aortic trunk vessels. Specifically important procedural considerations include access,

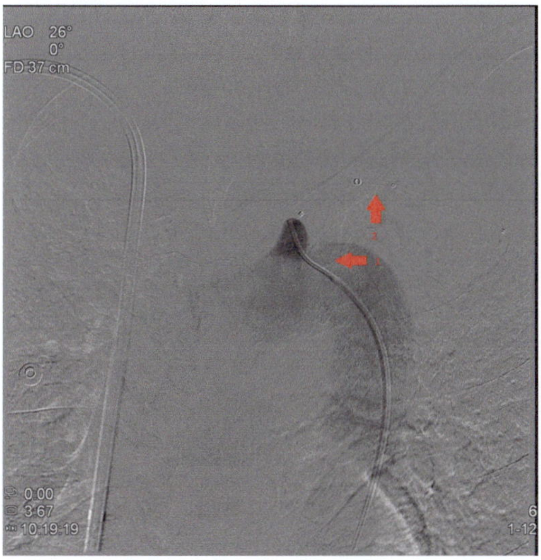

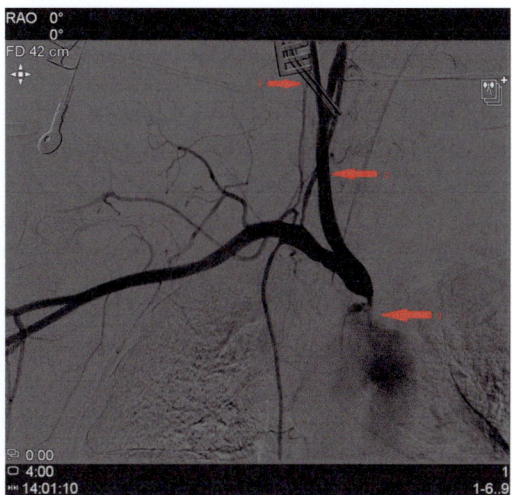

Fig. 17.4 Digital subtraction angiographic image demonstrating cannulation with a slightly angled catheter (arrow 1) of the proximal LSCA which is occluded just distal its orifice. Arrow 2 points out a catheter that has been introduced via a retrograde left brachial approach

Fig. 17.5 Digital subtraction angiographic imagine performed via open retrograde right common carotid artery access. A vascular clamp (arrow 1) is present to be used to occlude the distal common carotid artery during intervention to prevent distal atheroembolization. Vascular sheath is noted within proximal right common carotid artery (arrow 2). Focal severe stenosis of BCA (arrow 3)

therapeutic intervention, and distal thromboembolic protection measures.

Access options include an antegrade approach to the vessel via the femoral artery or retrograde approach via the carotid or brachial arteries. The femoral approach has advantages of familiarity with use for access, lack of need for surgical exposure, and lower access site complication rates compared to brachial artery access. Typically long sheaths are used to give adequate support. Once the vessel is accessed, the patient is anticoagulated with heparin, prior to manipulation of catheters within the aortic arch. A flush catheter is positioned in the ascending aorta and with a left anterior oblique projection of the c-arm to splay out the aortic arch; an arch angiogram is performed to define the anatomy (Fig. 17.3). Additional angiography in the right anterior oblique projection in many cases may help better define the right brachiocephalic artery bifurcation. A long slightly angled catheter is the first choice for selecting the arch vessels (Fig. 17.4). Due to its location, the left subclavian is usually the easiest to access. If unsuccessful with the first catheter, specialized double-curved catheters are utilized.

Retrograde access via either the brachial artery or common carotid artery offers the advantage of a shorter and straighter approach to the lesion which may allow for improved control of the response of catheters and wires to manipulation. A retrograde approach may also allow for distal clamping as a precaution against atheroembolization (Fig. 17.5) and may be the only option when the angle of the vessel or degree of disease prevents antegrade approach due to inability to cannulate or gain enough purchase within the artery to advance therapeutic devices. Queral and Criado [12] have reported on the successful use of open exposure of the common carotid artery with retrograde stenting. This technique involves clamping of the carotid artery distal to the access site during the intervention and "flushing" the artery to remove any possible embolic debris prior to restoring flow after the intervention. Since then others have reported successful use of this technique as well as combining it with carotid endarterectomy in the case of tandem lesions of the supra-aortic arch vessels and the carotid bifurcation [14, 15]. When retrograde brachial artery access is used, we prefer open exposure because of the larger size sheaths that are required (6 French and larger) to limit access site complications.

Once the lesion is crossed, depending on the degree of stenosis, pre-dilation with a smaller balloon may be required in order to successfully and safely pass the stent. Stent and final balloon sizing is based on preoperative cross-sectional imaging. If such imaging is not available, the diameter of the normal artery distal to the lesion on angiography is used as a guide for sizing. Both balloon angioplasty alone with provisional stenting [3, 5, 7, 9, 16] and primary stenting [8, 10–14, 17] have been reported. If primary stenting is not performed, it should be added to the procedure if there is residual stenosis greater than 30% after balloon angioplasty or a flow-limiting dissection. Typically primary stenting is used in cases with a heavily calcified lesion or a complete occlusion. Both balloon-expandable as well as self-expanding stents may be deployed. Balloon-expandable stents are generally chosen for orificial lesions secondary to the precise deployment which they allow. Generally when treating orificial lesions the stents are extended a few millimeters into the aorta. The authors of most current reports on the endovascular treatment of supra-aortic trunk pathology report the use of primary stenting over angioplasty alone [3, 8, 10–14, 17]. The current role of cover stents in the treatment of these lesions has not yet been defined.

Prevention of atheroembolism and stroke during these interventions is of great concern, but the role of available strategies to mitigate this has not been completely defined. Several series have demonstrated very low cerebrovascular event rates of 0–1.5% with the use of retrograde carotid access with distal clamping and flushing [12, 14], even with the addition of carotid endarterectomy [15]. Other series however have reported high neurologic event rates of up to 9–14.3% when retrograde stenting is combined with carotid endarterectomy [11, 18]. When transfemoral access is used, filter wires may be used for distal embolic protection of the carotid artery, but its role is not completely defined as some authors report routine use of protective devices when treating common or innominate arteries, while others use them only in select cases, and still others report never using such devices [3,

9, 13, 16]. Paukovits et al. describe the treatment of 77 innominate artery lesions all via a percutaneous femoral approach with a primary technical success rate of 93.5%, no death or major neurologic complications and a 2.6% rate of minor neurologic deficit (TIA) [9]. In the treatment of proximal common carotid artery lesions, Paukovits et al. reported on the treatment of 153 lesions, in which an embolic protection device was used in 16 of the cases with an overall 98.7% technical success, 2.0% major stroke rate, and 2.6% TIA rate [16].

Patients are treated with antiplatelet therapy postoperatively. Excellent technical success rates have been reported (92.3–98.7) [3, 10, 12, 14, 16, 17], though success rates are somewhat lower in cases of chronic total occlusions compared to stenotic lesions [10, 12]. Aziz et al. [19] published a review of the literature in 2011 where they report on the endovascular treatment of supra-aortic trunk lesions in 26 studies comprising 1305 patients. A technical success rate for stenotic lesions was 94% (73–100%) and for occlusions 64% (0–83%). The procedure is associated with low morbidity and mortality with several studies reporting less than 3% combined 30 day stroke and death rates [3, 10, 12, 14, 16, 17]. Access site complications are reported from 0 to 15% [3, 10, 14, 16, 17]. Primary patency is reported at 90–100% at 1 year [3, 10, 16, 17] and greater than 70% after 4 years [10, 16, 17].

Open Surgical Therapy

Extra-thoracic Arterial Reconstructions

Extra-thoracic arterial reconstructions for the treatment of supra-aortic branch pathology have played a substantial role due to the relative ease of exposure and elimination of the morbidity of a transthoracic exposure. All extra-thoracic reconstructions require at least one disease-free arch vessel to serve as the donor vessel. In the long term, as atherosclerosis is a progressive disease, the donor vessel is always at risk of stenosis itself which may eventually lead to decreased durability of the extra-thoracic repairs. However, many patients requiring arterial reconstruction of supra aortic branch pathology are poor candidates to tolerate major invasive operations secondary to deabilitation, advanced age and significant comorbidities such as coronary artery disease and chronic obstructive pulmonary disease, chronic obstructive pulmonary disease, and debilitation, and are of advanced age for which a more invasive procedure would not be as well tolerated. These operations include bypass between the carotid and subclavian arteries, transposition of the subclavian artery onto the carotid artery and vice versa, carotid-carotid artery bypass, and axillo-axillary bypass. Despite the maturation of endovascular techniques which has led to the decrease in number of open arterial reconstructions required for symptomatic occlusive disease of the aortic arch branch vessels, there has been an increase in the number of these extra-thoracic arterial reconstructions being performed in our practice as a means of "debranching" the aortic arch to create a satisfactory proximal landing zone for thoracic stent grafting in the treatment of aortic pathology.

Carotid Subclavian Bypass/ Transposition Operations

After general anesthesia is induced with the patient in a supine position, a rolled up sheet is placed underneath the patient's shoulder and the table positioned with the head and torso raised approximately 30°. The neck is extended and rotated slightly to the contralateral side. The ipsilateral arm is adducted with slight downward pull to depress the shoulder.

Starting approximately 1–2 cm above the clavicle and 1 cm lateral to the midline, a transverse incision is made which is continued laterally approximately 6–8 cm. The platysma muscle is divided with electric cautery, and flaps are developed superiorly approximately 5 cm and inferiorly to the clavicle. The sternocleidomastoid muscle is mobilized along its lateral border, and if necessary, more often in the case of subclavian artery transposition, the clavicular head of the sternocleidomastoid muscle is freed off of the clavicle to allow for extended medial exposure.

The sternocleidomastoid muscle is mobilized medially and anteriorly exposing the carotid sheath. Once the carotid sheath is identified, it is incised taking care not to injure the structures within it. Next the internal jugular vein and vagus nerve which run parallel with the carotid artery are mobilized anteriorly and medially to expose the artery. This will also be the pathway through which the transposed subclavian artery or the bypass graft will traverse. Approximately 5–6 cm of the common carotid artery is exposed to allow sufficient room to clamp the artery and to perform the anastomosis. When the planned operation is for treatment of proximal LCCA occlusive disease with transposition to the LSCA, dissection of the LCCA as proximally as possible is required to allow for adequate length to transpose to the LSCA. Continuing exposure of the subclavian artery, the omohyoid muscle is encountered and divided, furthering exposure of the anterior scalene fat pad. Starting on the medial edge of the anterior scalene muscle, the fat pad is separated from the internal jugular vein and then its inferior border mobilized. This allows for the fat pad to be retracted laterally and superiorly. During this dissection, all lymphatics are carefully ligated as they are divided. On the left side, care is taken not to injure the thoracic duct; however if injured or divided, it is meticulously oversewn with fine monofilament polypropylene suture.

The anterior scalene muscle is then exposed along with the phrenic nerve which runs lateral to medial, anterior to, and within the investing fascia of the muscle. The nerve is carefully mobilized off the muscle, incising the fascia a few millimeters on either side of it. The edges of the anterior scalene muscle are then freed, and the muscle is divided exposing the subclavian artery and brachial plexus. For cases in which carotid artery to subclavian artery bypass is planned, only enough of the subclavian artery needs to be exposed to allow for application of vascular clamps for proximal and distal control as well as allow for an area to perform the anastomosis. The site on the subclavian artery chosen for this is typically at its apex directly behind the anterior scalene muscle. A second approach for exposing the subclavian artery in cases of planned bypass

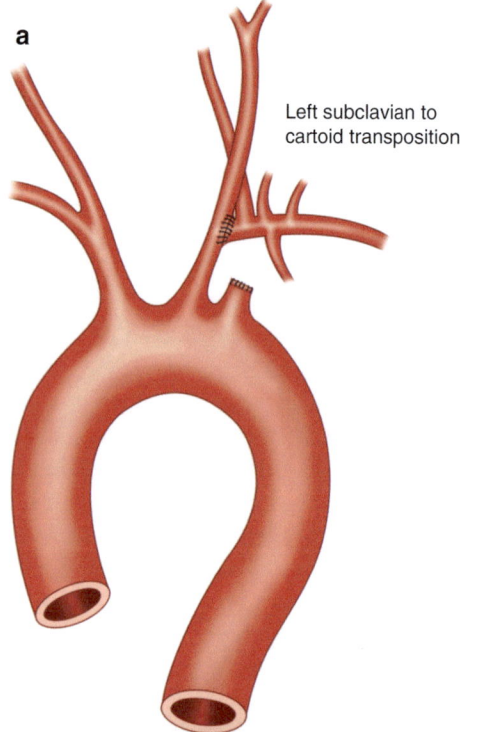

Left subclavian to
cartoid transposition

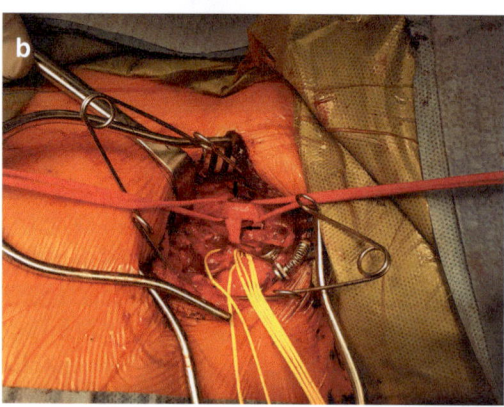

Fig. 17.6 (**a**) Illustration depicting LSCA transposed onto LCCA with oversewn proximal LSCA. (**b**) Intraoperative photo demonstrating mobilized LSCA (arrow 1) positioned for anastomosis to LCCA (arrow 2)

is exposure between the lateral border of the anterior scalene muscle and the brachial plexus which avoids mobilization of most of the anterior scalene fat pad and complete division of the anterior scalene muscle.

When subclavian artery to carotid artery transposition (Fig. 17.6) is planned, more proximal dissection of the subclavian artery is required.

Dissection is continued medially identifying and mobilizing the internal mammary and vertebral arteries. The vertebral vein is often encountered superficial to the subclavian artery and is divided to facilitate exposure. An adequate length of the subclavian artery proximal to the vertebral artery to allow for safe clamping and oversewing of the proximal stump, as well as sufficient length to reach the common carotid artery, needs to be exposed. Consideration may be made to ligating the internal mammary artery to allow for increased mobilization of the subclavian artery. Mobilization of the proximal vertebral artery for 1–2 cm is often required to allow for transposition of the subclavian artery; however excessive mobilization may lead to arterial kinking.

Once exposure is complete, the artery is palpated, and assessment is made to ensure that the artery can be successfully clamped and oversewn while still leaving adequate length for transposition to the carotid artery. If there is uncertainty, subclavian artery transposition should be abandoned in favor of performance of a carotid subclavian bypass.

Having made the decision to proceed with subclavian artery to carotid artery transposition, the patient is systemically anticoagulated with heparin (100 units/Kg) with its effect monitored using ACT (>250 s). After adequate anticoagulation is achieved, vascular clamps are applied to the subclavian artery and its branches. The subclavian artery is divided proximal to the vertebral artery, and the proximal stump is carefully oversewn with monofilament polypropylene suture. Prior to cutting the suture, the clamp is slowly released, and the arterial closure is inspected for hemostasis. Once hemostasis is ensured with the clamp completely removed, the sutures are cut. This is a critical point as the loss of control of the subclavian artery as it retracts back into the chest after ligation may lead to catastrophic bleeding which is very difficult to control.

Having controlled the proximal arterial stump, the distal end of the divided subclavian artery is swung over to the adjacent common carotid artery. The carotid artery is clamped proximally and distally with atraumatic vascular clamps. A number 11 blade knife is used to create an arte-

Fig. 17.7 Illustration depicting a LCCA to LSCA bypass with prosthetic graft with end-to-side anastomoses

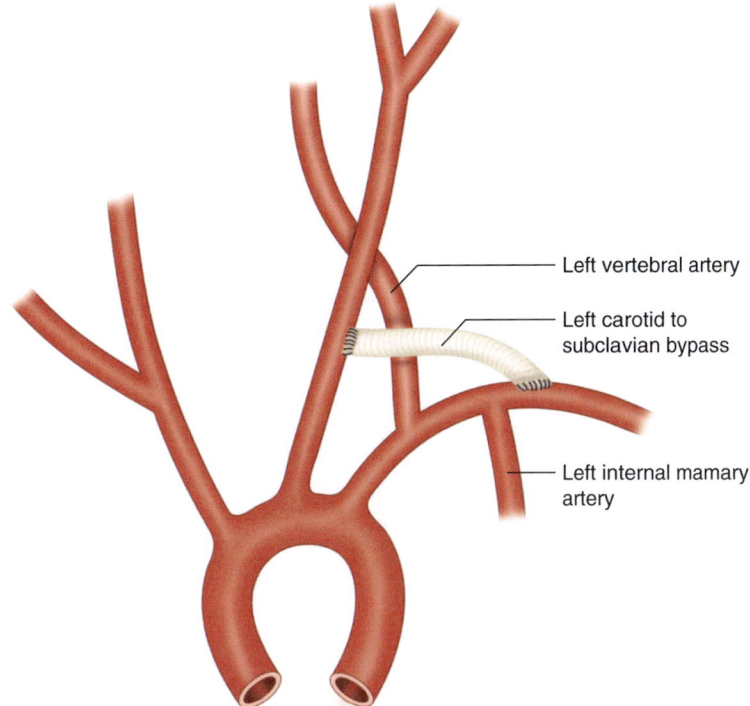

Left vertebral artery

Left carotid to subclavian bypass

Left internal mamary artery

riotomy which is lengthened in a longitudinal fashion on the lateral aspect of the carotid artery with a Potts scissors to a size that will accept the subclavian artery. An end of the subclavian artery to side of carotid artery anastomosis is then performed with running typically 5-0 or 6-0 monofilament polypropylene suture. Just prior to completion of the anastomosis, the vessels are vented. The anastomosis is completed and flow is restored. The distal perfusion is assessed with pulse examination and continuous wave Doppler interrogation. If found to be satisfactory, the heparin effect is reversed with protamine. We do not routinely monitor cerebral perfusion with EEG monitoring during this procedure.

The wound is inspected for bleeding as well as any sign of lymphatic leak. Having ensured hemostasis and ligation of any possible lymphatic leaks, the anterior scalene fat pad is re-approximated to its original position. A closed suction drain is placed within the wound and taken out through the skin via a separate inferior stab incision. The platysma is closed with interrupted 3-0 braided polyglactin sutures, and the skin is closed with running 4-0 braided polygla-

ctin suture. The drain is removed only after the patient has resumed normal oral intake without signs of chyle leak.

When carotid to subclavian artery bypass is planned (Fig. 17.7), having completed adequate dissection and initiated anticoagulation as described above, one is ready to proceed with performance of the bypass operation. Typically a prosthetic graft is chosen. The author prefers a Dacron graft due to ease of handling and reduced needle hole bleeding. While the size of the graft is ultimately determined by the size of the donor and recipient vessels, a graft 6–8 mm in diameter is typically chosen.

Technically it is easier to perform the subclavian artery anastomosis first, followed by the carotid artery anastomosis. The mid and most apical portion of the subclavian artery is typically the site chosen for the anastomosis. Atraumatic clamps are applied proximally and distally while allowing adequate space for the anastomosis. One should be aware that the subclavian artery is more fragile than the typically encountered common femoral artery. Manipulation should be minimized, including the clamping and unclamp-

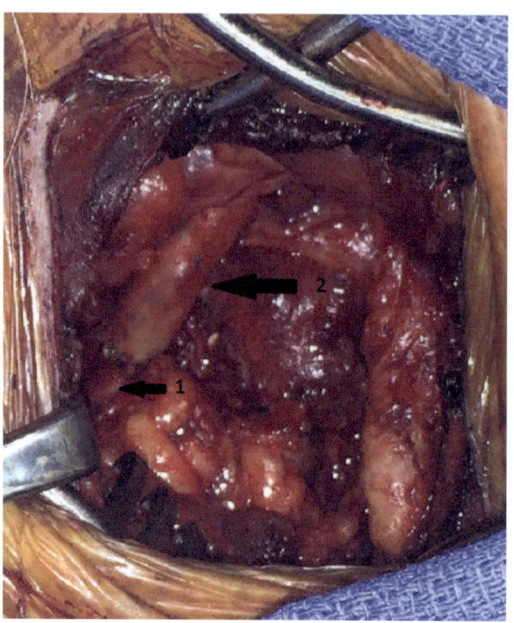

Fig. 17.8 Intraoperative photograph demonstrating the apex of the LSCA (arrow 1) anastomosed to the transposed LCCA (arrow 2)

ing of the artery, as well as significant caution exercised if considering endarterectomizing the artery. Clamps should be applied in a deliberate and gentle manner. Once the artery is controlled, an arteriotomy is created with a #11 blade knife and extended appropriately with a Potts scissors. The end of the graft is cut in a beveled fashion and sewn end to side to the artery with running monofilament polypropylene 5-0 or 6-0 suture. Once the anastomosis is completed, the proximal and distal arteries are vented through the graft, and the anastomosis is tested for hemostasis. After ensuring hemostasis, the graft is brought over to the carotid artery. The graft is then cut so as not to be redundant or under tension when anastomosed to the carotid artery. The anastomosis is performed as described above for the carotid artery to subclavian transposition as is closure of the wound.

In operations when the carotid artery is transposed to the subclavian artery (Fig. 17.8), obtaining adequate proximal length of the common carotid is essential. As well, the same care is required in ligation of the proximal stump. The carotid artery will usually be anastomosed to the retro-anterior scalene subclavian artery.

When a concomitant procedure is planned for the more distal carotid artery such as carotid endarterectomy, this portion of the carotid artery may be exposed through a separate incision along the anterior border of the sternocleidomastoid muscle. The graft to the subclavian artery anastomosis is performed first, followed by the carotid bifurcation/internal carotid artery endarterectomy. If a carotid shunt is required during the endarterectomy, it may be placed, the endarterectomy is performed, and then prior to patch closure of the artery, a second arteriotomy is created on the lateral aspect of the common carotid artery for the bypass graft anastomosis. Once the carotid-graft anastomosis is completed, the patch closure of the carotid artery may be performed and the shunt removed just prior to completion of the patch closure.

Both subclavian to carotid artery transposition and carotid to subclavian artery bypass have low morbidity and mortality, along with excellent long-term patency (75%–90% at 5 years for bypass and almost 100% for transposition) [19–25]. Complications include injury to adjacent nerves (brachial plexus, phrenic nerve, and sympathetic chain) and lymphatic structures (thoracic and accessory thoracic ducts). Nerve injuries are usually self-limited. Lymphatic injuries can be problematic, and, if drainage is significant or persistent, early reexploration and thoracic duct ligation are advised.

Carotid-Carotid Artery Bypass

Carotid-carotid artery bypass is an additional option that a vascular surgeon has for revascularizing the supra-aortic trunk vessels in appropriate situations. This type of reconstruction is less common for occlusive disease but may be a necessary option in patients who do not have an ipsilateral donor vessel and are not candidates for a transthoracic approach. Or as is becoming more common in modern day vascular surgery, this operation is used as a debranching operation of the aortic arch to allow extension of thoracic endografts into zone 1 of the aortic arch which covers the origins of the left carotid and subclavian arteries.

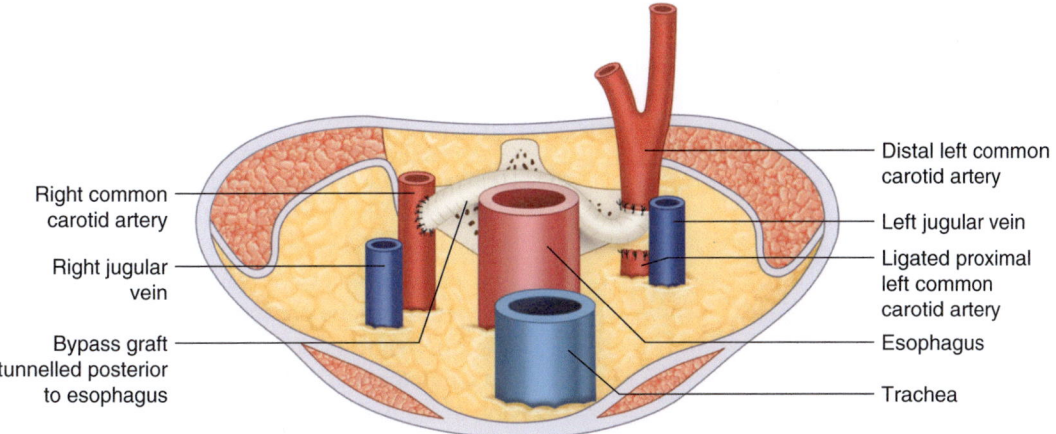

Fig. 17.9 Illustration of a RCCA to LCCA bypass with a prosthetic graft coursing in the retropharyngeal space over the vertebral body

This operation is performed under general anesthesia, and the patient must be positioned, prepped, and draped in a manner which allows access to both sides of the neck. The common carotid arteries are exposed bilaterally in the standard manner. The tunnel connecting them will be in the retropharyngeal space (Fig. 17.9). This tunnel is created by dissecting below the common carotid arteries over the vertebral bodies palpated behind the pharynx. The space behind the pharynx is entered and developed bilaterally using finger dissection. The shiny prevertebral fascia is visualized. Within this space a short tunnel is created between the two common carotid arteries through which to pass the graft. The graft is then anastomosed to the donor vessel in an end of graft to side of artery fashion, taken through the tunnel and anastomosed to the recipient vessel in an end-to-end fashion.

Ozsvath et al. [26] reported on 24 carotid-carotid artery bypass with no perioperative mortality and 1 stroke. Three-year primary patency was 88% and secondary patency 92%, with a stroke-free survival at 4 years of 94%. In a review of carotid-carotid bypass procedures by Aziz et al. [19], 4 studies were identified with a total of 67 patients. Perioperative mortality rate was 0–0.7%, and stroke rate was 0–6.2%. Patency at 5 years reported in two studies was 70 and 94%.

Axillo-axillary Bypass

Axillo-axillary bypass is an additional option that a vascular surgeon has for revascularizing the supra-aortic trunk vessels provided the contralateral axillo-subclavian artery is widely patent (Fig. 17.10). Advantages to this operation include both the safety and technical ease in which it can be performed compared to some of the other available surgical options. In situations of a hostile neck and/or mediastinum, it may be a good option. Disadvantages include that the graft does produce a noticeable bulge across the sternum and its superficial position leads to concern for skin erosion and infection. Also some report poor long-term patency of this bypass compared to other types of reconstructions for supra-aortic arch branch disease [27].

The operation is generally performed under general anesthesia. The patient is placed in a supine position with the arms along the side of the body with the elbows slightly flexed, and the upper body elevated about 15°. The operating table can then be tilted side to side depending on which side is being worked on so that the skin overlying the infraclavicular fossa is in the horizontal plane. The incision is 1–2 cm below the clavicle overlying the deltopectoral groove starting just lateral to the sternal head of the clavicle and extending lateral about 7–8 cm toward the coracoid process. The incision is ended laterally

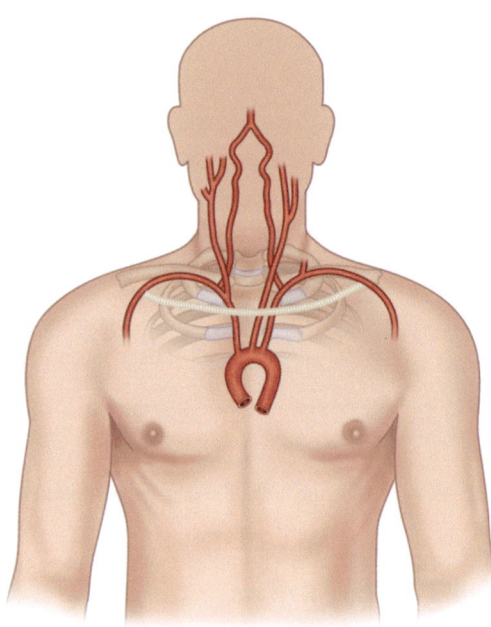

Fig. 17.10 Illustration depicting course of axillary to axillary artery bypass

slightly more inferiorly (2 cm below clavicle) roughly paralleling the muscles of the pectoralis major muscle. The fascia of the pectoralis major muscle is incised and the muscle fibers split. The clavipectoral fascia is incised. If necessary the pectoralis minor muscle fibers which are at the lateral limits of the dissection may be divided to improve exposure. Arterial branches of the thoracoacromial trunk and accompanying veins may be encountered and require ligation and division. The axillary vein is mobilized and retracted to expose the axillary artery.

The axillary artery is exposed for 3–4 cm and encircled with vessel loops. After completing this dissection bilaterally, a subcutaneous tunnel is then created superficial to the sternum at the level of the first interspace. This can often be accomplished with finger dissection alone. Once the tunnel is completed, the patient is systemically anticoagulated, and the anastomosis is performed. Prosthetic grafts of 7–8 mm diameter are typically chosen for conduit. The grafts are usually cut at a 30°–45° angle for their anastomosis to the artery. Once the artery is controlled with atraumatic vascular clamps, an appropriate

length longitudinal arteriotomy is created removing a small ellipse of the artery, which is usually on the anterior medial aspect of the artery. The donor side anastomosis is performed first in a running fashion usually with running 5-0 or 6-0 polypropylene suture. Once the anastomosis is completed, the proximal and distal arteries are vented, and the graft is arterialized. After insuring the anastomosis is hemostatic, the graft is taken through the previously created tunnel taking care not to twist or kink it. After creation of an arteriotomy in the recipient artery in like fashion to the donor artery, the graft is cut in a beveled fashion so as not to be redundant or under tension. The outflow anastomosis is then completed in like fashion. Just prior to completion of the anastomosis, the artery and graft are vented, then the anastomosis is completed, and flow is restored. Distal flow in the upper extremities is accessed by pulse exam and continuous wave Doppler evaluation. Once flow is noted to be satisfactory, the heparin effect is reversed with protamine, hemostasis within the wounds is insured, and they are closed.

Overall this operation can be performed with minimal morbidity and mortality. A review of the literature regarding axillo-axillary bypass by Aziz et al. [19] found 16 studies containing 426 patients. Perioperative mortality averaged 0.5% (0–3%). Perioperative stroke averaged 1.1% (0–10%). Five-year patency of 90% was reported in one study, and 87% patency was reported at 10 years in one study.

Transthoracic Arterial Reconstruction

Transthoracic supra-aortic trunk reconstruction has become less common with the advancement of endovascular techniques. However there remain some patients with multivessel disease, or in situations where complete arch debranching in preparation for thoracic aortic endografting, anatomic (transthoracic) revascularization may be the preferred or only option for revascularization. Thus the vascular surgeon should be facile with the approaches needed to treat such lesions. At the author's institution, these cases are performed with collaboration between the vascular surgery and cardiac surgery services. Preoperative cardiopulmonary assessment is important prior to proceeding with aortic arch reconstruction. It is important to evaluate for any cardiac dysfunction, valvular disease, or coronary ischemia. Noninvasive studies such as transthoracic echo and myocardial perfusion scans are useful in this evaluation. However, given the need for median sternotomy, to ensure no other cardiac intervention may be indicated, there is a low threshold for obtaining catheter-based coronary angiography prior to proceeding with aortic BCA bypass operations.

Severe cardiopulmonary disease, a heavily calcified aortic arch, or prior sternotomy places patients at higher risk, makes the operation more difficult, and may preclude them as candidates for the operation.

Details of Procedure

Procedures are performed under general anesthesia. Appropriate preoperative antibiotics are administered within 1 h prior to incision. Preoperative discussion with the anesthesiology team in regard to arterial line placement and venous access is important. Considerations include which arteries are diseased, which arteries are going to be clamped, and are any concomitant procedures such as carotid endarterectomy planned.

The patient is positioned with a posterior shoulder roll to extend the neck and elevate the sternal notch after general anesthesia is induced. Median sternotomy or in some cases hemisternotomy is performed often with a slight cervical extension to the right to better expose the right common carotid and subclavian arteries as the BCA bifurcation is often the site of one of the distal anastomosis. Having divided the sternum, a self-retaining retractor is place. Next the pericardium is divided in the midline, and stay sutures are then placed on both edges of the pericardium to elevate the mediastinal structures and create a pericardial well. The thymus is typically incised

along the intralobar cleft. The left brachiocephalic vein is dissected out circumferentially and encircled with a vessel loop which may be used to retract the vein superiorly or inferiorly as needed to provide exposure to the underlying structures. The ascending aorta is exposed dissecting it free from the main pulmonary trunk laterally and the right pulmonary artery inferiorly in order to provide additional mobility and excellent proximal control.

Distally the proximal right subclavian artery and right common carotid arteries are isolated taking care not to injure the recurrent laryngeal nerve as it courses under the right subclavian artery and behind the left common carotid artery origin before entering the larynx. When the left carotid and/or left subclavian arteries are to be bypassed, they are dissected from their origins distally until a non-disease soft segment is found typically 3–5 cm from their origin. Division of the left brachiocephalic vein may offer improved exposure of the left subclavian artery via an anterior median sternotomy.

Once dissection is complete, the patient is systemically heparinized. The anesthesiology team is then asked to drop the systolic blood pressure and maintain at approximately 100 mmHg. Once this is achieved, to a previously chosen disease-free site usually slightly laterally and to the right of the ascending aorta, a side-biting clamp is applied for partial exclusion of the artery. Typically a Lemole-Strong clamp is used for this (Fig. 17.11). Prior to incising the aorta, the excluded portion is aspirated with a needle to insure that there is no clamp leak. An arteriotomy is then created in the aorta. An appropriate size graft is then brought to the field which is typically 10–12 mm for a bypass to the BSA. The graft is beveled appropriately to lay comfortably to the right of the ascending aorta. The proximal anastomosis is performed with 4-0 polypropylene in a continuous running fashion.

Once completed, any slack within the suture line is removed and the suture tied. The patient is then temporarily placed in Trendelenburg position as the clamp is released to check for bleeding. The Trendelenburg position is to protect against air trapped in the anastomosis emboliz-

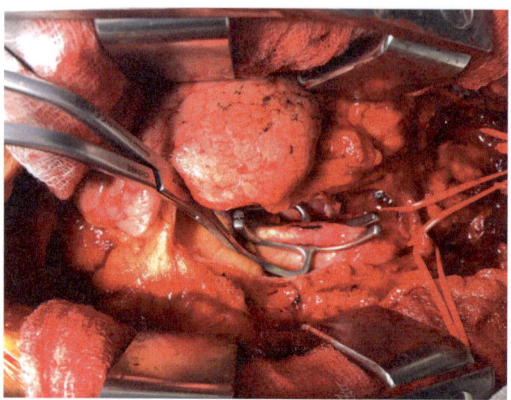

Fig. 17.11 Intra operative photograph demonstrating placement of side-biting aortic clamp (Lemole-Strong) partially occluding the ascending aorta in preparation for performance of proximal anastomosis

ing into the carotid system. Side branches to the left carotid artery or subclavian artery should come off the main graft as proximal as possible (3–4 cm) from the graft origin so as to exit the chest from the left side of the trachea as opposed to in front of it. Inverted bifurcated grafts are typically not used as the main bodies when cut tangentially for end-to-side anastomosis require larger aortotomy and when the graft is distended and the chest is closed occupy too much space and can lead to graft compression and kinking.

Distal anastomoses are then performed. For bypass of the BSA, the site of anastomosis is typically to the bifurcation of the artery or separately to the subclavian and common carotid arteries. Ideally the right subclavian and common carotid arteries are controlled separately as opposed to clamping the distal innominate artery as plaque may extend to this area and there also may lead to great chance of injuring the recurrent laryngeal nerve. The proximal ends of the arteries are oversewn. The graft is beveled appropriately in order to lay comfortably under the innominate vein without causing compression. The anastomosis is then performed with 5-0 polypropylene suture in a continuous running fashion.

The same technique can be applied to bypass the left carotid artery or the left subclavian artery

when they are involved. If more than one artery is involved, then side branch grafts can be anastomosed to the larger main graft ideally prior to starting the bypass (Fig. 17.12). Commercially available branched grafts are available that are designed for bypassing more than one arch vessel. Depending on the anatomy of the left subclavian artery, specifically how lateral and posterior it is positioned, adequate exposure for performing arterial reconstruction via a median sternotomy may not be possible. If revascularization of this vessel is required, an extra anatomic reconstruction may be considered after direct revascularization of the left carotid artery.

For focal BSA plaque, not involving the BSA origin/plaque not extending into the aorta, endarterectomy may be considered. In this case, a side-biting clamp is placed on the aorta over the origin of the innominate artery. Longitudinal arteriotomy is then created in the BSA and endarterectomy is performed followed by primary or patch closure.

Having completed the arterial reconstruction, the heparin effect is reversed with protamine. Hemostasis is insured. Typically one large bore drainage tube is used to drain the mediastinum. It is exteriorized inferiorly and sutured to the skin. The sternal incision is closed in the standard fashion.

Reported outcomes for transthoracic supra-aortic arch vessel reconstructions are limited, and most report on patients treated over two decades ago. Generally excellent patency rates are reported, but with significant morbidity and mortality. Average postoperative lengths of stay are reported at 7–14 days [4, 28, 29]. Early complications typically involve cardiopulmonary events or stroke. Mortality rates range from 2.7 to 8%. Stroke rates from 2.7 to 11%, and myocardial infarction rates from 1.5 to 3%, have been reported [4–6, 28–31]. Survival rates at 5 and 10 years are 77.5–87% and 51.9–81%, respectively. Graft patency at 5 and 10 years is reported from 94 to 98% and 88 to 96%, respectively [28, 30, 31].

Fig. 17.12 Illustration depicting an ascending aorta to BSA bypass with side branch to LCCA

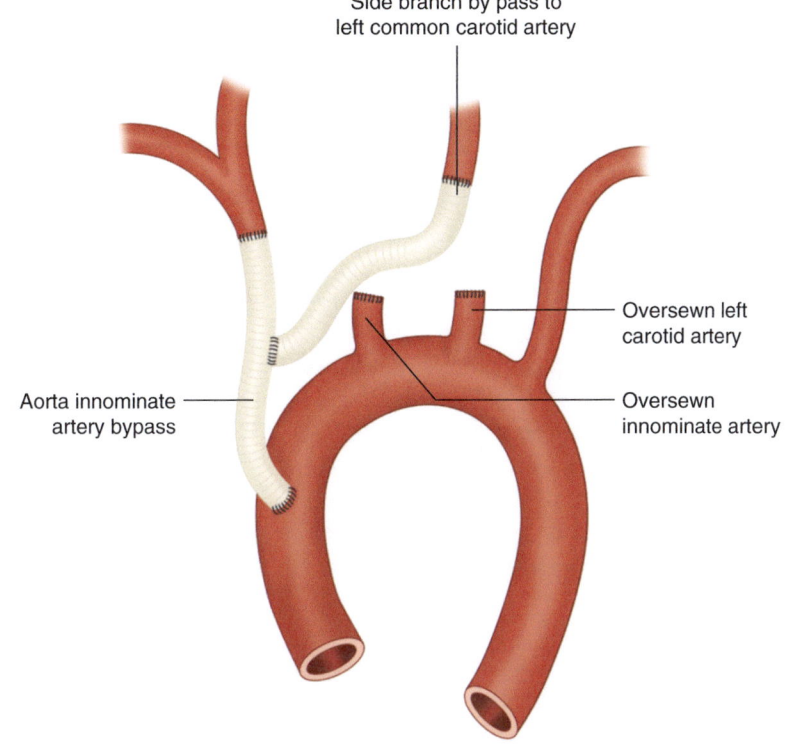

Side branch by pass to left common carotid artery

Aorta innominate artery bypass

Oversewn left carotid artery

Oversewn innominate artery

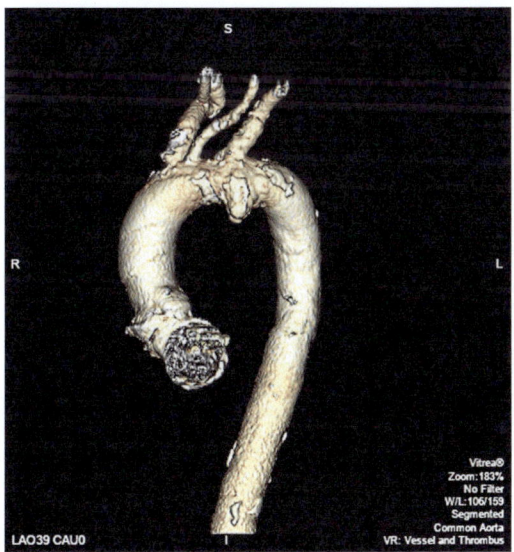

Fig. 17.13 A 3-D reconstruction computed tomography image of the aortic arch of the patient described in Question 1

Review Questions

1 A 71-year-old gentleman presents with chest and back pain. Past medical history includes coronary artery disease for which he has undergone coronary bypass graft surgery with a left internal mammary artery to left anterior descending artery bypass, as well as chronic obstructive pulmonary disease. A CT scan of the chest is obtained with 3D reconstruction shown below (Fig. 17.13). The most appropriate next step in management is:

A. Repeat CT scan in 3 months

B. Open repair of the thoracic aorta

C. Endovascular stent graft repair of the thoracic aorta with left subclavian revascularization if symptoms develop

D. Left carotid artery to subclavian artery bypass followed by endovascular repair of thoracic aorta

E. Sternotomy with complete debranching of the aortic arch followed by endovascular repair of the thoracic aorta

Answer: D

2. A 36-year-old female presents with progressive right upper extremity ischemia. She reports a prolonged febrile illness the previous year. On physical exam there is no right brachial pulse, and the right arm blood pressure is 50 mmHg compared to 120 mmHg on the left side. Her erythrocyte sedimentation rate is normal. CT angiography demonstrates an innominate artery occlusion and moderate stenosis of the left common carotid and subclavian arteries. The best treatment option for this patient is:
   A. Innominate artery endarterectomy
   B. Steroid therapy
   C. Axillary-axillary bypass
   D. Innominate artery stenting
   E. Aorto-innominate bypass

Answer: E

3. A 65-year-old female is sent from her primary care physician for evaluation of blood pressure discrepancy between the right and left arms. The right arm blood pressure is 120 mmHg systolic, and the left arm is 70 mmHg systolic. A duplex exam reveals hemodynamically significant stenosis in the proximal left subclavian artery. The patient has no symptoms of effort fatigue in the left upper extremity or symptoms of vertebrobasilar insufficiency. The best treatment option for this patient is:
   A. Left carotid subclavian bypass
   B. Left carotid subclavian transposition
   C. Left subclavian artery stenting
   D. Right axillary to left axillary bypass

E. Observation with risk factor modification for peripheral vascular occlusive disease

Answer: E

4. All of the following are acceptable indications for surgical intervention of supra-aortic trunk vessels except:
   A. A 67-year-old male with recurrent right hemispheric TIAs and an 80% innominate artery stenosis
   B. A 72-year-old male with history of coronary artery disease, status post coronary artery bypass surgery including use of left internal mammary artery who now has recurrent chest pain and a proximal severe left subclavian artery stenosis
   C. A 66-year-old female with right upper extremity ischemia from atheroembolism and findings of 60% atherosclerotic innominate artery stenosis
   D. A 79-year-old male with vertebrobasilar symptoms with use of left upper extremity and an 80% stenosis of the proximal left subclavian artery
   E. A 64-year-old female with finding of proximal left subclavian artery occlusion on workup for discrepancy in blood pressure between arms

Answer: E

5. When using endovascular techniques to treat supra-aortic trunk vessel, occlusive disease factors that affect both procedural and long-term outcome include:
   A. Degree of calcification
   B. Length of lesion
   C. Stenosis verse occlusion
   D. All of the above
   E. None of the above

Answer: D

References

1. Hass WK, Fields WS, North RR, Kricheff II, Chase NE, Bauer RB. Joint study of extracranial arterial occlusion II. Arteriography, techniques, sites, and complications. JAMA. 1968;203(11):961–8. https://doi.org/10.1001/jama.1968.03140110053011.
2. Wylie EJ, Effeney DJ. Surgery of the aortic arch branches and vertebral arteries. Surg Clin North Am. 1979;59(4):669–80.
3. Ben Ahmed S, Benezit M, Hazart J, Brouat A, Daniel G, Rosset E. Outcomes of the endovascular treatment for the supra-aortic trunks occlusive disease: a 14-year monocentric experience. Ann Vasc Surg. 2016;33:55–66.
4. Azakie A, McElhinney DB, Higashima R, Messina LM, Stoney RJ. Innominate artery reconstruction: over 3 decades of experience. Ann Surg. 1998;228(3):402–10.
5. Przewlocki T, Kablak-Ziembicka A, Pieniazek P, Musialek P, Kadzielski A, Zalewski J, Kozanecki A, Tracz W. Determinants of immediate and long-term results of subclavian and innominate artery angioplasty. Catheter Cardiovasc Interv. 2006;67:519–26.
6. Rhodes JM, Cherry KJ, Clark RC, Panneton JM, Bower C, Gloviczki P, Hallett JW, Pairolero PC. Aortic-origin reconstruction of the great vessels: risk factors of early and late complications. J Vasc Surg. 2000;31(2):260–9.
7. Hüttl K, Nemes B, Simonffy Á, Entz L, Bérczi V, et al. Angioplasty of the innominate artery in 89 patients: experience over 19 years. Cardiovasc Intervent Radiol. 2002;25(2):109–14.
8. Brountzos EN, Petersen D, Binkert C, Panagiotou I, Kaufman JA. Primary stenting of subclavian and innominate artery occlusive disease: a single center's experience. Cardiovasc Intervent Radiol. 2004;27(6):616–23.
9. Paukovits TM, Lukács L, Bérczi V, Hirschberg K, Nemes B, Hüttl K. Percutaneous endovascular treatment of innominate artery lesions: a single-centre experience on 77 lesions. Eur J Vasc Endovasc Surg. 2010;40(1):35–43.
10. Soga Y, Tomoi Y, Fujihara M, Okazaki S, Yamauchi Y, Shintani Y, Suzuki K, Investigators SCALLOP. Perioperative and long-term outcomes of endovascular treatment for subclavian artery disease from a large multicenter registry. J Endovasc Ther. 2015;22(4):626–33.
11. Sullivan TM, Gray BH, Bacharach JM, Perl J II, Childs MB, Modzelewski L, Beven EG. Angioplasty and primary stenting of the subclavian, innominate, and common carotid arteries in 83 patients. J Vasc Surg. 1998;28(6):1059–65.
12. Queral LA, Criado FJ. The treatment of focal aortic arch branch lesions with Palmaz stents. J Vasc Surg. 1996;23(2):368–75.
13. Takach TJ, Duncan JM, Livesay JL, Krajcer Z, et al. Brachiocephalic reconstruction II: operative and endovascular management of single-vessel disease. J Vasc Surg. 2005;42(1):55–61.
14. Payne DA, Hayes PD, Bolia A, Fishwick G, Bell PRF, Naylor AR. Cerebral protection during open retrograde angioplasty/stenting of common carotid and innominate artery stenoses. Br J Surg. 2006;93:187–90.
15. Sfyroeras GS, Karathanos C, Antoniou GA, Saleptsis V, Giannoukas AD. A meta-analysis of combined endarterectomy and proximal balloon angioplasty for tandem disease of the arch vessels and carotid bifurcation. J Vasc Surg. 2011;54(2):534–40.
16. Paukovits TM, Haász J, Molnár A, Szeberin Z, Nemes B, Varga D, Hüttl K, Bérczi V. Transfemoral endovascular treatment of proximal common carotid artery lesions: a single-center experience on 153 lesions. J Vasc Surg. 2008;48(1):80–7.
17. AbuRahma AF, Robinson pA, Jennings TG. Carotid-subclavian bypass grafting with polytetrafluoroethylene grafts for symptomatic subclavian artery stenosis or occlusion: a 20-year experience. J Vasc Surg. 2000;32(3):411–9.
18. Clouse WD, Ergul EA, Cambria RP, Brewster DC, et al. Retrograde stenting of proximal lesions with carotid endarterectomy increases risk. J Vasc Surg. 2016;63(6):1517–23.
19. Aziz F, Gravett MH, Comerota AJ. Endovascular and open surgical treatment of brachiocephalic arteries. Ann Vasc Surg. 2011;25(4):569–81.
20. Aiello F, Morrissey NJ. Open and endovascular management of subclavian and innominate arterial pathology. Semin Vasc Surg. 2011;24(1):31–5.
21. Ziomek S, Quiñones-Baldrich WJ, Busuttil RW, Baker JD, Machleder HI, Moore WS. The superiority of synthetic arterial grafts over autologous veins in carotid-subclavian bypass. J Vasc Surg. 1986;3:140–5.
22. AbuRahma AF, Bates MC, Stone PA, Dyer B, Armistead L, Scott Dean L, Scott Lavigne P. Angioplasty and stenting versus carotid-subclavian bypass for the treatment of isolated subclavian artery disease. J Endovasc Ther. 2007;14(5):698–704.
23. Law MM, Colburn MD, Moore WS, Quinones-Baldrich WJ, Machleder JI, Gelabert HA. Carotid-subclavian bypass for brachiocephalic occlusive disease. Choice of conduit and long-term follow-up. Stroke. 1995;26:1565–71.
24. Cinà CS, Safar HA, Laganà A, Arena G, Clase CM. Subclavian carotid transposition and bypass grafting: consecutive cohort study and systematic review. J Vasc Surg. 2002;35(3):422–9.
25. Berguer R, Morasch MD, Kline RA, Kazmers A, Friedland MS. Cervical reconstruction of the supra-aortic trunks: a 16-year experience. J Vasc Surg. 1999;29(2):239–48.
26. Ozsvath KJ, Roddy SP, Darling RC, Byrne J, et al. Carotid-carotid crossover bypass: is it a durable procedure? J Vasc Surg. 2003;37(3):582–5.
27. AbuRahma AF, Robinson PA, Khan MZ, Khan JH, Boland JP. Brachiocephalic revascularization: a comparison between carotid-subclavian artery bypass and axilloaxillary artery bypass. Surgery. 1992;112:84–91.

28. Berguer R, Morasch MD, Kline RA. Transthoracic repair of innominate and common carotid artery disease: immediate and long-term outcome for 100 consecutive surgical reconstructions. J Vasc Surg. 1998;27(1):34–41. discussion 42

29. Ligush J, Criado E, Keagy BA. Innominate artery occlusive disease: management with central reconstructive techniques. Surgery. 1997;121:556–62.

30. Takach TJ, Reul GJ, Cooley DA, Duncan JM, et al. Brachiocephalic reconstruction I: operative and long-term results for complex disease. J Vasc Surg. 2005;42(1):47–54.

31. Kieffer E, Sabatier J, Koskas F, Bahnini A. Atherosclerotic innominate artery occlusive disease: early and long-term results of surgical reconstruction. J Vasc Surg. 1995;21:326–37.

Vertebral Artery Reconstruction

Mark D. Morasch

Indications

Atherosclerosis is the most common disease affecting the vertebral artery. Uncommon pathologic processes include trauma, fibromuscular dysplasia, Takayasu's disease, osteophyte compression, dissections, and aneurysms [1, 2], all of which can lead to symptoms of posterior circulation ischemia. Approximately 25% of all ischemic strokes occur in the vertebrobasilar territory. One half of patients will present initially with stroke, and 26% of patients present with transient ischemic symptoms rapidly followed by stroke [3]. For patients who experience vertebrobasilar TIAs, disease in the vertebral arteries portends a 22–35% risk of stroke over 5 years [4–6]. The mortality associated with a posterior circulation stroke is 20–30% which is higher than that for an anterior circulation event [7–9].

Ischemia affecting the temporo-occipital areas of the cerebral hemispheres or segments of the brainstem and cerebellum characteristically produces bilateral symptoms. The classic symptoms of vertebrobasilar ischemia are dizziness, vertigo, drop attacks, diplopia, perioral numbness, alternating paresthesia, tinnitus, dysphasia, dysarthria, and ataxia.

M. D. Morasch
Division of Vascular and Endovascular Surgery,
Department of Cardiac, Thoracic and Vascular
Surgery, Billings Clinic, Billings, MT, USA

In general, the ischemic mechanisms can be broken down into those that are hemodynamic and those that are embolic. Hemodynamic symptoms occur as a result of transient "end-organ" (brainstem, cerebellum, and/or occipital lobes) hypoperfusion and rarely result in infarction. Symptoms tend to be transient, repetitive, and more of a nuisance than a danger. For hemodynamic symptoms to occur, occlusive pathology must be present in both of the paired vertebral vessels and in the basilar artery. In addition, compensatory contribution from the carotid circulation via the circle of Willis must be incomplete. Alternatively, hemodynamic ischemic symptoms may follow proximal subclavian artery occlusion and the syndrome of subclavian/vertebral artery steal.

Up to one third of vertebrobasilar ischemic episodes are caused by embolization from plaques or mural lesions of the subclavian, vertebral, and/or basilar arteries [10]. Actual infarctions in the vertebrobasilar distribution are most often the result of embolic events.

Surgical reconstruction is not indicated in an asymptomatic patient with stenotic or occlusive vertebral lesions as these patients are well compensated from the carotid circulation through the posterior communicating vessels. The minimal anatomic requirement to justify vertebral artery reconstruction for patients with true hemodynamic symptoms is stenosis greater than 60% diameter in both vertebral arteries if both are patent and complete or the same degree of stenosis in the dominant vertebral artery if the opposite vertebral artery is hypoplastic, ends in a posteroinferior cerebellar artery, or is occluded. A single, normal vertebral artery is sufficient to adequately perfuse the basilar artery, regardless of the patency status of the contralateral vertebral artery. Conversely, patients with symptomatic vertebrobasilar ischemia due to emboli are candidates for surgical revascularization regardless of the condition of the contralateral vertebral artery. Surgical intervention is not indicated in asymptomatic patients who harbor suspicious radiographic findings.

Duplex ultrasound is an excellent tool for detecting lesions in the carotid artery, but it has significant limitations when used to detect vertebral artery pathology. The usefulness of duplex ultrasound lies in its ability to confirm reversal of flow within the vertebral arteries and detect flow velocity changes consistent with a proximal stenosis [11].

Contrast-enhanced magnetic resonance angiography (MRA) with 3D reconstruction and maximum image intensity (MIP) imaging techniques provide full imaging of the vessels including the supra-aortic trunks and the carotid and vertebral arteries better than CT; transaxial MRI images can readily diagnose both acute and chronic posterior fossa infarcts.

The most common site of disease, the vertebral artery origin, may not be well imaged with ultrasound or MRA and often can only be displayed with catheter-based angiography that employs oblique projections that may not be part of standard arch evaluation. Patients with suspected vertebral artery compression should also undergo dynamic angiography, which incorporates provocative positioning. Lastly, delayed imaging should be performed in order to demonstrate reconstitution of the extracranial vertebral arteries through cervical collaterals, such as the occipital artery or via collaterals from the ipsilateral subclavian artery via branches of the thyrocervical trunk (Fig. 18.1) [12].

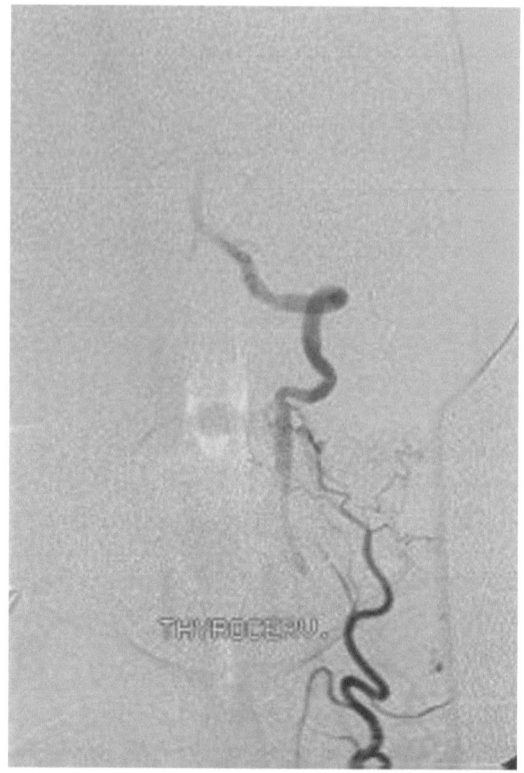

Fig. 18.1 V3 segment reconstitution via thyrocervical collateral. From: Morasch MD. Vertebral artery reconstruction. In: Hans SS, Shepard AD, Weaver MR, Bove P, Long GW. Endovascular and open vascular reconstruction: a practical approach. Copyright © 2017, CRC Press, reproduced by permission of Taylor & Francis Books UK

Operative Strategy and Technique

Surgical Anatomy of the Vertebral Artery

The surgical anatomy of the paired vertebral arteries is divided into four segments: V1, the origin of the vertebral artery arising from the subclavian artery to the point at which it enters the C6 transverse process; V2, the segment of the artery buried deep within intertransversarii muscles and the cervical transverse processes of C6–C2; V3, the surgically accessible extracranial segment between the transverse process of the C2 and the base of the skull before it enters the foramen magnum; and V4, the intracranial portion beginning at the atlanto-occipital membrane and terminating as the two vertebrals converge to form the basilar artery (Fig. 18.2). The location of disease will dictate the type of surgical reconstruction that is required. With rare exceptions, most reconstructions of the vertebral artery are performed to relieve either an orificial stenosis (V1 segment) or stenosis, dissection, or occlusion of its intraspinal component (V2 and V3 segments).

Stenosing ostial lesions in V1 [13] are best managed surgically with transposition of the proximal vertebral artery onto the adjacent carotid artery. More distal pathology usually requires bypass from the common carotid to the V3 segment vertebral artery between C_1 and C_2.

Exposure and Transposition of the Vertebral Artery into the Common Carotid Artery

The approach to the proximal vertebral artery is the same as the approach for a subclavian to carotid transposition. The patient is positioned in a slight chair position to decrease venous pressure. The incision is placed transversely just above the clavicle and directly over the two heads of the sternocleidomastoid muscle. Subplatysmal skin flaps are created to provide for adequate exposure. Dissection follows between the two bellies of the sternocleidomastoid after the omohyoid muscle is divided. The jugular vein is retracted laterally, and the carotid sheath is entered. The vagus nerve is retracted medially with the common carotid artery (Fig. 18.3). The remainder of

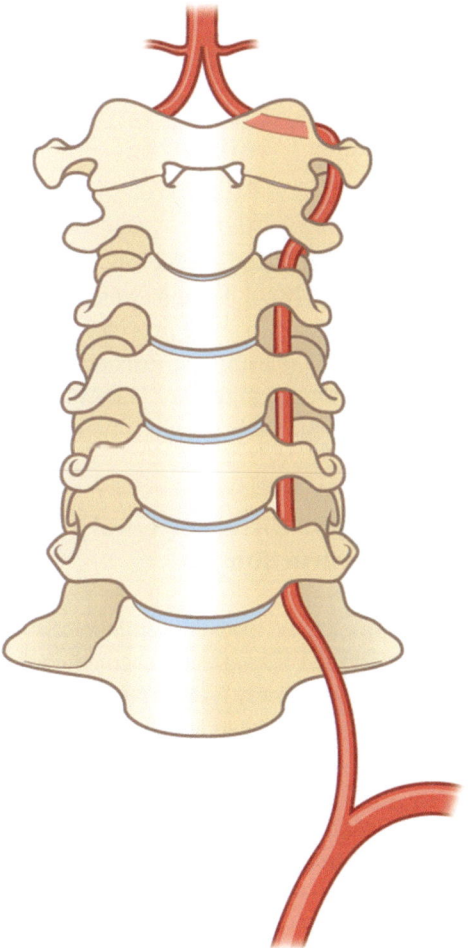

Fig. 18.2 Vertebral artery anatomy: V1–V4 segments. From: Morasch MD. Vertebral artery reconstruction. In: Hans SS, Shepard AD, Weaver MR, Bove P, Long GW. Endovascular and open vascular reconstruction: a practical approach. Copyright © 2017, CRC Press, reproduced by permission of Taylor & Francis Books UK

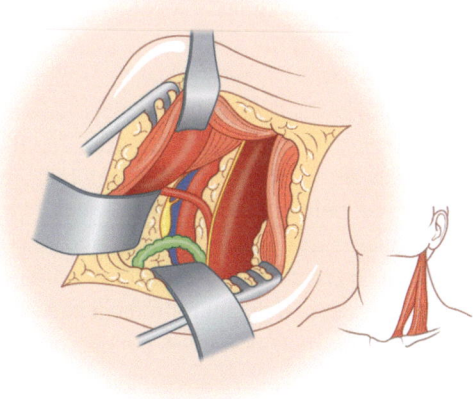

Fig. 18.3 Surgical approach to the V1 segment of the vertebral artery. The jugular vein is retracted laterally and the carotid sheet is entered. The vagus nerve is retracted medially with the common carotid artery. From: Morasch MD. Vertebral artery reconstruction. In: Hans SS, Shepard AD, Weaver MR, Bove P, Long GW. Endovascular and open vascular reconstruction: a practical approach. Copyright © 2017, CRC Press, reproduced by permission of Taylor & Francis Books UK

the dissection is carried out between the jugular vein and the carotid artery in the base of the neck.

On the left side, the thoracic duct is encircled with a right-angled clamp and then divided between ligatures. Accessory lymph ducts, often seen on the right side of the neck, are also identified, ligated, and divided. The entire dissection is confined medial to the prescalene fat pad that covers the scalenus anticus muscle and phrenic nerve. These structures are left unexposed lateral to the field. The inferior thyroid artery runs transversely across the field, and it is ligated and divided.

The vertebral vein should be identified as it emerges from the angle formed by the longus colli and scalenus anticus. The vein invariably overlies the proximal vertebral artery and, at the bottom of the field, the subclavian artery. It is ligated and divided. The vertebral and subclavian vessels lie immediately deep to the vein. It is important to identify and avoid injury to the adjacent sympathetic chain. The vertebral artery is exposed from its origin at the posteromedial aspect of the subclavian artery distally to the tendon of the longus coli muscle where it enters the transverse foramen of C6. The vertebral artery is freed from the sympathetic trunk resting on its anterior surface without damaging the trunk or the ganglionic rami.

Once the artery is fully exposed, an appropriate site for carotid reimplantation is identified. The patient is given systemic heparin. The distal portion of the V1 segment of the vertebral artery is clamped below the edge of the longus colli with a microclip avoiding any axial twisting. The proximal vertebral artery is ligated with 5-0 polypropylene transfixion suture immediately above its origin. The artery is divided, pulled from under the sympathetic chain, and brought over to the common carotid artery. The free end is spatulated for anastomosis (Fig. 18.4). The carotid artery is cross-clamped. An elliptical 5–7 mm arteriotomy is created in the posterolateral wall of the common carotid artery with an aortic punch. The anastomosis is performed in parachute fashion with continuous 7-0 polypropylene suture. Upon completion of the anastomosis, the suture slack is tightened, standard flushing maneuvers per-

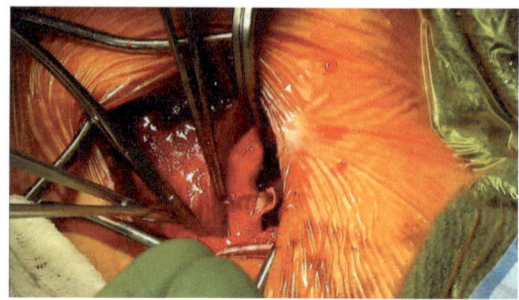

Fig. 18.4 Surgical approach to the V1 segment of the vertebral artery. The distal portion of the V1 segment is clamped, and the proximal vertebral artery is ligated immediately above its origin. The artery is then divided, pulled from under the sympathetic chain, and brought over the common carotid artery. The free end is spatulated for anastomosis. From: Morasch MD. Vertebral artery reconstruction. In: Hans SS, Shepard AD, Weaver MR, Bove P, Long GW. Endovascular and open vascular reconstruction: a practical approach. Copyright © 2017, CRC Press, reproduced by permission of Taylor & Francis Books UK

formed, suture tied, clamps removed, and flow reestablished (Fig. 18.5). A drain, which can be removed the following morning provided there is no chylous leak, is placed. The incision is then closed by reapproximating the platysma and closing the skin with a subcuticular stitch.

V3 Exposure and Distal Vertebral Artery Reconstruction

Saphenous vein bypass from the common carotid or subclavian to the V3 vertebral segment is the technique most commonly used to perform a distal reconstruction [12]. Alternatively, radial artery can be utilized as conduit in the absence of suitable vein. The distal portion of the reconstruction is generally completed at the C1–C2 spinal level.

The skin incision is placed anterior to the sternocleidomastoid muscle, the same as in a carotid operation, and is carried superiorly immediately below the earlobe. The dissection proceeds in a retrojugular plane between vein and the anterior edge of the sternocleidomastoid. The spinal accessory nerve will be encountered and should gently be dissected over a 5 cm length so that it can safely be retracted. The nerve is followed

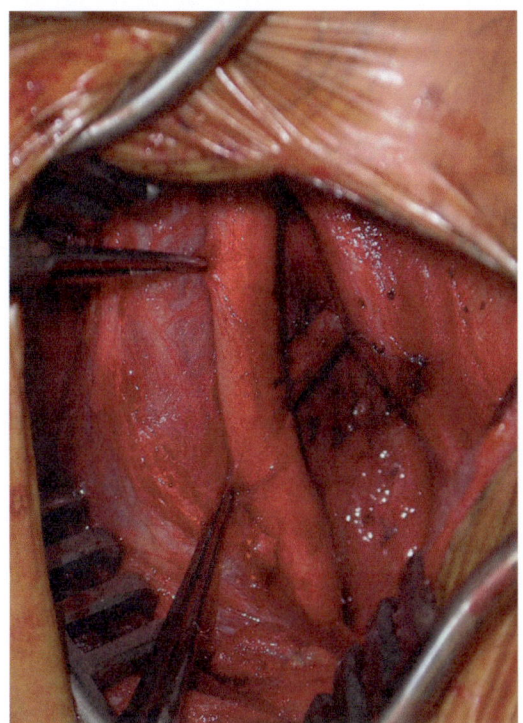

Fig. 18.5 Completed proximal vertebral-to-common carotid artery bypass. From: Morasch MD. Vertebral artery reconstruction. In: Hans SS, Shepard AD, Weaver MR, Bove P, Long GW. Endovascular and open vascular reconstruction: a practical approach. Copyright © 2017, CRC Press, reproduced by permission of Taylor & Francis Books UK

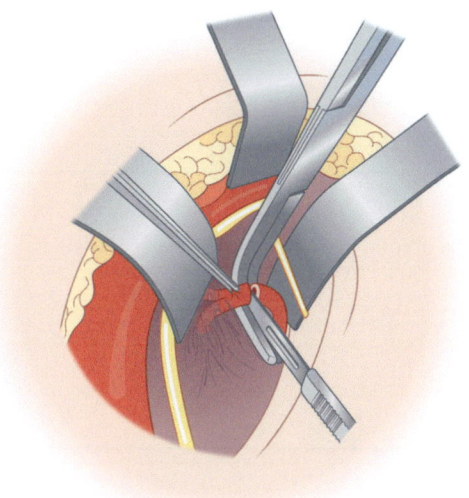

Fig. 18.6 Transection of the C2 nerve root and the V3 segment of the vertebral artery, which lies just deep to this structure. The C2 ramus should be cut before it branches. From: Morasch MD. Vertebral artery reconstruction. In: Hans SS, Shepard AD, Weaver MR, Bove P, Long GW. Endovascular and open vascular reconstruction: a practical approach. Copyright © 2017, CRC Press, reproduced by permission of Taylor & Francis Books UK

proximally as it crosses in front of the jugular vein and the transverse process of C1. The first cervical vertebrae can be easily felt by the finger palpation.

The levator scapula muscle is exposed by removing of the fibrofatty tissue overlying it. Once the anterior edge of the levator scapula is identified, the anterior ramus of C2 becomes visible. With the ramus as a guide, a right-angle clamp is slid under the levator scapula and then divided. The C2 ramus divides into three branches after crossing the vertebral artery. The ramus should be cut (Fig. 18.6) before it branches. This will expose the V3 segment of the vertebral artery which can then be freed from the surrounding venous plexus over a 1–2 cm length.

Once the vertebral artery is adequately exposed, the distal common carotid artery should be prepared as inflow for the bypass graft. There

is no need to dissect the carotid bifurcation, and the location selected for the proximal anastomosis should not be too close to the bifurcation as cross-clamping at this level may fracture underlying atheroma.

A suitable conduit of appropriate length is harvested and prepared. A valveless segment of vein facilitates back-bleeding of the vertebral artery after completion of the distal anastomosis. The patient is given intravenous heparin. The vertebral artery is elevated by gently pulling on an encircling vessel loop and is occluded with a small J-clamp. This isolates a short segment for an end-to-side anastomosis. The vertebral artery is opened longitudinally over a short length adequate to accommodate the spatulated end of the vein graft. The end-to-side anastomosis is done with continuous 7-0 polypropylene and fine needles. A vascular clamp is placed in the vein graft proximal to the anastomosis, and the vertebral J-clamp is removed.

The proximal end of the graft is passed behind the jugular vein and in proximity to the side of

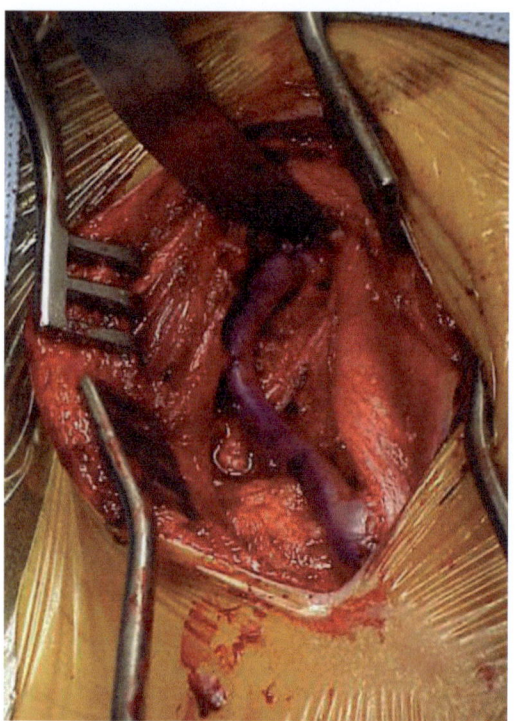

Fig. 18.7 Completed common carotid artery-to-V# segment vertebral artery bypass using reverse greater saphenous vein as conduit. From: Morasch MD. Vertebral artery reconstruction. In: Hans SS, Shepard AD, Weaver MR, Bove P, Long GW. Endovascular and open vascular reconstruction: a practical approach. Copyright © 2017, CRC Press, reproduced by permission of Taylor & Francis Books UK

struction. Reparable technical flaws may be identified, and repair can prevent reconstruction failure.

Surgical Results

Combined death and stroke rates for open surgery range from 1% in proximal reconstructive efforts to 4% in distal revascularizations [14, 15]. Risk is generally increased when patients undergo a combination of both vertebral and carotid revascularization. Surgical morbidity includes immediate thrombosis (1.4%), vagus and recurrent laryngeal nerve palsy (2%), Horner's syndrome (8.4–28%), lymphocele (4%), and chylothorax (5%) [15]. Long-term outcomes of open revascularization for vertebral artery disease are generally excellent with high stroke-free survival rates and patency as high as 90% at 10 years [16]. While the number of studies is limited and these reports consist of only medium-sized case series, the results seen with open vertebral reconstruction should be considered benchmarks upon which endoluminal therapy should be compared.

Potential Postoperative Complications

The perioperative complication rates differ for proximal versus distal vertebral artery repairs. Perioperative complications that can follow any reconstruction include stroke, bleeding, thrombosis, and nerve injury.

Stroke is usually the result of prolonged clamp time or to immediate postop thrombosis of vertebral arteries or conduits. Completion angiography may be helpful in preventing these complications. Distal reconstructions have a combined stroke and death rate of 3–4% and have a higher stroke and death rates than operations on the proximal vertebral artery.

Nerve injury—Complications that are particular to proximal reconstruction include vagus and recurrent laryngeal nerve palsy (2%) and Horner's syndrome (8.4–28%). Complications that may follow distal reconstruction include

the common carotid artery. The common carotid artery is then cross-clamped, an elliptical arteriotomy is made in its posterior wall with an aortic punch, and the proximal vein graft is anastomosed end-to-side to the common carotid artery (Fig. 18.7). Before the anastomosis is completed, standard flushing maneuvers are performed, suture is tied, and flow is reestablished. The vertebral artery is occluded with a clip placed immediately below the anastomosis to create a functional end-to-end anastomosis and so as to avoid competitive flow or the potential for recurrent emboli. The wound is closed without a drain, by reapproximating the platysma and closing skin with a subcuticular stitch.

Intraoperative completion imaging using digital angiography is useful and should be considered for all types of vertebral artery recon-

vagus (1%) and spinal accessory nerve (2%) injuries. Most patients who undergo proximal vertebral reconstruction will experience at least a short-lived Horner's syndrome. Often times it is not noticeable to the patient but can be seen by other observers. The treatment is expectant. Most, if not all, will resolve in time. Vagus nerve injuries manifest as hoarseness and are most often the result of traction on the vagus itself during exposure of the deep neck structures during proximal vertebral transposition or during mobilization of the common carotid during a distal bypass. Since this rarely is the result of cutting the recurrent nerve, usually time and patience are all that are required. If a vocal cord palsy persists beyond 3 months, cord medialization may be warranted. A spinal accessory nerve injury results from undo traction. Most neuropraxia-type injuries will resolve in time.

Conservative management is appropriate initially for a chylous or significant lymphatic leak as most will resolve. This includes local compression, dietary manipulation, and administration of octreotide. Leaks that persist beyond 3 days require re-exploration of the surgical wound and attempt direct suture repair. A purse-string placement of a small-gauge monofilament suture works best to control a large lymphatic or thoracic duct leak. If all else fails, ligation of the thoracic duct using video-assisted thoracotomy surgery can be considered.

Endovascular Treatment

In the last decade, endovascular treatment of vertebral artery disease, usually with stent placement, has gained favor as an alternative to surgery. Endovascular access to the vertebral artery is relatively straightforward. The procedure can be performed under local anesthesia, enabling continuous neurological monitoring of the patient. Most cases are performed from a femoral approach, although trans-brachial and trans-radial access has also been used. The stenotic lesions are crossed and treated with 0.014 or 0.018 in. guidewires and small coronary-diameter balloons and stents. Procedures can be performed with or without the assistance of embolic protection devices. Periprocedural risks include embolization, rupture, thrombosis, arterial dissection, and stent malposition or fracture.

In their series of 105 patients who underwent endovascular stenting for symptomatic vertebral artery disease, Jenkins et al. achieved 100% radiographic improvement (residual stenosis ≤30%) [17]. The authors reported immediate (30-day) periprocedural risk of death of 1% and periprocedural complication rate of 4.8%. Complications included transient ischemic attack, flow-limiting dissection, hematoma, and catheter-access-site problems. At 1 year of follow-up, six patients had died and five had experienced a vertebrobasilar stroke [17].

A recent Cochrane review identified 313 endovascular interventions for vertebral artery stenosis, with just over half of the interventions using stent placement as part of the treatment of vertebrobasilar stenosis. The 30-day risk of TIA or stroke was 3.2% and death rate was also 3.2% [18]. The technical success rate was 95%. Overall, retrospective reviews suggest that vertebral artery stenting is reasonably safe, although a selection bias exists.

Despite high technical success rates, endovascular treatment of vertebral artery disease appears to have unacceptably high rates of restenosis, especially when angioplasty is performed alone. Adjuvant stent placement seems to add to the clinical durability but adds inherent morbidity such as malposition and potential stent fracture. Eighteen patients with extracranial vertebral artery disease in The Stenting of Symptomatic Atherosclerotic Lesions in the Vertebral or Intracranial Arteries (SSYLVIA) trial underwent angioplasty and stenting. Technical success (determined as less than 50% residual stenosis following treatment) was achieved in 17 (94%) of the 18 patients [19]. There were no periprocedural neurological complications. The investigators, however, reported 6-month restenosis rates of 50%. These recurrences were symptomatic in 39% of cases [19]. Jenkins et al. reported in their series that at approximately 2.5 years of follow-up, 70% of patients remained symptom-free, but 13% of patients had restenosis requiring retreatment [17].

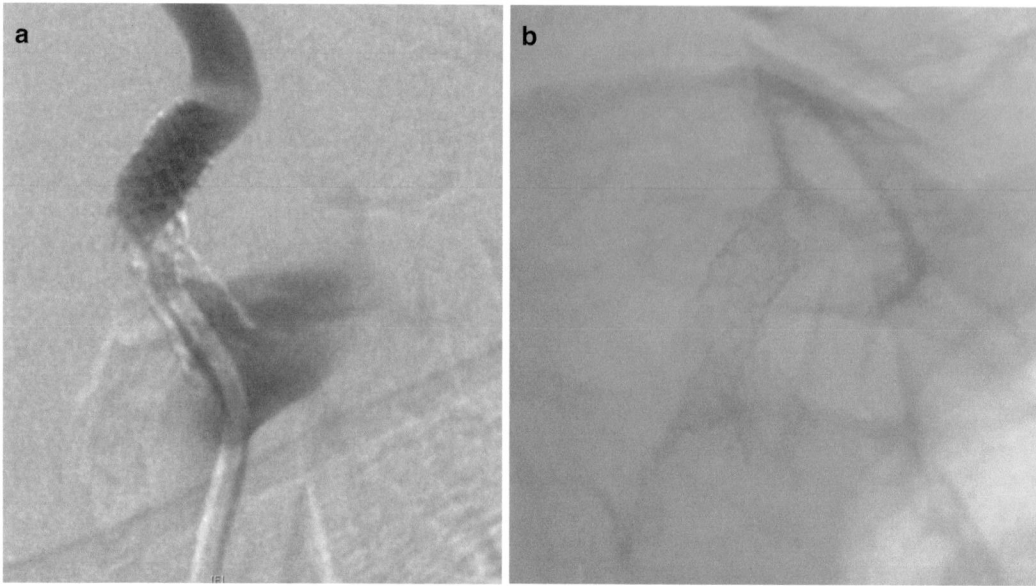

Fig. 18.8 (**a**, **b**) Angiography of 69-year-old man (case example) showing vertebral stent fracture and recurrent high-grade vertebral artery stenosis at the site of the stent damage. V1 segment stent fracture with symptomatic in-stent restenosis. From: Morasch MD. Vertebral artery reconstruction. In: Hans SS, Shepard AD, Weaver MR, Bove P, Long GW. Endovascular and open vascular reconstruction: a practical approach. Copyright © 2017, CRC Press, reproduced by permission of Taylor & Francis Books UK

Late stent fracture with concomitant in-stent restenosis appears to also be a problem plaguing endoluminal therapies that target lesions at the vertebral artery origin. Recall that the vertebral takes origin from the subclavian artery at a near right angle. In addition, the first portion of the subclavian artery has relative mobility while the vertebral becomes fixed as it passes into the transverse foramen of C6. This particular anatomy may create unique mechanical forces that make stent fracture more likely than other parts of the body (Fig. 18.8).

The use of drug-eluting stents to impede neointimal hyperplasia and prevent restenosis has been well established in the coronary arteries [20]. Ogilvy et al. reported a series of patients with the longest follow-up thus far (21 months) in whom drug-eluting stents were used in vertebral artery origin stenoses. They found decreased incidence of in-stent restenosis (>50% diameter) from 38% in patients who received non-drug-eluting stents to 17% in those who received drug-eluting stents [21]. Other reports also suggest decreased restenosis rates with drug-eluting stents; however, majority of the studies have mean patient follow-up times less than 1 year [22, 23]. Treatment with drug-eluting stents requires long-term dual antiplatelet therapy; it remains unclear to date whether differing stent makeup will have a significant impact in the outcomes of patients who undergo interventions of the vertebral artery.

As with open surgical techniques, only retrospective case series exist for endoluminal therapies for the treatment of vertebral artery disease. There are currently no level I data to support the routine application of angioplasty and stenting of the vertebral artery over best medical therapy. A subset of 16 patients treated within the Carotid and Vertebral Artery Transluminal Angioplasty Study (CAVATAS 2001) represents the only report of a randomized controlled trial comparing endoluminal therapy with best medical care for symptomatic vertebral stenosis. There were no 30-day strokes or deaths in either group, although two of eight patients who underwent endoluminal therapy experienced transient ischemic symptoms. Furthermore, with a mean follow-up of 4.5 years, there were no posterior circulation strokes noted in either group. Currently underway is a single multicenter randomized trial prospectively analyzing the impact of percutaneous vertebral interventions over medical therapy, the Vertebral Artery Stenting Trial (VAST), for stenting of intracranial or extracranial vertebral artery stenosis [24].

While vertebral artery angioplasty and stenting may be a relatively safe and effective approach that avoids the morbidity associated with major surgery, most available data on the efficacy of this therapy is limited to single-center retrospective reports that carry inherent selection bias. The only randomized data available is underpowered, and definitive conclusions on the effectiveness of endovascular therapy for vertebral disease cannot be drawn. At present, the technique should be reserved for select cases until indications for its routine application become clearer.

Conclusion

Atherosclerotic vertebral artery disease is an underdiagnosed cause of posterior circulation ischemia. Revascularization of the vertebral artery is often a viable option and should be considered in symptomatic patients in whom medical therapy has failed. Both surgical and endoluminal approaches to treating vertebral artery pathology may be considered, and the choice between the two is often determined by the anatomic location of the lesion being intervened upon. Such consideration requires a complete understanding of the vertebrobasilar anatomy using appropriate imaging studies. Open techniques for revascularization of the vertebral artery have proven clinical durability and acceptable surgical morbidity in experienced hands. Endoluminal techniques, which have gained momentum over the past decade, have shown clinically feasible but have yet to deliver on durability benchmarks set

by open surgical revascularization. As such, vertebral artery stenting should be reserved to select centers with high volume experience that have established acceptable outcomes in both clinical success and safety. For each individual patient who suffers from medically refractive vertebrobasilar ischemia, practitioners must carefully balance the risks of surgery versus the limitations of endoluminal intervention before recommending intervention.

Review Questions

1. In patients experiencing TIA in the distribution of vertebrobasilar territory, stroke risk over 5 years is:
   A. 5–15%
   B. 16–20%
   C. 21–33%
   D. >33%

   Answer: C

2. Patient develops chylous leak following vertebral artery transposition into the common carotid artery. Initial management should consist of:
   A. Dietary manipulation and octreotide
   B. Local operative exploration
   C. Thoracic duct embolization
   D. Video-assisted thoracotomy and thoracic duct ligation

   Answer: A

3. High-grade stenotic ostial lesion of V1 segment of the vertebral artery in a symptomatic patient with contralateral vertebral occlusion should be treated with:
   A. Balloon angioplasty
   B. Anticoagulation with Coumadin
   C. Vertebral artery endarterectomy
   D. Transposition of proximal vertebral artery into the common carotid artery

   Answer: D

References

1. Morasch MD, Phade SV, Hurie JH, Naughton PA, Garcia-Toca M, Escobar G, Berguer R. Primary extracranial vertebral artery aneurysms. Ann Vasc Surg. 2013;27(4):418–23.
2. Sultan S, Morasch M, Colgan MP, Madhavan P, Moore D, Shanik G. Operative and endovascular management of extracranial vertebral artery aneurysm in Ehlers-Danlos syndrome: a clinical dilemma, case report and literature review. Vasc Endovasc Surg. 2002;36:389–92.
3. Wityk RJ, Chang HM, Rosengart A, et al. Proximal extracranial vertebral artery disease in the New England Medical Center Posterior Circulation Registry. Arch Neurol. 1998;55(4):470–8.
4. Cartlidge NE, Whisnant JP, Elveback LR. Carotid and vertebral-basilar transient cerebral ischemic attacks. A community study, Rochester, Minnesota. Mayo Clin Proc. 1977;52(2):117–20.
5. Heyman A, Wilkinson WE, Hurwitz BJ, et al. Clinical and epidemiologic aspects of vertebrobasilar and nonfocal cerebral ischemia. In: Berguer R, Bauer RB, editors. Vertebrobasilar arterial occlusive disease. Medical and surgical management. New York: Raven Press; 1984. p. 27–36.
6. Whisnant JP, Cartlidge NE, Elveback LR. Carotid and vertebral-basilar transient ischemic attacks: effect of anticoagulants, hypertension, and cardiac disorders on survival and stroke occurrence—a population study. Ann Neurol. 1978;3(2):107–15.
7. Jones HR Jr, Millikan CH, Sandok BA. Temporal profile (clinical course) of acute vertebrobasilar system cerebral infarction. Stroke. 1980;11(2):173–7.
8. McDowell FH, Potes J, Groch S. The natural history of internal carotid and vertebral-basilar artery occlusion. Neurology. 1961;11(4 Pt2):153–7.
9. Patrick BK, Ramirez-Lassepas M, Synder BD. Temporal profile of vertebrobasilar territory infarction. Prognostic implications. Stroke. 1980;11(6):643–8.
10. Caplan LR, Wityk RJ, Glass TA, et al. New England Medical Center posterior circulation registry. Ann Neurol. 2004;56(3):389–98.
11. Berguer R, Higgins R, Nelson R. Noninvasive diagnosis of reversal of vertebral-artery blood flow. N Engl J Med. 1980;302(24):1349–51.
12. Berguer R. Distal vertebral artery bypass: technique, the "occipital connection," and potential uses. J Vasc Surg. 1985;2(4):621–6.
13. Edwards WH, Mulherin JL Jr. The surgical approach to significant stenosis of vertebral and subclavian arteries. Surgery. 1980;87(1):20–8.
14. Berguer R. Complex carotid and vertebral revascularizations. In: Pearce WH, Matsumura JS, Yao JST, editors. Vascular surgery in the endovascular era. Evanston: Greenwood Academic; 2008. p. 344–52.
15. Berguer R, Morasch MD, Kline RA. A review of 100 consecutive reconstructions of the distal vertebral artery for embolic and hemodynamic disease. J Vasc Surg. 1998;27(5):852–9.
16. Berguer R, Flynn LM, Kline RA, Caplan L. Surgical reconstruction of the extracranial vertebral artery: management and outcome. J Vasc Surg. 2000;31(1 Pt 1):9–18.
17. Jenkins JS, Patel SN, White CJ, et al. Endovascular stenting for vertebral artery stenosis. J Am Coll Cardiol. 2010;55(6):538–42.
18. Coward LJ, Featherstone RL, Brown MM. Percutaneous transluminal angioplasty and stenting for vertebral artery stenosis. Cochrane Database Syst Rev. 2005;2:CD000516.
19. SSYLVIA Study Investigators. Stenting of symptomatic atherosclerotic lesions in the vertebral or intracranial arteries (SSYLVIA): study results. Stroke. 2004;35(6):1388–92.
20. Stone GW, Ellis SG, Cox DA, et al. A polymer-based, paclitaxel-eluting stent in patients with coronary artery disease. N Engl J Med. 2004;350(3):221–31.
21. Ogilvy CS, Yang X, Natarajan SK, et al. Restenosis rates following vertebral artery origin stenting: does stent type make a difference? J Invasive Cardiol. 2010;22(3):119–24.
22. Steinfort B, Ng PP, Faulder K, et al. Midterm outcomes of paclitaxel-eluting stents for the treatment of intracranial posterior circulation stenoses. J Neurosurg. 2007;106(2):222–5.
23. Vajda Z, Miloslavski E, Guthe T, et al. Treatment of stenoses of vertebral artery origin using short drug-eluting coronary stents: improved follow-up results. AJNR Am J Neuroradiol. 2009;30(9):1653–6.
24. Compter A, van der Worp HB, Schonewille WJ, et al. VAST: vertebral artery stenting trial. Protocol for a randomised safety and feasibility trial. Trials. 2008;9:65.

Fibromuscular Dysplasia, Carotid Kinks, and Other Rare Lesions

19

Ahmed Kayssi and Dipankar Mukherjee

Fibromuscular Dysplasia

Definition

Fibromuscular dysplasia (FMD) is a non-atherosclerotic, noninflammatory arteriopathy that primarily affects middle-sized vessels such as the extracranial cerebrovascular and renal arteries [1]. It was first described in 1938 by Leadbetter and Burkland in a patient with hypertension secondary to renal artery disease [2]. In that same year, McCormick et al. coined the term "fibromuscular dysplasia" to describe this condition, also in the renal arteries [3]. Connett and Lansche were the first to describe FMD in the cerebrovascular circulation when they published the case of a 34-year-old woman who presented to a hospital with a transient ischemic attack and angiographic evidence of internal carotid artery (ICA) aneurysmal degeneration [4]. Extracranial cerebrovascular FMD most often involves the ICA at the levels C1–C2 and is usually bilateral [5]. Vertebral artery involvement, while described, is far less common [6]. FMD has also been reported in arteries throughout the body, including the mesenteric, external iliac, and brachial arteries [7].

Prevalence

Estimating the prevalence of FMD in the general population is challenging for two reasons. Firstly, the majority of patients with FMD are asymptomatic, which complicates its detection, and, secondly, FMD reports have relied largely on renal transplant donor reports, retrospective audits of angiograms, and sub-studies of renal artery stenting clinical trials [8]. Analyses of angiograms performed in patients with neurological conditions have suggested a 0.3–3.2% prevalence of cerebrovascular FMD in those patients [9]. Due to the rarity of this condition and the lack of robust epidemiological data, several centers in the United States partnered in 2008 to create the US Registry for Fibromuscular Dysplasia. The Registry began enrolling in 2009 and now includes 13 active centers that prospectively collect and share clinical data. The Registry's first report on 447 patients was published in 2012 and found that extracranial carotid and renal artery involvement were equally prevalent in FMD patients [10].

Etiology

While the exact etiology of FMD is unknown, it is clear that it affects females by a greater than 9:1 ratio compared to men [11]. The relationship between female gender and risk of FMD is

A. Kayssi
Vascular Surgery, University of Toronto, Toronto, ON, Canada

D. Mukherjee (✉)
Vascular Surgery, Inova Fairfax Hospital, Falls Church, VA, USA

© The Editor(s) (if applicable) and The Author(s) 2018
S. S. Hans (ed.), *Extracranial Carotid and Vertebral Artery Disease*,
https://doi.org/10.1007/978-3-319-91533-3_19

not understood, however, and no link has been identified between FMD and estrogen levels, contraceptives, or pregnancy [12]. Numerous investigators have suggested a genetic predisposition to FMD. Rushton et al. analyzed 20 families in which at least one member had FMD [13]. They found that 12 of those families (60%) had between 1 and 11 relatives with clinical evidence of FMD and concluded that the condition likely had an autosomal dominant inheritance pattern with variable penetrance. Mettinger and Ericson further assessed 37 patients with FMD and found that 30% had a first-degree relative with a history of stroke, hypertension, migraine, or impaired hearing and also suggested a dominant inheritance pattern with reduced penetrance [14]. Perdu et al. used high-resolution echo tracking of the carotid artery of 47 relatives of 13 cases from six families to generate a semiquantitative arterial score and compared their results with 47 controls [15]. The authors found that FMD cases had a significantly higher score compared with the controls and concluded that the condition was likely a result of a major genetic defect.

Pathology and Classification

FMD is classified according to the affected arterial wall layer (Table 19.1). Regardless of the affected arterial segment, the same classification system is used throughout the body [16]. The most common type of FMD impacts the medial

Table 19.1 Pathologic classification of fibromuscular dysplasia

Type	Prevalence	Radiological appearance
Medial fibroplasia	80–90%	"String-of-beads" appearance secondary to alternating thinned and thickened medial ridges
Intimal fibroplasia	10%	Long, concentric stenotic lesion secondary to intimal collagen deposits
Perimedial fibroplasia	<1%	Similar to medial hyperplasia but typically presents with smaller and fewer beads
Adventitial fibroplasia	Unknown	Similar to intimal fibroplasia

layer and includes medial fibroplasia, perimedial fibroplasia, and medial hyperplasia. The majority of FMD (80–90%) presents as medial fibroplasia, which is characterized by thinned media, thickened collagen-containing medial ridges, and a characteristic "string-of-beads" appearance on angiography (Fig. 19.1a, b) [12]. This appearance is secondary to stenotic webs that cause sequential stenoses and dilations in the arterial wall. These dilations may eventually lead to the aneurysmal degeneration seen in FMD patients. Medial fibroplasia is more common in females and in the pediatric population [18].

Intimal fibroplasia is the next most common form of FMD (10%). It is characterized by an irregular accumulation of subendothelial mesenchymal cells within a loose matrix of fibrous connective tissue [18]. Angiographically, intimal fibroplasia appears as long, irregular tubular stenoses in younger patients and as smooth, focal stenoses in older patients (Fig. 19.1c, d). Unlike

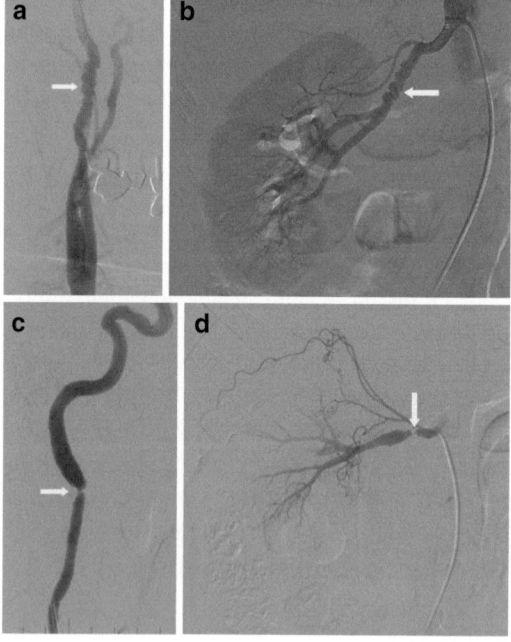

Fig. 19.1 Fibromuscular dysplasia in the internal carotid (**a**) and renal (**b**) arteries with the classic string-of-beads appearance of medial fibroplasia. The less common intimal fibroplasia presents as a focal, bandlike narrowing in the internal carotid (**c**) and renal (**d**) arteries. From: Poloskey et al. [17]. Reprinted with permission from Wolters Kluwer Health, Inc

medial fibroplasia, intimal fibroplasia affects both genders equally. Other forms of FMD such as medial hyperplasia, perimedial dysplasia, and adventitial fibroplasia are very rare.

Differential Diagnosis

Atherosclerosis

Patients with FMD are typically younger and have fewer cardiovascular risk factors than patients with atherosclerotic vascular disease. Furthermore, atherosclerotic lesions usually occur at the origin or within the proximal portion of the artery, while FMD occurs in the middle or distal portion of the artery [19]. It is important to keep in mind, however, that FMD and atherosclerotic disease can present concurrently [20–22].

Connective-Tissue Disease and Other Disorders

Several reports have documented an association between FMD and connective-tissue diseases such as Marfan's and Ehlers-Danlos type IV [23, 24]. Furthermore, FMD has been associated with segmental arterial mediolysis and neurofibromatosis type I [25, 26].

Vasculitis

FMD, by definition, is noninflammatory, which helps to distinguish it from vasculitis. Patients with FMD will thus have normal inflammatory serological markers. However, like vasculitis, FMD can occur in multiple vascular territories and may be associated with TIAs, stroke, hypertension, and renal failure [12]. FMD has also been described in patients with Takayasu's arteritis [27].

Clinical Presentation

Most patients with cerebrovascular FMD are asymptomatic, middle-aged women who are otherwise healthy, but patients can be of any age or gender [28]. Patients may present with non-specific symptoms such as headaches or dizziness or have a carotid bruit on physical exam

[11]. The presence of asymptomatic cerebrovascular FMD, however, is not a reliable predictor of future complications. Corrin et al. followed 79 asymptomatic patients with angiographically diagnosed cerebrovascular FMD for up to 18 years and reported only 3 (4%) incidents of cerebral ischemic events [29].

Symptomatic cerebrovascular FMD may present in a variety of different ways. Patients may develop cerebral ischemia secondary to a thromboembolic event originating from a diseased arterial segment or a low-flow state [30]. Furthermore, patients with FMD may present with dissections, and up to 15% of patients with cervical artery dissections have evidence of FMD on angiography [31, 32]. Most patients with carotid or vertebral artery FMD also present with headaches [14]. The presence of extracranial cerebrovascular FMD places patients at a higher risk of intracranial aneurysms. In a well-conducted meta-analysis, Cloft et al. reported a 7.3% prevalence of cerebral aneurysms in patients presenting with internal carotid or vertebral artery FMD [33]. Consequently, patients with FMD may present with subarachnoid hemorrhage secondary to intracranial aneurysm rupture. Of note, subarachnoid hemorrhage has also been described in patients without evidence of aneurysms on angiography but whose autopsy revealed evidence of microaneurysmal degeneration of the basilar artery [34]. Other rare, but morbid, complications of cerebrovascular FMD include Horner's syndrome, carotid-cavernous fistulas, and vertebral arteriovenous fistulas [14, 35, 36].

Investigations

The work-up of patients with suspected FMD is radiological. As the condition is noninflammatory, there is little use in measuring serological markers such as erythrocyte sedimentation rate (ESR) or C-reactive protein (CRP), except to rule out vasculitis. Available imaging modalities include ultrasound, computerized tomography angiography (CTA), magnetic resonance angiography (MRA), and digital subtraction angiography (DSA) (Table 19.2). While there

Table 19.2 Assessment of different imaging modalities for the work-up of FMD

	Advantages	Disadvantages
Ultrasound	Easy access, cheap, safe, hemodynamic data, high sensitivity for detection of significant stenosis	Operator-dependent, poor specificity
CTA	High sensitivity, high specificity, high spatial resolution, short acquisition time	Iodine injection (risk of allergies or renal failure), radiation exposure, no hemodynamic data
MRA	Safety, moderate sensitivity and specificity	Specific contraindications, moderate spatial resolution, no hemodynamic data
Digital subtraction angiography	High spatial resolution, short acquisition time	Iodine injection (risk of allergies or renal failure), radiation exposure, invasive procedure

Data from Varennes et al. [37]

are no validated imaging diagnostic criteria for FMD, the presence of a "string-of-beads" sign or a "web-like" defect at the origin of the ICA on CTA or MRA in the extracranial cerebrovascular circulation is suggestive of FMD [38].

Ultrasound

Diagnostic duplex ultrasound is cheap, noninvasive, and widely available. It is also considered a standard first-line modality in the work-up of extracranial cerebrovascular pathology. The evidence for the utility of diagnostic ultrasound in diagnosing FMD stems primarily from the renal literature [39, 40]. While the "string of beads" may on occasion be visualized, ultrasound studies of FMD will typically demonstrate evidence of turbulence, tortuosity, and a velocity shift in the middle and distal portions of the affected arteries, as well as vascular loops, ectasia, intimal flap, or aliasing [12].

Unlike in patients with carotid artery stenosis secondary to atherosclerotic disease, the degree of arterial stenosis in FMD patients cannot be determined by Doppler velocity shifts. In FMD patients, the multiple areas of stenosis and dilation result in unique flow characteristics that cannot be judged according to atherosclerotic carotid disease criteria. As such, ultrasound is insufficient in diagnosing FMD, and patients with concerning features on ultrasound should undergo cross-sectional imaging. On Doppler ultrasound report, Olin and Sealove recommend a statement of maximum velocity as well as the presence of turbulence or tortuosity, rather than an estimation of degree of stenosis [12].

CTA

This imaging modality is widely available and less resource-intensive compared with MRA. It allows for a thorough evaluation of the cerebrovascular vasculature and three-dimensional reconstructions that help in the diagnosis and treatment of any concerning lesions.

MRA

We are not aware of any studies that have demonstrated an advantage for MRA in the diagnosis of cerebrovascular FMD when compared with CTA or DSA. However, MRA may be helpful in assessing any concurrent arterial dissection through simultaneously acquired T1 fat-saturation images with a time-of-flight or gadolinium-enhanced imaging protocol [41]. Furthermore, an MRA should be obtained in patients with carotid or vertebral FMD to rule out a concurrent intracranial aneurysm.

DSA

Given advances in modern imaging technologies, the use of DSA in the diagnosis of FMD is largely reserved for cases in which there is a high degree of clinical suspicion and otherwise equivocal CTA or MRA studies. DSA studies provide a high degree of anatomical detail and are very helpful in operative planning (Fig. 19.2). However, visual inspection of an arteriogram does not accurately determine the degree of carotid artery stenosis in FMD patients. Indeed, up to a third of patients with no angiographic stenosis after angioplasty will have evidence of residual stenosis by pressure gradient or intravascular ultrasound (IVUS) imaging [12].

Fig. 19.2 Angiography of the right carotid artery. Medial fibromuscular dysplasia of right internal carotid artery with the typical "string-of-beads" sign. From: Jahnlova and Veselka [42]. Reprinted with permission from Thieme

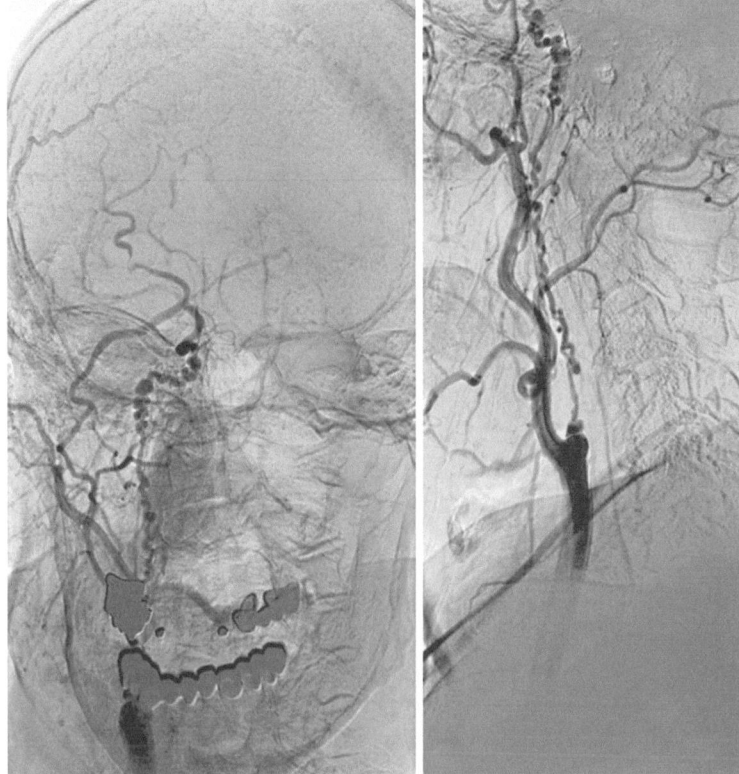

Medical Management

FMD is a chronic, non-curable condition that requires patient education and lifelong follow-up. Due to its occurrence in multiple arterial beds and the diversity of its potential complications, FMD should be treated by multidisciplinary teams that include vascular surgeons, interventional radiologists, nephrologists, neurosurgeons, and neurologists. Most FMD patients are asymptomatic on presentation and, as such, should not require any interventions. However, patients with carotid or vertebral artery FMD should receive a daily regimen of low-dose aspirin (81 mg/day) and undergo surveillance with an ultrasound study every 6–12 months to rule out any aneurysmal degeneration that would require intervention [12]. Blood pressure management is also important, and any evidence of increasing blood pressure that is refractory to antihypertensive medications should warrant work-up of renal artery FMD.

Patients with extracranial cerebrovascular FMD should be referred to a neurosurgeon to rule out any concurrent intracranial lesions that may require monitoring or intervention. A "head to pelvis" CTA should also be performed at the time of diagnosis, regardless of the initial site of the FMD, due to the incidence of asymptomatic aneurysms and dissections in FMD patients [43]. Patients who present with spontaneous carotid dissection should first be managed with anticoagulation using a weight-based regimen of unfractionated heparin, followed by oral anticoagulation using warfarin or a novel oral anticoagulation agent for 3–6 months to prevent thromboembolic complications [44].

Surgical Management

Interventions for cerebrovascular FMD should be considered in patients who fail non-operative management. In most cases, angioplasty alone will be enough to resolve FMD-related stenosis and restore a normal pressure gradient across a lesion. As with endovascular interventions for other indications, stents should only be considered if the lesion does not adequately respond to angioplasty alone or when complications such as dissection or perforation occur.

Patients with FMD-related ICA dissections who continue to have symptoms while on an anticoagulation regimen should be evaluated for carotid artery stent placement [45]. If the patient is not suitable for stent placement, then consideration should be given to open surgical repair, although this is very rarely required. A recent report of the US Registry for FMD by Kadian-Dodov et al. demonstrated that 40% of carotid artery and 10% of vertebral artery dissection FMD patients will eventually require a therapeutic intervention [43].

There are no guidelines for the management of FMD-related carotid or vertebral artery aneurysms. Kadian-Dodov et al. reported 35% of the patients in the US Registry have undergone an intervention for carotid artery aneurysms and 5% for vertebral artery aneurysms [43]. A variety of different treatment approaches have been described, including coiling, stenting, or open surgery, as determined by the location of the aneurysm, its size, and the patient's fitness for endovascular versus open repair [7].

Olin et al. have described their use of angioplasty to treat FMD patients with severe, debilitating headaches [12]. Those patients were evaluated by a neurologist, and other causes of headache were ruled out. Interestingly, all four patients in their series experienced relief of their headaches immediately after balloon angioplasty of the FMD lesion in the ICA. All patients in the report were symptom-free on follow-up for up to 3 years. The authors do not advocate this approach for all FMD patients with headaches, however, and have reserved it for those with the most debilitating and refractory disease.

Prognosis

While the progression of renal artery FMD has been well-described, the same could not be said for cerebrovascular FMD [46]. Studies have reported an ischemic stroke risk of 0–5% per year, but the study populations in those reports were a heterogeneous mixture of symptomatic and asymptomatic patients who were not treated in a standardized fashion [9, 47]. Due to the uncommon and commonly asymptomatic nature of cerebrovascular FMD, it is currently not possible to determine its natural history.

Carotid Kinks

Definition

Structural abnormalities have been described in the carotid arteries since the early twentieth century [48]. These conditions are related to the embryological development of the fetus as well as atherosclerotic degeneration in later life. The ICA is normally coiled, and straightening occurs when the fetal heart and great vessels descend into the mediastinum [49]. If the descent is incomplete, then coiling of the carotid artery occurs (Fig. 19.3). Conversely, kinking occurs

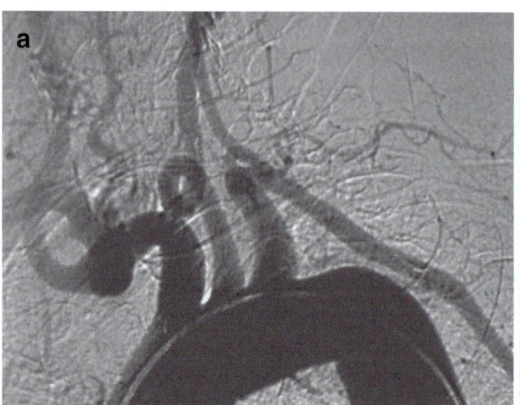
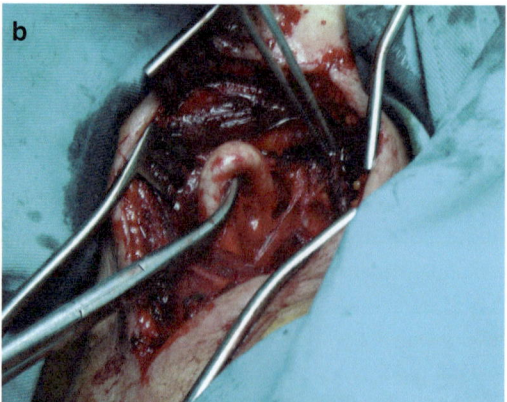

Fig. 19.3 (**a**) Left common carotid artery coiling; (**b**) intraoperative photograph of the coiling. From: Milic et al. [50]. Reprinted with permission from Elsevier

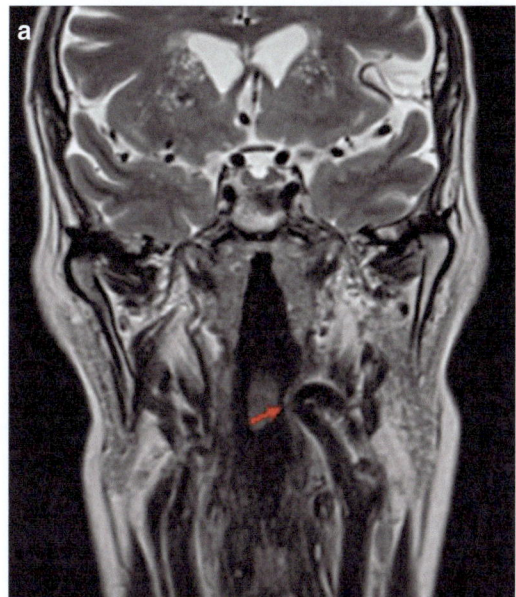

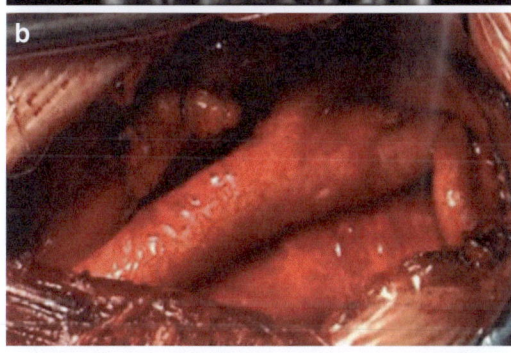

Fig. 19.4 (**a**) Left internal carotid artery kinking (arrow) demonstrated by MRA; (**b**) intraoperative photograph of the kinking. From: Stilo et al. [51]. Reprinted with permission from Elsevier

when a tortuous carotid artery develops an acute angulation (Fig. 19.4). Other terms for carotid artery tortuosity include elongation, redundancy, undulation, and "S-shaped curve" [52].

Prevalence and Risk Factors

The true incidence of carotid kinks is unknown, because most patients are asymptomatic. However, it has been estimated to affect 10–16% of the general population based on angiography studies [53, 54]. Hypertension is present in 80–85% of patients with carotid kinks, and atherosclerosis is present in almost all patients

[55]. Carotid kinks are equally likely to occur in women and men, although it is more frequently bilateral than unilateral [56, 57]. Other risk factors include advanced age and hyperlipidemia.

Pathology and Classification

As noted above, the current understanding of carotid tortuosity is based on a developmental etiology. However, kinking of the ICA usually occurs in atherosclerotic vessels and is characterized by subintimal deposits, loss of elasticity, elongation, and, in some cases, aneurysmal degeneration [58]. Ballotta et al. performed a histopathological assessment of 92 patients with symptomatic coiling or kinking of the ICA and noted 3 main lesions at the carotid bifurcation [59]:

1. Non-specific medial degeneration that is characterized by elastic fragmentation and disorganization, fibrosis, cystic medial necrosis, or medionecrosis (44% of patients)
2. Medial hyperplasia and thickening (39% of patients) (Fig. 19.5)
3. Fibromuscular hyperplasia suggestive of FMD (17% of patients)

Intraoperative inspection of the ICA reveals ulceration of the plaque on the medial wall of the carotid bulb immediately proximal to the kink in the vessel, likely caused by turbulence and hemodynamic changes that result from the carotid artery kinking [49].

In 1965, Weibel et al. classified elongated carotid artery abnormalities as tortuosity, coiling, or kinking [56]. Metz et al. from London attempted to quantify the degree of kinking according to the acuity of the angle [60]. They defined a kink as an angle of less than or equal to 90° between two segments of a carotid artery and proposed three grades of kinking according to angiographic features: Grade I between 90° and 60° of angulation, Grade II between 60° and 30°, and Grade III less than 30° (Fig. 19.6). However, this classification system has not been associated with clinical outcomes and is not widely used today.

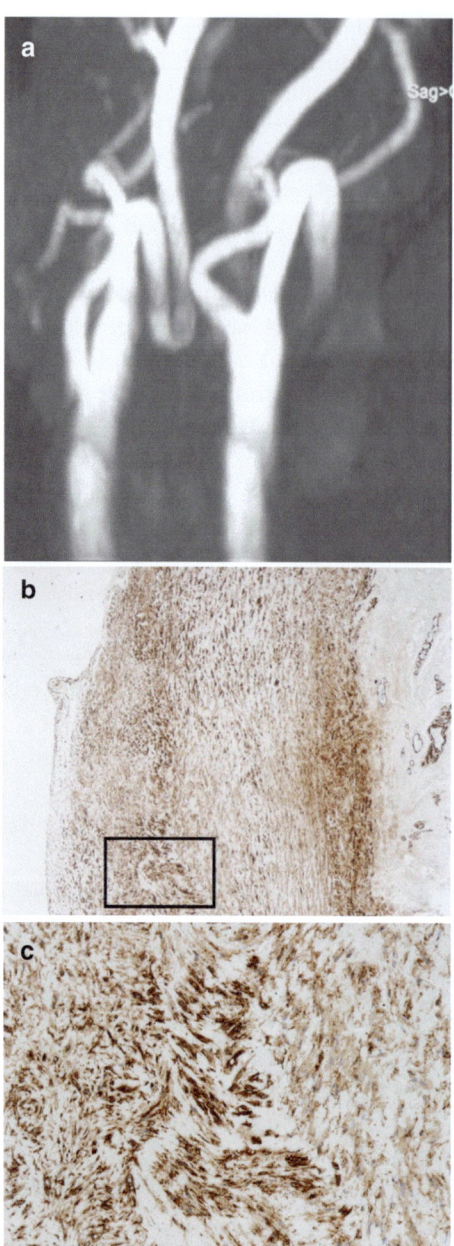

Fig. 19.5 (**a**) Angiographic picture of bilateral carotid elongation with kinking causing right hemispheric symptoms; (**b**) transparietal section of the carotid artery at its origin showing the tunica media hyperplasia characterized by increased extracellular matrix surrounding variously oriented smooth muscle cells. Immunohistochemical staining with anti-α actin antibody for the identification of smooth muscle cells (in brown). Note the high number of variously oriented smooth muscle cells within the tunica media; (**c**) close-up of (**b**). Original magnifications: **b** = 8×; **c** = 31×. From: Ballotta et al. [59]. Open Access, STM Signatory Elsevier

Clinical Presentation

Most carotid kinks and structural abnormalities are asymptomatic and noted incidentally, while patients are being worked up for an unrelated condition. Patients may complain of dizziness or light headedness and have a history of position-related transient ischemic attacks, previous stroke, or ongoing global cerebrovascular ischemia [49]. On physical examination, patients may have evidence of an ipsi- or contralateral mid-neck bruit. Patients may also present with clinical evidence of hypoglossal nerve palsy due to extrinsic nerve compression [61]. Leipzig and Dorhmann have catalogued an extensive list of other abnormal clinical presentations in this patient population, including subjective mastoid bruit, tinnitus, sudden vertigo, fainting sensation, nausea and sweating, loss of consciousness, seizures, neck aches, shoulder stiffening, personality changes, and progressive mental deterioration [52]. Patients also have a higher than normal incidence of abdominal aortic aneurysms compared with the general population [49].

Investigations

Patients who are asymptomatic and present with an incidentally noted lesion require no further investigations. However, if a carotid structural abnormality is suspected based on clinical findings, then a duplex ultrasound should be the initial investigative modality. Del Corso et al. reported that 83% of carotid abnormalities were associated with hemodynamic changes on duplex in the vascular bed distal to the abnormalities [55]. Due to the rarity of this condition, however, there are no specific duplex diagnostic criteria.

CTA and MRA both provide excellent anatomical details for the diagnosis of carotid structural abnormalities and are often sufficient for operative planning. While DSA remains the gold standard for diagnosis, it should be noted that, as with FMD, there tends to be a discrepancy between angiographic findings and intraoperative characteristics of the elongated vessels. Angiography tends to underestimate both the degree of stenotic disease and tortuosity [49].

Fig. 19.6 Tracings of lateral carotid angiograms to illustrate the classification of kinks according to severity

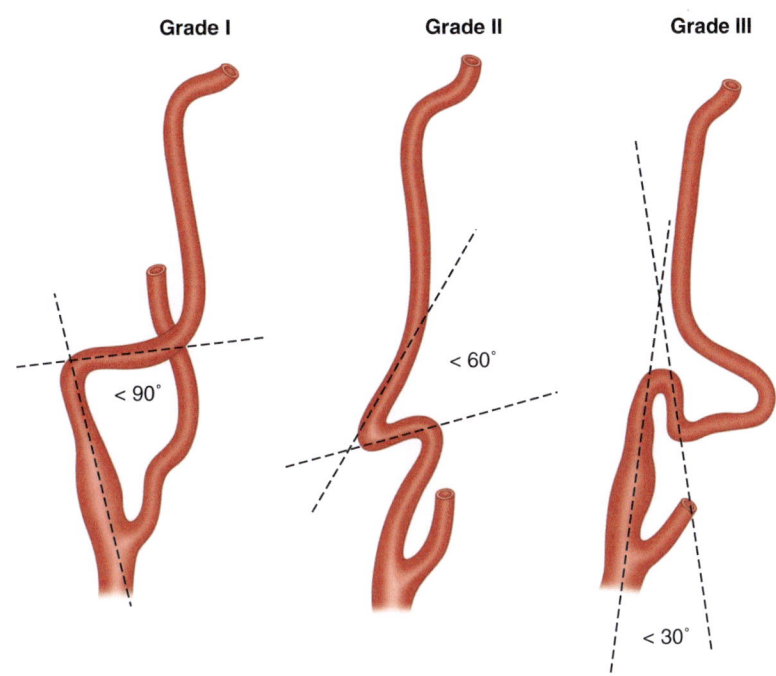

Medical Management

There are no published guidelines for treating asymptomatic carotid kinks or coils. However, as with FMD, consideration should be given to starting patients on a low dose (81 mg) daily aspirin regimen to prevent thromboembolic complications. Patients do not require routine monitoring, as there is little evidence to suggest disease progression. Those who present with dissections, aneurysmal degeneration, or symptoms refractory to non-operative management should initially be managed medically as discussed in the FMD section above.

Surgical Management

Patients with symptomatic carotid kinks or coils who fail medical therapy should be considered for surgery. Ballotta et al. conducted a prospective clinical study in which patients with symptomatic carotid elongation underwent medical versus surgical repair and found that surgical correction of symptomatic isolated carotid elongations with coiling or kinking is better for stroke prevention than medical treatment [59].

Kinks and coils are a contraindication for endovascular interventions due to the danger associated with passing a wire through a sharply angulated arterial segment. Numerous variations for surgical repair of carotid elongation abnormalities have been described (Fig. 19.7). The first approach, published by Riser et al. from France in 1951, entailed tacking a kinked ICA to the sternocleidomastoid muscle [62]. The limitation of this approach, however, is that it does not remove the diseased segment of artery despite addressing the underling hemodynamic abnormality. Other approaches include resecting the kinked or coiled arterial segment and performing an end-to-end anastomosis, resecting the common carotid artery and retracting the redundant internal carotid artery to form an end-to-end anastomosis, creating an interposition graft using saphenous vein, and resecting and reimplanting the internal carotid artery onto a proximal segment of common carotid artery [58].

The results of most approaches are excellent, with few long-term complications and a low risk of recurrence. Lepidi et al. reported a complete resolution of hemispheric symptoms with surgery and no mortality in their series with symptomatic carotid lesions [63]. Similarly, a single-institution

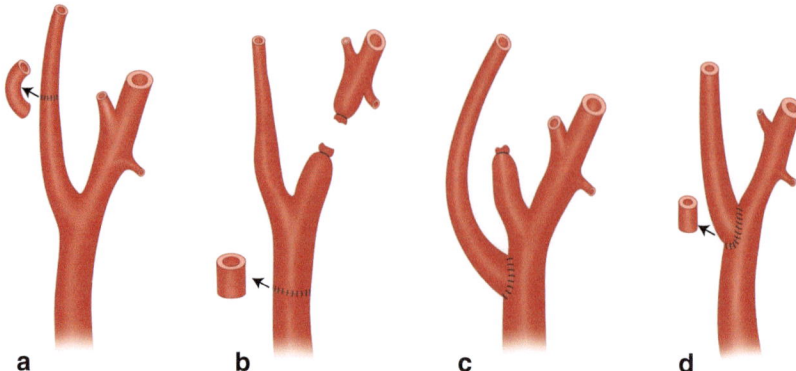

Fig. 19.7 Tortuous internal carotid artery (ICA) sutured to the sternocleidomastoid muscle; (**a**) redundant ICA resected and reanastomosed; (**b**) kinked ICA straightened by resecting the common carotid artery segment; (**c**) reimplantation of ICA without resection; and (**d**) segmental resection and reimplantation of the ICA

review by Mukherjee et al. showed no evidence of postoperative neurological dysfunction in their series of symptomatic carotid kinks and coils who underwent operative repair [49].

Rare Cerebrovascular Lesions

Takayasu's Arteritis

Takayasu's is a rare, chronic, granulomatous, large-vessel vasculitis occurring predominantly in females in the second or third decades of life [64]. Patients typically present with a history or clinical findings of absent or diminished pulses, loss of blood pressure, or bruits. Takayasu's can result in carotid artery stenosis, occlusion, and aneurysmal degeneration. Additionally, common carotid artery dissection has also been reported in patients with Takayasu's [65].

Carotid artery involvement has been reported in 45–84% of patients with Takayasu's disease [66]. In addition to serological evidence of systemic inflammation, Doppler ultrasound studies will show evidence of long-segmental or diffuse circumferential thickening with isoechogenicity or hyperechogenicity of the arterial wall [66]. On CTA, patients will have evidence of mural thickening and a low-attenuation ring between the outer wall and the intraluminal opacified blood [67]. Patients with active Takayasu's dis-

ease should receive steroid therapy, and surgical interventions should be limited to those who are refractory to non-operative management.

Extracranial carotid artery aneurysms develop in 1.8–3.9% of patients with Takayasu's (Fig. 19.8) [69–71]. Tabata et al. from Tokyo described their experience managing six extracranial carotid artery aneurysms in patients with Takayasu's disease [68]. All six patients presented with a painless neck mass and current or previous serological evidence of active systemic inflammation, as defined by a positive CRP or an ESR greater than 20 mm/h. The authors caution that all extracranial carotid aneurysms in Takayasu's arteritis have a risk of rupture, even in the noninflammatory stage, and recommend surgical repair for all these patients. Furthermore, the authors recommend the use of an autologous conduit in repairing the aneurysmal segment, as an anastomotic aneurysm developed in the single patient who was treated with a prosthetic graft.

Giant-Cell Arteritis

Giant-cell arteritis (GCA) is a rare condition that affects medium and large arteries [72]. It can involve all the major branches of the aorta and the extracranial carotid circulation, including the temporal arteries [73]. While the exact etiology of GCA has not been determined, histopathological lesions involve all layers of the arte-

Fig. 19.8 Carotid artery aneurysm in patient with Takayasu's arteritis. (**a**) CT image of the neck, showing aneurysm of the right common carotid artery with prominent intraluminal thrombus. (**b**) Angiographic appearance of the right common carotid aneurysm. Arrow indicates aneurysm. From: Tabata et al. [68]. Open Access, STM Signatory Elsevier

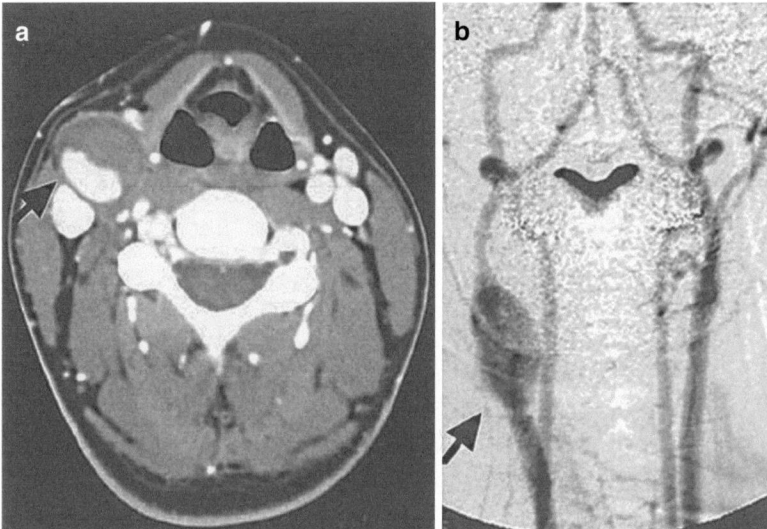

rial wall and are associated with multinucleated giant cells, fragmented internal elastic lamina, and polymorphic cellular infiltrates, leading to intimal hyperplasia and luminal obstruction that results in ischemic manifestations [74].

Patients with GCA may present with temporal headaches, pulselessness, and carotidynia [75]. Unlike Takayasu's, GCA tends to occur more frequently in individuals older than 50 years of age, and its incidence increases with age. The management of GCA is similar to Takayasu's disease and is largely based on temporizing the active phase of the disease with steroid therapy. Furthermore, there is some evidence for the efficacy of antiplatelet therapy in preventing cephalic ischemic complications [76]. Surgery is very rarely indicated for the management of this condition.

Marfan's Syndrome

Marfan's is an autosomal dominant connective-tissue disease that is caused by mutations in the gene FBN1 [77]. Patients typically present with abnormalities of the ocular, skeletal, and cardiovascular systems, with aortic aneurysmal degeneration being the most important and potentially lethal complication. The treatment of Marfan's is primarily medical with adequate blood pressure control using β-blocker therapy and angiotensin

II receptor blockers [78]. As the patient's prognosis is determined primarily by the incidence of aortic complications, surgery is indicated when the aortic root diameter is greater than 5 cm.

Cerebrovascular manifestations of Marfan's include carotid artery dissection and aneurysm formation [79–81]. Due to the rarity of this condition, the absence of guidelines for its treatment, and its unpredictable natural history, most authors have elected to intervene early on patients with carotid artery aneurysms or refractory symptomatic dissections. However, there is some evidence that carotid artery aneurysms in Marfan's patients do not progress at the same rate as aortic aneurysms [82].

Ehlers-Danlos

Ehlers-Danlos syndrome is caused by a disorder in the metabolism of fibrillary collagen, resulting in abnormalities in the skin, joints, hollow organs, and blood vessels [83]. Vascular Ehlers-Danlos, previously known as Ehlers-Danlos type IV, is a rare autosomal dominant collagen vascular disorder that results from mutations in the COL3A1 gene, which encodes type III procollagen [84]. The syndrome's vascular subtype has the worst prognosis because the affected arteries and hollow organs are at a higher risk of rupture at a young age [85].

Ehlers-Danlos can have several cerebrovascular manifestations, including ischemic stroke, cervical artery dissection, carotid-cavernous fistula, intracranial dissection, aneurysms, and arterial rupture [86]. Surgical interventions are notoriously perilous in those patients because of the highly fragile nature of the tissues. According to Eagleton, vascular clamps should be avoided in patients undergoing surgery, if possible, and balloon occlusion should be sparingly used because of the potential for vessel rupture [83]. Suturing should be carried out with utmost care, and pledgets should be used to prevent suture material from slicing through the arterial wall. Finally, vessel ligation should be carried out using umbilical tapes or vascular patch material to prevent the risk of rupture.

Review Questions

1. All of the following is true about fibromuscular dysplasia (FMD), except:
    A. It is a complication of atherosclerotic disease.
    B. It is noninflammatory.
    C. It primarily affects middle-sized vessels.
    D. It is chronic and non-curable.

   Answer: A

2. The relationship between gender distribution and FMD is best reflected by which statement?
    A. FMD is associated with higher estrogen levels.
    B. FMD is associated with the use of contraceptives.
    C. The relationship between female gender and FMD is not well understood.
    D. FMD is associated with pregnancy.

   Answer: C

3. The majority of fibromuscular dysplasia (FMD) presents as:
    A. Medial hyperplasia
    B. Medial fibroplasia
    C. Intimal fibroplasia
    D. Perimedial fibroplasia

   Answer: B

4. All of the following statements about carotid kinks are true, except:
    A. Is defined as angle of less than or equal to 90° between two segments of a carotid artery.
    B. Atherosclerosis is a strong predictive factor for developing carotid kinks.
    C. Carotid kinks are more frequently bilateral than unilateral.
    D. Carotid kinks affect women more than men.

   Answer: D

5. Takayasu's arteritis is a rare condition characterized by which of the following?
    A. Occurs predominantly in females.
    B. Is a form of small vessel vasculitis.
    C. First-line treatment is a course of antiplatelet therapy.
    D. Extracranial carotid artery aneurysms occur in 5–15% of patients.

   Answer: A

References

1. Luscher TF, Lie JT, Stanson AW, Houser OW, Hollier LH, Sheps SG. Arterial fibromuscular dysplasia. Mayo Clin Proc. 1987;62(10):931–52.
2. Leadbetter WF, Burkland CE. Hypertension in unilateral renal disease. J Urol. 1938;39:611–26.
3. McCormack LJ, Hazard JB, Poutasse EF. Obstructive lesions of the renal artery associated with remediable hypertension. Am J Pathol. 1938;34:582.
4. Connett MC, Lansche JM. Fibromuscular hyperplasia of the internal carotid artery: report of a case. Ann Surg. 1965;162:59–62.
5. Begelman SM, Olin JW. Fibromuscular dysplasia. Curr Opin Rheumatol. 2000;12(1):41–7.
6. So EL, Toole JF, Dalal P, Moody DM. Cephalic fibromuscular dysplasia in 32 patients: clinical findings and radiologic features. Arch Neurol. 1981;38(10):619–22.
7. Brinza EK, Gornik HL. Fibromuscular dysplasia: advances in understanding and management. Cleve Clin J Med. 2016;83(11 Suppl 2):S45–51.
8. Shivapour DM, Erwin P, Kim E. Epidemiology of fibromuscular dysplasia: a review of the literature. Vasc Med. 2016;21(4):376–81.
9. Touze E, Oppenheim C, Trystram D, Nokam G, Pasquini M, Alamowitch S, et al. Fibromuscular dysplasia of cervical and intracranial arteries. Int J Stroke. 2010;5(4):296–305.

10. Olin JW, Froehlich J, Gu X, Bacharach JM, Eagle K, Gray BH, et al. The United States registry for fibromuscular dysplasia: results in the first 447 patients. Circulation. 2012;125(25):3182–90.

11. Olin JW, Pierce M. Contemporary management of fibromuscular dysplasia. Curr Opin Cardiol. 2008;23(6):527–36.

12. Olin JW, Sealove BA. Diagnosis, management, and future developments of fibromuscular dysplasia. J Vasc Surg. 2011;53(3):826–36.e1.

13. Rushton AR. The genetics of fibromuscular dysplasia. Arch Intern Med. 1980;140(2):233–6.

14. Mettinger KL, Ericson K. Fibromuscular dysplasia and the brain. I. Observations on angiographic, clinical and genetic characteristics. Stroke. 1982;13(1):46–52.

15. Perdu J, Boutouyrie P, Bourgain C, Stern N, Laloux B, Bozec E, et al. Inheritance of arterial lesions in renal fibromuscular dysplasia. J Hum Hypertens. 2007;21(5):393–400.

16. Harrison EG Jr, McCormack LJ. Pathologic classification of renal arterial disease in renovascular hypertension. Mayo Clin Proc. 1971;46(3):161–7.

17. Poloskey SL, Olin JW, Mace P, Gornik HL. Fibromuscular dysplasia. Circulation. 2012;125(18):e636–9.

18. Stanley JC, Gewertz BL, Bove EL, Sottiurai V, Fry WJ. Arterial fibrodysplasia. Histopathologic character and current etiologic concepts. Arch Surg. 1975;110(5):561–6.

19. Slovut DP, Olin JW. Fibromuscular dysplasia. N Engl J Med. 2004;350(18):1862–71.

20. Aqel R, Gupta R, Zoghbi G. Coexistent fibromuscular dysplasia and atherosclerotic renal artery stenosis. J Invasive Cardiol. 2005;17(10):572–3.

21. Aqel R, AlJaroudi WW, Hage FG, Nanda NC. Renal artery fibromuscular dysplasia is a cause of refractory hypertension in the elderly. Echocardiography. 2009;26(1):109–10.

22. Jayawardene S, Reidy J, Scoble J. Clinical picture: ipsilateral atherosclerotic and fibromuscular renal artery stenosis. Lancet. 2000;356(9248):2138.

23. Schievink WI, Bjornsson J, Piepgras DG. Coexistence of fibromuscular dysplasia and cystic medial necrosis in a patient with Marfan's syndrome and bilateral carotid artery dissections. Stroke. 1994;25(12):2492–6.

24. Schievink WI, Limburg M. Angiographic abnormalities mimicking fibromuscular dysplasia in a patient with Ehlers-Danlos syndrome, type IV. Neurosurgery. 1989;25(3):482–3.

25. Slavin RE. Segmental arterial mediolysis: course, sequelae, prognosis, and pathologic-radiologic correlation. Cardiovasc Pathol. 2009;18(6):352–60.

26. Bol A, Missault L, Dewilde W. Renovascular hypertension associated with neurofibromatosis: a case report. Acta Clin Belg. 2007;62(1):61–3.

27. Janzen J, Vuong PN, Rothenberger-Janzen K. Takayasu's arteritis and fibromuscular dysplasia as causes of acquired atypical coarctation of the aorta: retrospective analysis of seven cases. Heart Vessels. 1999;14(6):277–82.

28. Sandok BA. Fibromuscular dysplasia of the internal carotid artery. Neurol Clin. 1983;1(1):17–26.

29. Corrin LS, Sandok BA, Houser OW. Cerebral ischemic events in patients with carotid artery fibromuscular dysplasia. Arch Neurol. 1981;38(10):616–8.

30. Abdul-Rahman AM, Abu S, Brun A, Kin H, Ljunggren B, Mizukami M, et al. Fibromuscular dysplasia of the cervico-cephalic arteries. Surg Neurol. 1978;9(4):217–22.

31. Hart RG, Easton JD. Dissections of cervical and cerebral arteries. Neurol Clin. 1983;1(1):155–82.

32. Grotta JC, Ward RE, Flynn TC, Cullen ML. Spontaneous internal carotid artery dissection associated with fibromuscular dysplasia. J Cardiovasc Surg. 1982;23(6):512–4.

33. Cloft HJ, Kallmes DF, Kallmes MH, Goldstein JH, Jensen ME, Dion JE. Prevalence of cerebral aneurysms in patients with fibromuscular dysplasia: a reassessment. J Neurosurg. 1998;88(3):436–40.

34. van de Nes JA, Bajanowski T, Trubner K. Fibromuscular dysplasia of the basilar artery: an unusual case with medico-legal implications. Forensic Sci Int. 2007;173(2–3):188–92.

35. Zimmerman R, Leeds NE, Naidich TP. Carotid-cavernous fistula associated with intracranial fibromuscular dysplasia. Radiology. 1977;122(3):725–6.

36. Reddy SV, Karnes WE, Earnest F, Sundt TM Jr. Spontaneous extracranial vertebral arteriovenous fistula with fibromuscular dysplasia. Case report. J Neurosurg. 1981;54(3):399–402.

37. Varennes L, Tahon F, Kastler A, Grand S, Thony F, Baguet JP, et al. Fibromuscular dysplasia: what the radiologist should know: a pictorial review. Insights Imaging. 2015;6(3):295–307.

38. Osborn AG, Anderson RE. Angiographic spectrum of cervical and intracranial fibromuscular dysplasia. Stroke. 1977;8(5):617–26.

39. Leung DA, Hoffmann U, Pfammatter T, Hany TF, Rainoni L, Hilfiker P, et al. Magnetic resonance angiography versus duplex sonography for diagnosing renovascular disease. Hypertension. 1999;33(2):726–31.

40. Carman TL, Olin JW, Czum J. Noninvasive imaging of the renal arteries. Urol Clin North Am. 2001;28(4):815–26.

41. Furie DM, Tien RD. Fibromuscular dysplasia of arteries of the head and neck: imaging findings. AJR Am J Roentgenol. 1994;162(5):1205–9.

42. Jahnlova D, Veselka J. Fibromuscular dysplasia of renal and carotid arteries. Int J Angiol. 2015;24(3):241–3.

43. Kadian-Dodov D, Gornik HL, Gu X, Froehlich J, Bacharach JM, Chi YW, et al. Dissection and aneurysm in patients with fibromuscular dysplasia: findings from the U.S. registry for FMD. J Am Coll Cardiol. 2016;68(2):176–85.

44. Schievink WI. Spontaneous dissection of the carotid and vertebral arteries. N Engl J Med. 2001;344(12):898–906.

45. Edgell RC, Abou-Chebl A, Yadav JS. Endovascular management of spontaneous carotid artery dissection. J Vasc Surg. 2005;42(5):854–60. Discussion 60.

46. Plouin PF, Perdu J, La Batide-Alanore A, Boutouyrie P, Gimenez-Roqueplo AP, Jeunemaitre X. Fibromuscular dysplasia. Orphanet J Rare Dis. 2007;2:28.

47. Stewart MT, Moritz MW, Smith RB 3rd, Fulenwider JT, Perdue GD. The natural history of carotid fibromuscular dysplasia. J Vasc Surg. 1986;3(2):305–10.

48. Edington GH. Tortuosity of both internal carotid arteries. Br Med J. 1901;2(2134):1526–7.

49. Mukherjee D, Inahara T. Management of the tortuous internal carotid artery. Am J Surg. 1985;149(5):651–5.

50. Milic DJ, Jovanovic MM, Zivic SS, Jankovic RJ. Coiling of the left common carotid artery as a cause of transient ischemic attacks. J Vasc Surg. 2007;45(2):411–3.

51. Stilo F, Catanese V, Casale M, Bernardini S, Montelione N, Spinelli F. Carotid-carotid bypass graft for internal carotid artery kinking causing dysphagia. Ann Vasc Surg. 2017;43:310.e5–7.

52. Leipzig TJ, Dohrmann GJ. The tortuous or kinked carotid artery: pathogenesis and clinical considerations. A historical review. Surg Neurol. 1986;25(5):478–86.

53. Cioffi FA, Meduri M, Tomasello F, Bonavita V, Conforti P. Kinking and coiling of the internal carotid artery: clinical-statistical observations and surgical perspectives. J Neurosurg Sci. 1975;19(1–2):15–22.

54. Poulias GE, Skoutas B, Doundoulakis N, Haddad H, Karkanias G, Lyberiadis D. Kinking and coiling of internal carotid artery with and without associated stenosis. Surgical considerations and long-term follow-up. Panminerva Med. 1996;38(1):22–7.

55. Del Corso L, Moruzzo D, Conte B, Agelli M, Romanelli AM, Pastine F, et al. Tortuosity, kinking, and coiling of the carotid artery: expression of atherosclerosis or aging? Angiology. 1998;49(5):361–71.

56. Weibel J, Fields WS. Tortuosity, coiling, and kinking of the internal carotid artery. I. Etiology and radiographic anatomy. Neurology. 1965;15:7–18.

57. Rowlands RP, Swan RH. Tortuosity of both internal carotid arteries. Br Med J. 1902;1(2141):76.

58. Vannix RS, Joergenson EJ, Carter R. Kinking of the internal carotid artery. Clinical significance and surgical management. Am J Surg. 1977;134(1):82–9.

59. Ballotta E, Thiene G, Baracchini C, Ermani M, Militello C, Da Giau G, et al. Surgical vs medical treatment for isolated internal carotid artery elongation with coiling or kinking in symptomatic patients: a prospective randomized clinical study. J Vasc Surg. 2005;42(5):838–46. Discussion 46.

60. Metz H, Murray-Leslie RM, Bannister RG, Bull JW, Marshall J. Kinking of the internal carotid artery. Lancet. 1961;1(7174):424–6.

61. Scotti G, Melancon D, Olivier A. Hypoglossal paralysis due to compression by a tortuous internal carotid artery in the neck. Neuroradiology. 1978;14(5):263–5.

62. Geraud JR, Ducoudray J, Ribaut L. Long internal carotid artery with vertigo syndrome. Rev Neurol (Paris). 1951;85(2):145–7.

63. Grego F, Lepidi S, Cognolato D, Frigatti P, Morelli I, Deriu GP. Rationale of the surgical treatment of carotid kinking. J Cardiovasc Surg. 2003;44(1):79–85.

64. Alibaz-Oner F, Direskeneli H. Update on Takayasu's arteritis. Presse Med. 2015;44(6 Pt 2):e259–65.

65. Hao R, Zhang J, Ma Z, Xiao M, Zhou L, Kang N, et al. Takayasu's arteritis presenting with common carotid artery dissection: a rare case report. Exp Ther Med. 2016;12(6):4061–3.

66. Park SH, Chung JW, Lee JW, Han MH, Park JH. Carotid artery involvement in Takayasu's arteritis: evaluation of the activity by ultrasonography. J Ultrasound Med. 2001;20(4):371–8.

67. Park JH, Chung JW, Im JG, Kim SK, Park YB, Han MC. Takayasu arteritis: evaluation of mural changes in the aorta and pulmonary artery with CT angiography. Radiology. 1995;196(1):89–93.

68. Tabata M, Kitagawa T, Saito T, Uozaki H, Oshiro H, Miyata T, et al. Extracranial carotid aneurysm in Takayasu's arteritis. J Vasc Surg. 2001;34(4):739–42.

69. Takagi A, Tada Y, Sato O, Miyata T. Surgical treatment for Takayasu's arteritis. A long-term follow-up study. J Cardiovasc Surg. 1989;30(4):553–8.

70. Matsumura K, Hirano T, Takeda K, Matsuda A, Nakagawa T, Yamaguchi N, et al. Incidence of aneurysms in Takayasu's arteritis. Angiology. 1991;42(4):308–15.

71. Kumar S, Subramanyan R, Mandalam KR, Rao VR, Gupta AK, Joseph S, et al. Aneurysmal form of aortoarteritis (Takayasu's disease): analysis of thirty cases. Clin Radiol. 1990;42(5):342–7.

72. Gonzalez-Gay MA, Barros S, Lopez-Diaz MJ, Garcia-Porrua C, Sanchez-Andrade A, Llorca J. Giant cell arteritis: disease patterns of clinical presentation in a series of 240 patients. Medicine (Baltimore). 2005;84(5):269–76.

73. Nesher G. The diagnosis and classification of giant cell arteritis. J Autoimmun. 2014;48-49:73–5.

74. Ly KH, Regent A, Tamby MC, Mouthon L. Pathogenesis of giant cell arteritis: more than just an inflammatory condition? Autoimmun Rev. 2010;9(10):635–45.

75. Shikino K, Yamashita S, Ikusaka M. Giant cell arteritis with carotidynia. J Gen Intern Med. 2017;32:1403.

76. Watelet B, Samson M, de Boysson H, Bienvenu B. Treatment of giant-cell arteritis, a literature review. Mod Rheumatol. 2017:1–8.

77. Canadas V, Vilacosta I, Bruna I, Fuster V. Marfan syndrome. Part 1: pathophysiology and diagnosis. Nat Rev Cardiol. 2010;7(5):256–65.

78. Canadas V, Vilacosta I, Bruna I, Fuster V. Marfan syndrome. Part 2: treatment and management of patients. Nat Rev Cardiol. 2010;7(5):266–76.

79. Alurkar A, Karanam LS, Oak S, Sorte S. Carotid dissection in Marfan's syndrome. Neurol India. 2013;61(2):206–7.

80. Ohyama T, Ohara S, Momma F. Aneurysm of the cervical internal carotid artery associated with Marfan's syndrome—case report. Neurol Med Chir (Tokyo). 1992;32(13):965–8.

81. Latter DA, Ricci MA, Forbes RD, Graham AM. Internal carotid artery aneurysm and Marfan's syndrome. Can J Surg. 1989;32(6):463–6.

82. Sztajzel R, Hefft S, Girardet C. Marfan's syndrome and multiple extracranial aneurysms. Cerebrovasc Dis. 2001;11(4):346–9.

83. Eagleton MJ. Arterial complications of vascular Ehlers-Danlos syndrome. J Vasc Surg. 2016;64(6): 1869–80.

84. Pepin M, Schwarze U, Superti-Furga A, Byers PH. Clinical and genetic features of Ehlers-Danlos syndrome type IV, the vascular type. N Engl J Med. 2000;342(10):673–80.

85. De Paepe A, Malfait F. The Ehlers-Danlos syndrome, a disorder with many faces. Clin Genet. 2012;82(1):1–11.

86. Debette S, Germain DP. Neurologic manifestations of inherited disorders of connective tissue. Handb Clin Neurol. 2014;119:565–76.

Cervical (Carotid and Vertebral) Artery Dissection

20

Vishal B. Jani and Richard D. Fessler

Introduction

Cervical artery dissection was first reported in an autopsy report by Fred Thomas in 1947 [1]. Cervical artery dissection (CAD) is a general term including both carotid and vertebral artery dissections. A CAD occurs when there is a tear in the intimal layer of a carotid or vertebral artery that leads to the development of an intramural hematoma. The hematoma can cause stenosis, occlusion, or aneurysmal dilation. Early detection is of paramount importance as the risk of recurrent stroke is highest during the first month following a CAD. CAD is now recognized as one of the most common causes of stroke in the young, accounting for up to 30% of stroke cases [2]. The present chapter will focus on the clinical features, diagnosis, and available treatment options for spontaneous (non-traumatic) CAD (Fig. 20.1).

Incidence and Epidemiology

CAD can occur spontaneously or after inciting trauma [3]. Spontaneous cervical artery dissection has an incidence rate of 2.6–2.9 per 100,000 people annually, with the highest incidence in autumn based on North American population-based studies [4]. CAD can also occur when there is major or minor trauma that causes the neck to hyperextend, laterally rotate, or have abnormal lateral displacement. True incidence is likely higher as many cases may go undiagnosed due to the fact that some patients only present with minor self-limiting clinical symptoms. In population-based studies, the median age for spontaneous CAD is around 45 years and in favor of the male gender (53% female to 57% male) [5, 6]. The most common location for CAD and accounting for 2.5% of all initial strokes is within the extracranial internal carotid artery, typically 2–3 cm above the carotid bifurcation [7].

Predisposing Factors

Extrinsic (Environmental) Risk Factors

The risk factors for CAD are distinct from other causes of stroke. CAD patients are more likely to have hypertension and less likely to have hypercholesterolemia compared to their matched healthy controls [8]. In addition, migraine particularly with aura [9, 10], hyperhomocysteinemia

V. B. Jani
Neurology in Stroke, Department of Neurology, Creighton University School of Medicine/CHI Health, Omaha, NE, USA

R. D. Fessler (✉)
Department of Surgery, St. John Hospital and Medical Centers, Detroit, MI, USA
e-mail: Richard.fessler2@ascension.org

© The Editor(s) (if applicable) and The Author(s) 2018
S. S. Hans (ed.), *Extracranial Carotid and Vertebral Artery Disease*,
https://doi.org/10.1007/978-3-319-91533-3_20

241

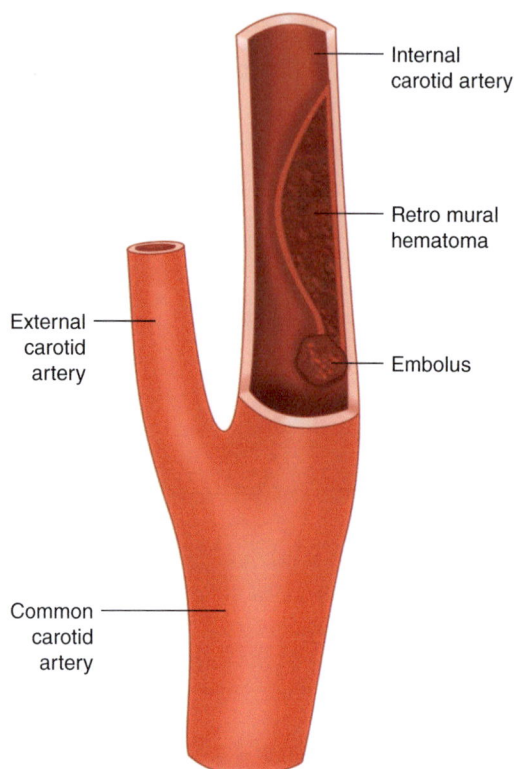

Internal carotid artery

Retro mural hematoma

External carotid artery

Embolus

Common carotid artery

Fig. 20.1 Carotid artery dissection

[11], aortic root dilatation [12], neck manipulation [12], oral contraceptive usage, and elevated high sensitivity C-reactive protein have all been identified as risk factors for the development of CAD. A history of recent infection (especially *Chlamydia pneumoniae*) is also a predisposing factor [13] and may partially explain the seasonal prevalence of dissection as described above. Atherosclerosis has not been shown to have any association with an increased risk of CAD [1].

Intrinsic (Genetic) Risk Factors

Genetic factors might have a role in the pathophysiology of CAD, mainly as part of a multifactorial predisposition. The prevailing theory is that CAD is a multifactorial disease caused by several genetic variants and environmental factors, each probably having a modest and potentially synergistic effect. Inherited connective tissue conditions such as Ehlers-Danlos syndrome, Marfan's syndrome, osteogenesis imperfecta, and fibromuscular dysplasia increase the risk of

CAD by 16- to 18-fold. Furthermore, there are case reports of CAD in patients with alpha 1 antitrypsin deficiency, hereditary hemochromatosis, Turner syndrome, and William's syndrome [14]. In the era of modern genetics, studies have reported associations with variants in three different candidate genes: *ICAM1* (encodes intercellular adhesion molecule 1), *COL3A1* (encodes collagen, type III, alpha 1), and *MTHFR* (encodes 5,10-methylenetetrahydrofolate reductase) [15–18]. Larger genetic studies of the relation of these genes and CAD are needed to further our understanding beyond this point.

Family History

Family history of arterial dissection has been shown to be a risk factor for recurrent arterial dissection. Five percent of CAD patients report a family history of spontaneous dissection of the aorta or its main branches [19]. Other familial associations with CAD that have been reported include bicuspid aortic valve and multiple cutaneous lentigines (a type of skin lesion) [1].

Pathogenesis

The overall pathogenesis of a CAD involves a hematoma that develops within the layers of the wall of a cervical artery (carotid or vertebral) due to [14] an intimal tear of the artery, direct bleeding into the arterial wall from ruptured vasa vasorum, or intramural hematoma expanding toward the intima or adventitia layers resulting in stenosis or aneurysmal dilatation of the cervical artery [14, 20]. Cervical arteries are susceptible to strain and dissection due to their limited mobility at the skull base, yet decent mobility within the neck region. The arteries are also prone to come in contact with bony structures like the styloid process and cervical vertebrae which potentially can cause additional damage. Significant tortuous intraosseous curvature of the vertebral artery puts a patient at higher risk for torsion-related dissection [20]. There are some studies which have tried to answer the clinical association of

Table 20.1 Presenting signs and symptoms

Dissection of carotid artery [4]	
Pain	78%
Headache	72%
Stroke or TIA	59%
Horner syndrome	25%
Pulsatile tinnitus	25%
Neck pain	19%
Taste impairment	10%
Retinal ischemia	3%
Asymptomatic	2.7%
Dissection of vertebral artery [1, 14, 22]	
Pain in posterior neck	50%
Headaches/thunderclap headache	66%
Posterior circulation stroke/TIA	90%
Cervical radicular signs and symptoms (usually C5–C6 distribution)	Rare

intramural hematoma and stroke; however, the pathophysiology of CAD is poorly understood. The challenge in understanding is due to the fact that most strokes (>90%) result from thromboembolic origin and not hemodynamic changes [1]. Experts believe CAD is a multifactorial event involving environmental factors and genetic factors that cause concomitant vasculopathy or arterial anomalies [1, 21].

Clinical Presentation

The classic triad of CAD includes unilateral pain of the head, neck, or face, partial Horner syndrome (ptosis, miosis), and cerebral or retinal ischemia. However, less than one-third of patients will present with all three components (Table 20.1) [1].

Diagnosis

History and physical findings with high probability for cervical artery dissection include a history of trauma, neck pain, partial Horner syndrome, and/or focal neurological signs and symptoms. If any of these are present, especially with a history of trauma, a high index of suspicion for CAD should be raised [1, 20]. The combination of magnetic resonance imaging (MRI) and mag-

netic resonance angiography (MRA) or computerized tomography angiography (CTA) is the best noninvasive modality for confirmation of arterial dissection [1, 23–26]. Color duplex and Doppler sonography are other noninvasive techniques used to screen for CAD. These screening methods should not be considered diagnostic tools as they are highly operator dependent and have a poor diagnostic yield for CAD located near the skull base and within the transverse foramina [27]. Conventional angiography is the most definitive test for accurately defining the exact level, arterial territory of dissection, and complications associated with dissection. Complications could include pseudoaneurysm, double lumen, or the presence of an intraluminal or distal clot. Conventional angiography is seldom necessary for extracranial dissections despite being the most sensitive testing due to its invasive nature [28–30]. The classic sign for dissection seen on neuroimaging is an enlarged artery with a crescent-shaped rim of hyper-intense signal from the hematoma that is surrounding the decreased lumen [14]. According to Debette et al., 41–75% of CAD cases present with the radiographical "rat's tail" or "string sign" which represents tapered stenosis on neuroimaging [14, 20]. These imaging methods are reviewed individually as follows.

MR Angiography

MRI with MRA offers excellent noninvasive imaging of cerebrovascular arterial dissection. Visualization of the brain and vasculature is commonly achieved with conventional T1- and T2-weighted and fluid attenuation inversion recovery (FLAIR) axial MRI with 3Dl time-of-flight (TOF) MRA. Characteristic imaging findings on MRI in extracranial carotid artery dissection include diminution or absence of signal flow void and crescent sign. The crescent sign is caused by the narrowing of the vessel and the intramural dissection of blood appearing in a semilunar fashion as a spiraling periarterial rim of intramural hematoma in cross section on T1-weighted and fluid attenuation inversion recovery axial MR image [31, 32].

Fig. 20.2 (a, b) CT angiography reveals a dissection along the medial aspect of the left internal carotid artery leading to severe stenosis and fusiform aneurysmal dilatation of the downstream artery

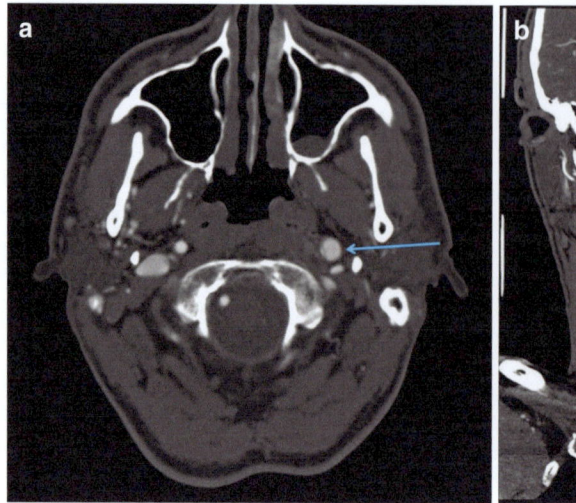

Contraindications and limitations of MRI/MRA in general include older pacemakers and other implanted metal, cost, prolonged scanning time, claustrophobia, body habitus, and susceptibility to motion artifacts. The specific limitations for MRI in vertebral artery dissection (VAD) include the tortuous course of the artery, variability in normal vessel caliber and frequent asymmetries, the small size of the mural hematoma, and the potential pitfalls caused by the adjacent perivertebral venous plexus [33].

CT Angiography (CTA)

CTA has high sensitivity and specificity and may also be used; however, it is associated with radiation exposure and potential technical challenges [34, 35]. In patients with CAD, a CTA can show the double lumen sign (true and false lumen) or a flame-like taper of the lumen. CTA offers more advantages over MR angiography in vertebral arteries as compared to MR imaging due to bony artifacts on MRI. CTA and MRA are less useful in the setting of metallic densities in the neck soft tissues (e.g., gunshot wound) (Fig. 20.2).

Ultrasonography

For practical purposes a carotid ultrasound is never a first-line imaging modality for diagnosis due to low sensitivity rates and poor visualization of intramural hematoma or dissection flap. This could be a good screening tool as 90% of patients with CAD will show altered flow dynamics, typically a patent carotid bifurcation and proximal internal carotid artery without major atherosclerotic plaque. In addition, many patients will have an absent or dampened systolic flow signal, which eventually will require some form of angiography to assess intramural hematoma and/or dissection flap [36]. General interpretation of a decrease or absence of flow velocities in the affected vessel, retrograde flow in supraorbital vessels, or bidirectional internal carotid artery flow suggests more distal obstruction or stenosis resulting from dissection [37]. Of significant importance, the transcranial Doppler test can detect cervical microemboli in greater than 50% of cases of acute CAD and may provide some guidance in the treatment strategy [14].

Catheter Angiography

Catheter angiogram should not be routinely used to diagnose dissection due to its inability to visualize intramural hematomas. Catheter angiography is also an invasive test that may potentially cause an iatrogenic dissection, especially in a patient population with underlying vessel wall weakness.

Treatment

The available evidence suggests that treatment with thrombolytic therapy should be used in eligible patients with very early acute ischemic stroke to prevent extracranial cervical artery thromboemboli. If a patient presents with an ischemic cerebrovascular accident or TIA caused by extracranial arterial dissection (carotid or vertebral artery), either antiplatelet agents or anticoagulation for at least 3–6 months should be initiated. If there is recurrence of symptoms despite this medical management, endovascular stenting can be considered, although it is not currently discussed in the guidelines. Finally, if endovascular treatment is contraindicated for the patient and symptoms remain persistent despite optimal medical management, surgical repair can be considered.

Medications

Anticoagulation and Antiplatelet Therapy

Antithrombotic therapy with either anticoagulation or antiplatelet drugs has been used as treatment for ischemic stroke and transient ischemic attack caused by cervical artery dissection. Anticoagulation may prevent occlusion of a stenotic vessel and minimize distal embolization. Extension of intramural hematoma in the presence of an anticoagulant is rare; however, the evidence suggests no advantage of anticoagulation over antiplatelet treatment [38].

Most of the evidence for antithrombotic treatment comes from meta-analyses and an open-label trial which was published in 2015. The open-label assessor-blind pilot trial (CADISS) involved 250 subjects with extracranial carotid and vertebral dissection. All subjects were randomly assigned to either antiplatelet or anticoagulant treatment for 3 months [39]. At the end of the trial, there was no significant difference between the two treatment groups. Ipsilateral ischemic stroke occurred in 2% of subjects in the antiplatelet group and 1% in the anticoagulation group (odds ratio of 0.34 and 95% CI 0.01–4.23).

There was no difference in outcome, and there were no deaths in either group. There was one major bleeding event, a subarachnoid hemorrhage, in a patient assigned to the anticoagulation group who had a vertebral artery dissection with intracranial extension. Due to the low stroke rate and rarity of outcome events, the CADISS trial was unable to establish which treatment is superior [40]. Antiplatelet therapy can be either aspirin 81–325 mg/day or clopidogrel 75 mg/day. If anticoagulation therapy is desired, unfractionated heparin followed by warfarin with a goal aPTT of 1.5–2 times controls with INR goal of 2.5 (range 2–3). Low molecular weight heparin can be substituted for unfractionated heparin in certain cases. The CADISS trial concluded that the risk of subsequent stroke after dissection in this study population was only 2%; treatment with anticoagulation was not found to lower the risk of subsequent stroke or death when compared to treatment with antiplatelet agents. There were some criticisms for the trial as well. CADISS likely studied a population of patients with mostly spontaneous dissections, which lead to recurrent stroke at lower rates than traumatic dissections. The study was also significantly underpowered to detect a statistically significant difference in outcome. The authors' own power analysis determined that 10,000 patients would be needed, which given the long recruitment period of this study would seem to be a nearly impossible sample size to reach. The high number of patients for which dissection was not confirmed on central review of radiographic imaging (20%) resulted in a per-protocol analysis. Study design also precluded patients with early severe subsequent stroke.

A 2012 meta-analysis of non-randomized studies included over 1600 patients with cervical artery dissection. The analysis concluded no significant difference in recurrent stroke risk or mortality between anticoagulation and antiplatelet therapy [41]. Similarly, a 2015 meta-analysis of non-randomized studies with over 1300 subjects who had acute carotid artery dissection also found no differences in outcome or complication rates when anticoagulation was used in place of antiplatelet therapy [42].

When a subarachnoid hemorrhage caused by the intracranial extension of CAD occurs, anticoagulation is contraindicated and thus should be excluded through imaging [22].

Concept of Transcranial Duplex and Microembolic Detection for Determination of Treatment

Carotid and vertebral artery dissections are frequently complicated by cerebral embolism. Detection of clinically silent circulating microemboli by transcranial Doppler sonography (TCD) is a known diagnostic tool in patients with CAD to identify patients at increased risk for stroke [43]. In the literature, a rapid decline in microembolic signal (MES) count has been reported in patients with symptomatic internal carotid artery dissection (ICAD) treated with anticoagulant therapy. Detection of MES may help to estimate the risk of recurrence, to monitor the effectiveness of antithrombotic therapy in patients with carotid artery dissection, and sometimes to choose the anticoagulation therapy if MES burden is too high [44].

Duration of Antithrombotic Therapy

There is no concrete data regarding optimal duration of antithrombotic therapy. The goal is to achieve healing of the vessel wall or resolution of vascular abnormalities which may be used as a marker to guide duration of initial treatment. Most arterial abnormalities stabilize in appearance or resolve by 3 months, and vessels that fail to reconstitute a normal lumen by 6 months are highly unlikely to recover at later time points [45]. After 3–6 months, repeated noninvasive imaging is suggested to assess vascular healing status. Multimodal CT or MRI, ultrasonography, or conventional angiography may be used, although serial noninvasive approaches are favored.

Cases Where Antiplatelets Are Preferred over Anticoagulation

Situations where antiplatelet therapy for extracranial cervical artery dissection is preferred over anticoagulation include a severe stroke in which the patient scores greater or equal to 15 on the National Institutes of Health Stroke Scale

(NIHSS); when neuroimaging is unavailable for the patient; when extracranial dissection is accompanied by intracranial dissection; a local compression syndrome without a cerebrovascular accident or TIA present; risk of bleeding due to any other concomitant health condition of the body; or in patients with limited intracranial collateral arterial circulation [46].

Thrombolytic Therapy

The major randomized trials of intravenous thrombolysis for acute ischemic stroke did not exclude patients with cervicocephalic arterial dissection. While thrombolysis in the setting of dissection may theoretically cause enlargement of the intramural hematoma, accumulating evidence suggests that the effectiveness and safety of thrombolysis for patients with ischemic stroke related to cervical artery dissection are similar to its effectiveness and safety for patients with ischemic stroke from other causes [47, 48]. A 2011 meta-analysis of individual patient data from 14 retrospective series and 22 case reports involving 180 patients with cervical artery dissection who were treated with thrombolysis and followed for a median of 3 months [38] compared these patients with matched historic controls from the observational SITS-ISTR registry of patients treated with intravenous alteplase for acute ischemic stroke. No major differences were found between groups for rates of symptomatic intracranial hemorrhage, mortality, excellent outcome, or favorable outcome.

Endovascular or Open Surgical Treatment

A variety of surgical interventions can be performed including endovascular stent angioplasty, direct carotid artery repair, carotid artery resection with a vein graft replacement, carotid ligation or clipping with or without extracranial to intracranial carotid artery bypass, thromboendarterectomy with a synthetic patch angioplasty, and carotid resection with a vein interposition graft [1, 20]. If there is persistence or recurrence of symptoms despite optimal medical management, endovascular stenting is recommended (ACCF/AHA

Class IIb, Level C; SIGN Grade D) [49]. In published systematic reviews of case reports and case series, stenting of carotid dissection reportedly results in a high level of arterial patency, 75–100% patency at 1-year follow-up [50] and around 11% stroke or TIA symptoms within 30 days post procedure. Finally, if endovascular treatment is contraindicated for the patient and symptoms remain persistent despite optimal medical management, consider surgical repair (weak recommendation, AHA/ASA Class IIb, Level C). Reasons for surgical carotid repair include a contradiction to anticoagulation and medical management, an expanding or symptomatic pseudoaneurysm, or significant compromise of cerebral blood flow due to a cervical dissection [20, 49].

American Heart Association/American Stroke Association Guideline Statement for Healthcare Professionals 2014 [51]

American Heart Association Treatment Recommendations for Stroke Patients with Arterial Dissections [51]

Thrombolysis with intravenous tPA is reasonably safe in the treatment of patients with acute ischemic stroke caused by CD within 4,5 h

For patients with TIA or ischemic stroke resulting from CD, antiplatelets or anticoagulant therapy for 3–6 month is reasonable

Endovascular therapy may be considered for patients with CD who experience definite recurrent cerebral ischemic events while on appropriate antithrombotic therapy

CD cervical artery dissection, *TIA* transient ischemic attack, *tPA* tissue-type plasminogen activator

---

Other Management

Blunt Cerebrovascular Injury

Blunt cerebrovascular injury (BCVI) is rare but potentially devastating, with a reported stroke rate of 3–59%, disproportionately affecting young adults. This is an extensive topic, but management

facts about BCVI will be briefly discussed. Blunt cerebrovascular injury is characterized as carotid or vertebral artery injuries due to blunt trauma. In the literature incidence is reported to be 1% of blunt trauma with mortality of 23–28% if untreated and morbidity of 48–58% if untreated [52, 53]. True BCVI was defined as any injury on initial imaging distinctly classified by the Denver criteria [54].

The treatment recommendations for BCVI by the Eastern Association for the Surgery of Trauma (EAST) are based on current treatment experience and comparing morbidity, mortality, and outcome with historic untreated patients. Based on the available literature low-grade (grade I or II) injuries or inaccessible lesions can be treated with anticoagulation (heparin without bolus goal aPTT 50–70 with transition to Coumadin) or antithrombotic (aspirin 325 mg or Plavix 75 mg) for 3–5 months [55], while higher-grade (grade III or IV) injuries are resistant to such therapy and may require more invasive therapy (surgery or angio-intervention) based on follow up non invasive survuilence imaging as these injuries rarely resolve with observation or heparinization. In children with ischemic neurologic event, consider aggressive management of intracranial hypertension including resection of ischemic brain tissue (may have improved outcomes as compared with adults). Follow-up angiography is recommended for grade I–III injuries at 7 days post injury [56].

Follow-Up

Noninvasive imaging of cervical arteries may be required to evaluate healing or progression of vascular lesions to tailor the treatment duration and to access any complications. Anticoagulation is usually maintained for ≤6 months, but antiplatelet therapy may be used long-term.

Outcome

In literature, complete resolution of arterial abnormality is estimated at around 46% for stenosis, 33% for occlusion, and 4% for dissecting aneurysm. Complete resolution is mostly seen in

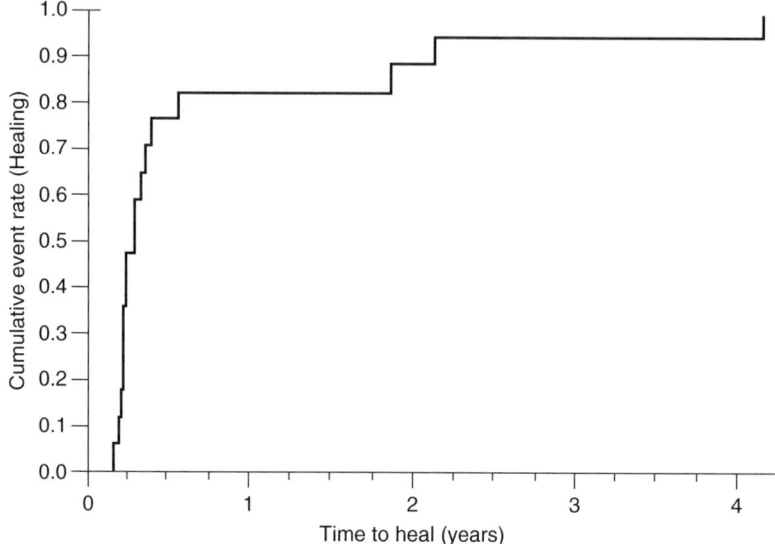

Fig. 20.3 Kaplan-Meier curve for healing in 19 dissected vessels in 17 patients with cervical artery dissection. The median time to healing is 0.29 years (95% CI, 0.23–0.4). From Lee et al. [4]. Reprinted with permission from Wolters Kluwer Health, Inc

patients who present with only local symptoms and signs [45]. Dissection cases typically do show significant improvement, complete resolution, or stable residual luminal irregularity within a median duration of 0.29 years and in 82% of the cases within the first year [4] (Fig. 20.3).

Recurrences

Recurrent ischemic events seem to be rare. Recurrent ischemic events usually occur during the first 4 weeks after the dissection [6, 57]. At 1 year, the rate of ischemic recurrences has been estimated to be between 0.4 and 13.3%. Factors associated with an increased risk of recurrent ischemic events are multiple dissections [6] and a history of hypertension [57]. Recurrences of dissections are also rare. They seem to be most frequent within the first 2 months after the initial event [58], and some dissections that were diagnosed as multiple might have occurred sequentially within a short time frame. Risk factors for recurrent CAD include younger age [59], family history of CAD [59], vascular Ehlers-Danlos syndrome [58], and fibromuscular dysplasia [60]. The prognosis of recurrent CAD has been described as benign.

Review Questions

1. Carotid and vertebral artery dissection (cervical artery) is responsible for:
   A. Less than 2% of initial stroke
   B. 2.5–3%
   C. Greater than 3–5%
   D. Greater than 5% of initial stroke

   Answer: B

2. The most common presenting symptom of cervical artery dissection is:
   A. Unilateral head, neck, and facial pain
   B. Stroke
   C. Horner Syndrome
   D. Pulsatile tinnitus

   Answer: A

3. The most commonly used initial treatment of carotid artery dissection is:
   A. Anticoagulation/antithrombotic therapy
   B. Thrombolytic therapy
   C. Stenting
   D. Open surgical repair

   Answer: A

References

1. Schievink WI. Spontaneous dissection of the carotid and vertebral arteries. N Engl J Med. 2001;344(12):898–906. https://doi.org/10.1056/NEJM200103223441206.

2. Ducrocq X, Lacour JC, Debouverie M, Bracard S, Girard F, Weber M. Cerebral ischemic accidents in young subjects. A prospective study of 296 patients aged 16 to 45 years. Revue Neurol. 1999;155(8):575–82. http://www.ncbi.nlm.nih.gov/pubmed/10486847.

3. Giroud M, Fayolle H, André N, Dumas R, Becker F, Martin D, et al. Incidence of internal carotid artery dissection in the community of Dijon. J Neurol Neurosurg Psychiat. 1994;57(11):1443. http://www.ncbi.nlm.nih.gov/pubmed/7964839.

4. Lee VH, Brown RD, Mandrekar JN, Mokri B. Incidence and outcome of cervical artery dissection: a population-based study. Neurology. 2006;67(10):1809–12. https://doi.org/10.1212/01.wnl.0000244486.30455.71.

5. Arnold M, Kappeler L, Georgiadis D, Berthet K, Keserue B, Bousser MG, Baumgartner RW. Gender differences in spontaneous cervical artery dissection. Neurology. 2006;67(6):1050–2. https://doi.org/10.1212/01.wnl.0000237341.30854.6a.

6. Touzé E, Gauvrit J-Y, Moulin T, Meder J-F, Bracard S, Mas J-L, Multicenter Survey on Natural History of Cervical Artery Dissection. Risk of stroke and recurrent dissection after a cervical artery dissection: a multicenter study. Neurology. 2003;61(10):1347–51. http://www.ncbi.nlm.nih.gov/pubmed/14638953.

7. Thanvi B, Munshi SK, Dawson SL, Robinson TG. Carotid and vertebral artery dissection syndromes. Postgrad Med J. 2005;81(956):383–8. https://doi.org/10.1136/pgmj.2003.016774.

8. Debette S, Metso T, Pezzini A, Abboud S, Metso A, Leys D, Cervical Artery Dissection and Ischemic Stroke Patients (CADISP) Group, et al. Association of vascular risk factors with cervical artery dissection and ischemic stroke in young adults. Circulation. 2011;123(14):1537–44. https://doi.org/10.1161/CIRCULATIONAHA.110.000125.

9. Pezzini A, Granella F, Grassi M, Bertolino C, Del Zotto E, Immovilli P, et al. History of migraine and the risk of spontaneous cervical artery dissection. Cephalalgia. 2005;25(8):575–80. https://doi.org/10.1111/j.1468-2982.2005.00919.x.

10. Tzourio C, Benslamia L, Guillon B, Aïdi S, Bertrand M, Berthet K, Bousser MG. Migraine and the risk of cervical artery dissection: a case-control study. Neurology. 2002;59(3):435–7. http://www.ncbi.nlm.nih.gov/pubmed/12177380.

11. Gallai V, Caso V, Paciaroni M, Cardaioli G, Arning E, Bottiglieri T, Parnetti L. Mild hyperhomocyst(e)inemia: a possible risk factor for cervical artery dissection. Stroke. 2001;32(3):714–8. http://www.ncbi.nlm.nih.gov/pubmed/11239192.

12. Grau AJ, Buggle F, Rubinstein SM, Peerdeman S, van Tulder M, Haldeman S. A systemic review of the risk factors for cervical artery dissection. Stroke. 2005;36(11):2340. https://doi.org/10.1161/01.STR.0000185695.67188.f7.

13. Grau AJ, Brandt T, Buggle F, Orberk E, Mytilineos J, Werle E, et al. Association of cervical artery dissection with recent infection. Arch Neurol. 1999;56(7):851–6. http://www.ncbi.nlm.nih.gov/pubmed/10404987.

14. Debette S, Leys D. Cervical-artery dissections: predisposing factors, diagnosis, and outcome. Lancet Neurol. 2009;8(7):668–78. https://doi.org/10.1016/S1474-4422(09)70084-5.

15. Arauz A, Hoyos L, Cantú C, Jara A, Martínez L, García I, et al. Mild Hyperhomocysteinemia and low folate concentrations as risk factors for cervical arterial dissection. Cerebrovasc Dis. 2007;24(2–3):210–4. https://doi.org/10.1159/000104479.

16. Longoni M, Grond-Ginsbach C, Grau AJ, Genius J, Debette S, Schwaninger M, et al. The ICAM-1 E469K gene polymorphism is a risk factor for spontaneous cervical artery dissection. Neurology. 2006;66(8):1273–5. https://doi.org/10.1212/01.wnl.0000208411.01172.0b.

17. Pezzini A, Del Zotto E, Archetti S, Negrini R, Bani P, Albertini A, et al. Plasma homocysteine concentration, C677T MTHFR genotype, and 844ins68bp CBS genotype in young adults with spontaneous cervical artery dissection and atherothrombotic stroke. Stroke. 2002;33(3):664–9. http://www.ncbi.nlm.nih.gov/pubmed/11872884.

18. von Pein F, Välkkilä M, Schwarz R, Morcher M, Klima B, Grau A, et al. Analysis of the COL3A1 gene in patients with spontaneous cervical artery dissections. J Neurol. 2002;249(7):862–6. https://doi.org/10.1007/s00415-002-0745-x.

19. Schievink WI, Mokri B, Piepgras DG, Kuiper JD. Recurrent spontaneous arterial dissections: risk in familial versus nonfamilial disease. Stroke. 1996;27(4):622–4. http://www.ncbi.nlm.nih.gov/pubmed/8614918.

20. Kim Y-K, Schulman S. Cervical artery dissection: pathology, epidemiology and management. Thromb Res. 2009;123(6):810–21. https://doi.org/10.1016/j.thromres.2009.01.013.

21. Brandt T, Orberk E, Weber R, Werner I, Busse O, Müller BT, et al. Pathogenesis of cervical artery dissections: association with connective tissue abnormalities. Neurology. 2001;57(1):24–30. http://www.ncbi.nlm.nih.gov/pubmed/11445623.

22. Brott TG, Halperin JL, Abbara S, Bacharach JM, Barr JD, Bush RL, et al. 2011 ASA/ACCF/AHA/AANN/AANS/ACR/ASNR/CNS/SAIP/SCAI/SIR/SNIS/SVM/SVS guideline on the Management of Patients with extracranial carotid and vertebral artery disease: executive summary. J Am Coll Cardiol. 2011;57(8):1002–44. https://doi.org/10.1016/j.jacc.2010.11.005.

23. Djouhri H, Guillon B, Brunereau L, Lévy C, Bousson V, Biousse V, et al. MR angiography for the long-term follow-up of dissecting aneurysms of the extracranial internal carotid artery. AJR Am J Roentgenol. 2000;174(4):1137–40. https://doi.org/10.2214/ajr.174.4.1741137.

24. Kasner SE, Hankins LL, Bratina P, Morgenstern LB. Magnetic resonance angiography demonstrates vascular healing of carotid and vertebral artery dissections. Stroke. 1997;28(10):1993–7. http://www.ncbi.nlm.nih.gov/pubmed/9341709.

25. Kirsch E, Kaim A, Engelter S, Lyrer P, Stock KW, Bongartz G, Radü EW. MR angiography in internal carotid artery dissection: improvement of diagnosis by selective demonstration of the intramural haematoma. Neuroradiology. 1998;40(11):704–9. http://www.ncbi.nlm.nih.gov/pubmed/9860118.

26. Leclerc X, Lucas C, Godefroy O, Nicol L, Moretti A, Leys D, Pruvo JP. Preliminary experience using contrast-enhanced MR angiography to assess vertebral artery structure for the follow-up of suspected dissection. AJNR Am J Neuroradiol. 1999;20(8):1482–90. http://www.ncbi.nlm.nih.gov/pubmed/10512235.

27. Provenzale JM. MRI and MRA for evaluation of dissection of craniocerebral arteries: lessons from the medical literature. Emerg Radiol. 2009;16(3):185–93. https://doi.org/10.1007/s10140-008-0770-x.

28. Lisovoski F, Rousseaux P. Cerebral infarction in young people. A study of 148 patients with early cerebral angiography. J Neurol Neurosurg Psychiatry. 1991;54(7):576–9. http://www.ncbi.nlm.nih.gov/pubmed/1895119.

29. Provenzale JM. Dissection of the internal carotid and vertebral arteries: imaging features. Am J Roentgenol. 1995;165(5):1099–104. https://doi.org/10.2214/ajr.165.5.7572483.

30. Shimoji T, Bando K, Nakajima K, Ito K. Dissecting aneurysm of the vertebral artery. J Neurosurg. 1984;61(6):1038–46. https://doi.org/10.3171/jns.1984.61.6.1038.

31. Clark W, Papamitsakis NIH. Stroke: pathophysiology, diagnosis, and management, 3rd ed. J Vasc Surg. 1999;30(6):769–86. https://doi.org/10.1016/S0741-5214(99)70063-7.

32. Stapf C, Elkind MSV, Mohr JP. Carotid artery dissection. Annu Rev Med. 2000;51(1):329–47. https://doi.org/10.1146/annurev.med.51.1.329.

33. Naggara O, Louillet F, Touzé E, Roy D, Leclerc X, Mas J-L, et al. Added value of high-resolution MR imaging in the diagnosis of vertebral artery dissection. AJNR Am J Neuroradiol. 2010;31(9):1707–12. https://doi.org/10.3174/ajnr.A2165.

34. Leclerc X, Godefroy O, Salhi A, Lucas C, Leys D, Pruvo JP. Helical CT for the diagnosis of extracranial internal carotid artery dissection. Stroke. 1996;27(3):461–6. http://www.ncbi.nlm.nih.gov/pubmed/8610314.

35. Vertinsky AT, Schwartz NE, Fischbein NJ, Rosenberg J, Albers GW, Zaharchuk G. Comparison of multidetector CT angiography and MR imaging of cervical artery dissection. AJNR Am J Neuroradiol. 2008;29(9):1753–60. https://doi.org/10.3174/ajnr.A1189.

36. Sturzenegger M, Mattle HP, Rivoir A, Rihs F, Schmid C. Ultrasound findings in spontaneous extracranial vertebral artery dissection. Stroke. 1993;24(12):1910–21. http://www.ncbi.nlm.nih.gov/pubmed/7902621.

37. Alecu C, Fortrat JO, Ducrocq X, Vespignani H, de Bray JM. Duplex scanning diagnosis of internal carotid artery dissections. A case control study. Cerebrovasc Dis. 2007;23(5–6):441–7. https://doi.org/10.1159/000101469.

38. Zinkstok SM, Vergouwen MDI, Engelter ST, Lyrer PA, Bonati LH, Arnold M, et al. Safety and functional outcome of thrombolysis in dissection-related ischemic stroke: a meta-analysis of individual patient data. Stroke. 2011;42(9):2515–20. https://doi.org/10.1161/STROKEAHA.111.617282.

39. CADISS Trial Investigators, Markus HS, Hayter E, Levi C, Feldman A, Venables G, Norris J. Antiplatelet treatment compared with anticoagulation treatment for cervical artery dissection (CADISS): a randomised trial. Lancet Neurol. 2015;14(4):361–7. https://doi.org/10.1016/S1474-4422(15)70018-9.

40. Kasner SE. CADISS: a feasibility trial that answered its question. Lancet Neurol. 2015;14(4):342–3. https://doi.org/10.1016/S1474-4422(14)70271-6.

41. Kennedy F, Lanfranconi S, Hicks C, Reid J, Gompertz P, Price C, CADISS Investigators, et al. Antiplatelets vs anticoagulation for dissection: CADISS nonrandomized arm and meta-analysis. Neurology. 2012;79(7):686–9. https://doi.org/10.1212/WNL.0b013e318264e36b.

42. Chowdhury MM, Sabbagh CN, Jackson D, Coughlin PA, Ghosh J. Antithrombotic treatment for acute extracranial carotid artery dissections: a meta-analysis. Eur J Vasc Endovasc Surg. 2015;50(2):148–56. https://doi.org/10.1016/j.ejvs.2015.04.034.

43. Droste DW, Junker K, Stögbauer F, Lowens S, Besselmann M, Braun B, Ringelstein EB. Clinically silent circulating microemboli in 20 patients with carotid or vertebral artery dissection. Cerebrovasc Dis. 2001;12(3):181–5. https://doi.org/10.1159/000047701.

44. Molina CA, Alvarez-Sabín J, Schonewille W, Montaner J, Rovira A, Abilleira S, Codina A. Cerebral microembolism in acute spontaneous internal carotid artery dissection. Neurology. 2000;55(11):1738–40. http://www.ncbi.nlm.nih.gov/pubmed/11113235.

45. Nedeltchev K, Bickel S, Arnold M, Sarikaya H, Georgiadis D, Sturzenegger M, et al. R2-recanalization of spontaneous carotid artery dissection. Stroke. 2009;40(2):499–504. https://doi.org/10.1161/STROKEAHA.108.519694.

46. Engelter ST, Brandt T, Debette S, Caso V, Lichy C, Pezzini A, Cervical Artery Dissection in Ischemic Stroke Patients (CADISP) Study Group, et al. Antiplatelets versus anticoagulation in cervical artery dissection. Stroke. 2007;38(9):2605–11. https://doi.org/10.1161/STROKEAHA.107.489666.

47. Engelter ST, Rutgers MP, Hatz F, Georgiadis D, Fluri F, Sekoranja L, et al. Intravenous thrombolysis in stroke attributable to cervical artery dissection. Stroke. 2009;40(12):3772–6. https://doi.org/10.1161/STROKEAHA.109.555953.

48. Georgiadis D, Baumgartner RW. Thrombolysis in cervical artery dissection. Front Neurol Neurosci. 2005;20:140–6. https://doi.org/10.1159/000088158.

49. Kernan WN, Ovbiagele B, Black HR, Bravata DM, Chimowitz MI, Ezekowitz MD, American Heart Association Stroke Council, Council on Cardiovascular and Stroke Nursing, Council on Clinical Cardiology, and Council on Peripheral Vascular Disease, et al. Guidelines for the prevention of stroke in patients with stroke and transient ischemic attack: a guideline for healthcare professionals from the American Heart Association/American Stroke Association. Stroke. 2014;45(7):2160–236. https://doi.org/10.1161/STR.0000000000000024.

50. Donas KP, Mayer D, Guber I, Baumgartner R, Genoni M, Lachat M. Endovascular repair of extracranial carotid artery dissection: current status and level of evidence. J Vasc Interv Radiol. 2008;19(12):1693–8. https://doi.org/10.1016/j.jvir.2008.08.025.

51. Biller J, Sacco RL, Albuquerque FC, Demaerschalk BM, Fayad P, Long PH, American Heart Association Stroke Council, et al. Cervical arterial dissections and association with cervical manipulative therapy: a statement for healthcare professionals from the American Heart Association/American Stroke Association. Stroke. 2014;45(10):3155–74. https://doi.org/10.1161/STR.0000000000000016.

52. Biffl WL, Moore EE, Ryu RK, Offner PJ, Novak Z, Coldwell DM, et al. The unrecognized epidemic of blunt carotid arterial injuries: early diagnosis improves neurologic outcome. Ann Surg. 1998;228(4):462–70. http://www.ncbi.nlm.nih.gov/pubmed/9790336.

53. Fabian TC, Patton JH, Croce MA, Minard G, Kudsk KA, Pritchard FE. Blunt carotid injury. Importance of early diagnosis and anticoagulant therapy. Ann Surg. 1996;223(5):513–22. http://www.ncbi.nlm.nih.gov/pubmed/8651742.

54. Burlew CC, Biffl WL, Moore EE, Barnett CC, Johnson JL, Bensard DD. Blunt cerebrovascular injuries: rede-

fining screening criteria in the era of noninvasive diagnosis. J Trauma Acute Care Surg. 2012;72(2):330–5. Discussion 336–7, quiz 539. https://doi.org/10.1097/TA.0b013e31823de8a0.

55. Miller PR, Fabian TC, Bee TK, Timmons S, Chamsuddin A, Finkle R, Croce MA. Blunt cerebrovascular injuries: diagnosis and treatment. J Trauma. 2001;51(2):279–85. http://www.ncbi.nlm.nih.gov/pubmed/11493785.

56. Bromberg WJ, Collier BC, Diebel LN, Dwyer KM, Holevar MR, Jacobs DG, et al. Blunt cerebrovascular injury practice management guidelines: the eastern association for the surgery of trauma. J Trauma. 2010;68(2):471–7. https://doi.org/10.1097/TA.0b013e3181cb43da.

57. Beletsky V, Nadareishvili Z, Lynch J, Shuaib A, Woolfenden A, Norris JW, Canadian Stroke Consortium. Cervical arterial dissection: time for a therapeutic trial? Stroke. 2003;34(12):2856–60. https://doi.org/10.1161/01.STR.0000098649.39767.BC.

58. Leys D, Bandu L, Hénon H, Lucas C, Mounier-Vehier F, Rondepierre P, Godefroy O. Clinical outcome in 287 consecutive young adults (15 to 45 years) with ischemic stroke. Neurology. 2002;59(1):26–33. http://www.ncbi.nlm.nih.gov/pubmed/12105303.

59. Schievink WI, Mokri B, O'Fallon WM. Recurrent spontaneous cervical-artery dissection. N Engl J Med. 1994;330(6):393–7. https://doi.org/10.1056/NEJM199402103300604.

60. Dziewas R, Konrad C, Dräger B, Evers S, Besselmann M, Lüdemann P, et al. Cervical artery dissection—clinical features, risk factors, therapy and outcome in 126 patients. J Neurol. 2003;250(10):1179–84. https://doi.org/10.1007/s00415-003-0174-5.

Carotid Body Tumors

21

Frank M. Davis, Andrea Obi,
and Nicholas Osborne

Introduction

The carotid body is located in the adventitia of the common carotid artery at its bifurcation and consists of neural crest cell-derived chemoreceptors. These receptors detect changes in oxygen, carbon dioxide, and pH concentration and are involved in neurogenic physiologic adaptation to changes in these parameters. When tumors develop from these cells, they are referred as extra-adrenal neuroendocrine neoplasms. Carotid body tumors (CBTs), also known as cervical paragangliomas, chemodectomas, or glomus caroticum tumors, are the most common head and neck paraganglioma arising from both mesodermal and neuroectodermal origin. A recent review of CBTs demonstrated a mean age of 55 years (range, 18–94 years) at time of diagnosis and a male-to-female ratio of 1:1.9. More tumors (57%) were on the right side, whereas 25% were on the left, 17% were bilateral, and 4.3% were malignant [1]. CBTs tend to be sporadic but are familial in 10–20% of cases [2].

F. M. Davis
Vascular Surgery, University of Michigan,
Ann Arbor, MI, USA

A. Obi · N. Osborne (✉)
Vascular Surgery, University of Michigan,
Ann Arbor, MI, USA

Vascular Surgery, Ann Arbor Veterans Medical
Center, Ann Arbor, MI, USA
e-mail: nichosbo@med.umich.edu

Pathogenesis

CBTs have been reported to be more prevalent in conditions that lead to chronic hypoxemia, including high altitudes, smoking, and chronic obstructive pulmonary disease [2–4]. The majority of cases are sporadic; however approximately 10% occur along familial lines. Recently published research has identified mutations in succinate dehydrogenase subunit D (SDHD), an enzyme that plays a role in oxidative phosphorylation of the Krebs cycle, to be associated with patients with head and neck paragangliomas [5–7]. Germ-line mutations have been identified to involve the subunits A, B, C, and D and the assembly factor 2 (AF2) of the SDH enzyme complex; the most prevalent ones noted involve the B and D subunits. However, to date, recommendations for genetic testing for mutations of the SDH subunit genes in patients with head and neck paragangliomas for hereditary paraganglioma-pheochromocytoma syndrome have not been established.

CBTs characteristically splay the carotid bifurcation and, depending on their size, can encapsulate the external or internal carotid artery, or both. The bulk of the tumor is generally located at and, more often, deep to the bifurcation and can extend over the common carotid artery proximal to the bifurcation. These tumors grow quite slowly, with a reported median doubling time of 4.2 years, with large and small tumors growing at a slower rate than intermediate-sized ones [8]. CBTs are characteristically extremely vascular, secrete catecholamines on rare occasions, and are usually benign. Microscopically, the tumors reproduce the architecture of the normal carotid body, which is composed of granular epithelioid chief cells and sustentacular supporting cells. When malignant, CBTs metastasize to the local lymph nodes, liver, lung, and bone, although metastases occur in no more than 5% of cases.

Clinical Presentation

CBTs usually manifest as an asymptomatic anterior neck mass. In larger tumors, they can be associated with the myriad of presenting symptoms of a space-occupying lesion in this location, such as fullness, pain, dysphagia, odynophagia, hoarseness, and stridor. Tumors that are at least 3 cm may be appreciated on physical examination as a bulging lump in the anterior triangle of the neck. The tissue is often rubbery, firm, and noncompressible. The mass may be displaced laterally but not vertically (Fontaine's sign). Generally, a palpable thrill or bruit is absent. Historically, cranial nerve deficits were present in approximately 10% of patients secondary to nerve compression; however with improved imaging modalities, CBTs are

detected earlier at smaller sizes, and thereby cranial nerve compromise is rare currently. Lastly, a rare functional CBT may produce neuroendocrine secretions causing catecholamine-related symptoms, such as palpitations, headaches, hypertension, tachycardia, or flushing.

Diagnosis and Preoperative Planning

CBTs are usually identified by clinical examination or found incidentally on imaging studies [9]. Color-flow carotid duplex is the ideal screening test for CBTs, and these tumors are characteristically a well-defined hypoechoic mass that splay the carotid bifurcation. With color Doppler imaging, a hypervascularity with low-resistance flow pattern is evident (Fig. 21.1). Historically, angiography was the "gold standard" diagnostic procedure for CBTs to confirm diagnosis and provide accurate delineation of the vascular supply. However with improvements in high-resolution imaging, cross-sectional imaging (such as CT angiography (CTA) or MRA) is the preferred modality for surgical planning of tumor resection because it best defines the relationship of the tumor with the artery bifurcation and the likely location of the cranial nerves (Fig. 21.2). CTA is

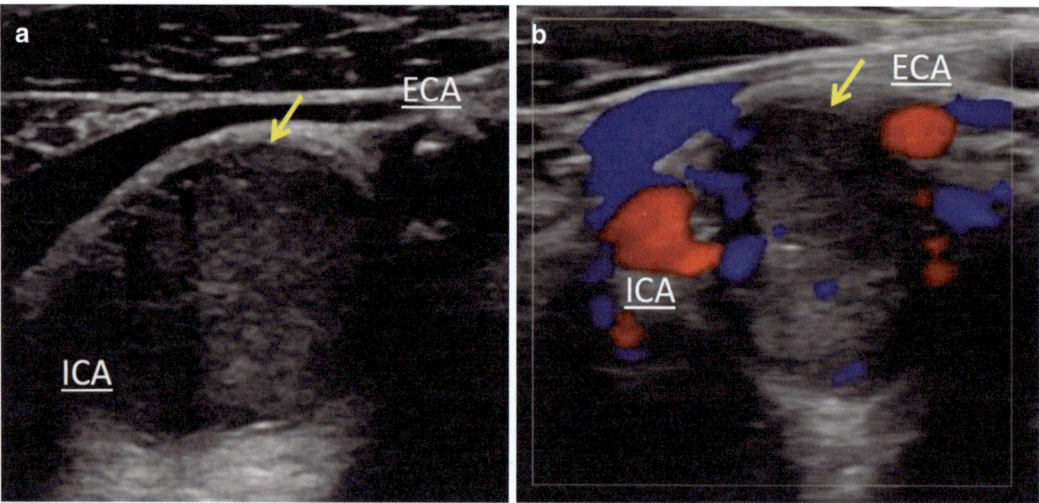

Fig. 21.1 (a) Gray scale, (b) color flow. Duplex ultrasound of carotid body tumor (arrow) splaying of the internal (ICA) and external carotid artery (ECA)

Fig. 21.2 (**a**) Computed tomography angiography (CTA) demonstrating right carotid body tumor splaying the bifurcation of the right internal (large arrow) and external (small arrow) carotid arteries. (**b**) CTA 3D reformatted images of right carotid body tumor

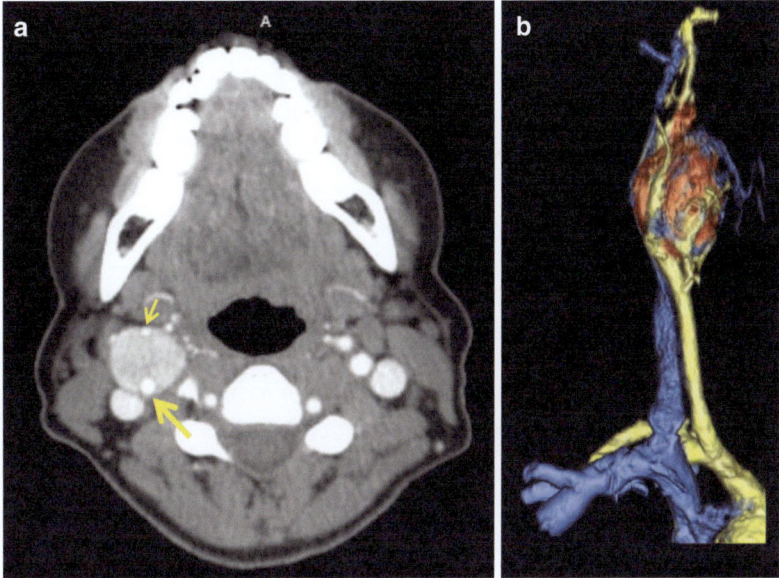

able to define the size of the tumor and its relation to bone landmarks, which can modify surgical approach. It can also easily identify contralateral tumors and other head/neck paragangliomas. Finally, CTA is especially helpful in classifying the Shamblin group (Fig. 21.2b). Shamblin classification divides CBTs into three groups that related to the difficulty of resection and the risk of neurovascular complications (Fig. 21.3). Type I tumors are small lesions at the carotid bifurcation and can generally be removed without difficulty. Type II tumors are larger and significantly splay the carotid bifurcation, but do not circumferentially encase the carotid arteries. Type III tumors are large, encapsulate the internal and/or external carotid arteries, and often adhere or incorporate the adjacent cranial nerves. MRA with gadolinium enhancement is also helpful at characterizing CBTs and associated vessel encasement. Finally, if there is clinical suspicion for the rare occurrence of a tumor that is functional and secreting catecholamines, biochemical evaluation is recommended [10]. This is undertaken with a plasma or a 24-h urinary collection for metanephrines and the catecholamines, epinephrine, and norepinephrine, with the former being the more sensitive test.

Preoperative Embolization

One controversy surrounding surgical excision of CBTs has been the role of preoperative embolization of the tumor's blood supply. Since these tumors are highly vascular, some surgeons advocate for highly selective embolization of the ascending pharyngeal branch of the external carotid artery to reduce intraoperative blood loss. Although several retrospective studies demonstrated no difference in blood loss or perioperative morbidity between embolized and non-embolized groups [11], others have found reduced intraoperative bleeding after embolization of tumors of more than 3 cm in diameter [12, 13]. Preoperative embolization procedure is not without its own inherent risks as the polyvinyl alcohol particles used for embolization have resulted in strokes in several studies [9, 11, 12]. Ultimately, if preoperative embolization is conducted, expeditious surgical resection should be performed, preferably within 24 h and no later than 48 h, to avoid additional surgical challenges from a post-embolization inflammatory response.

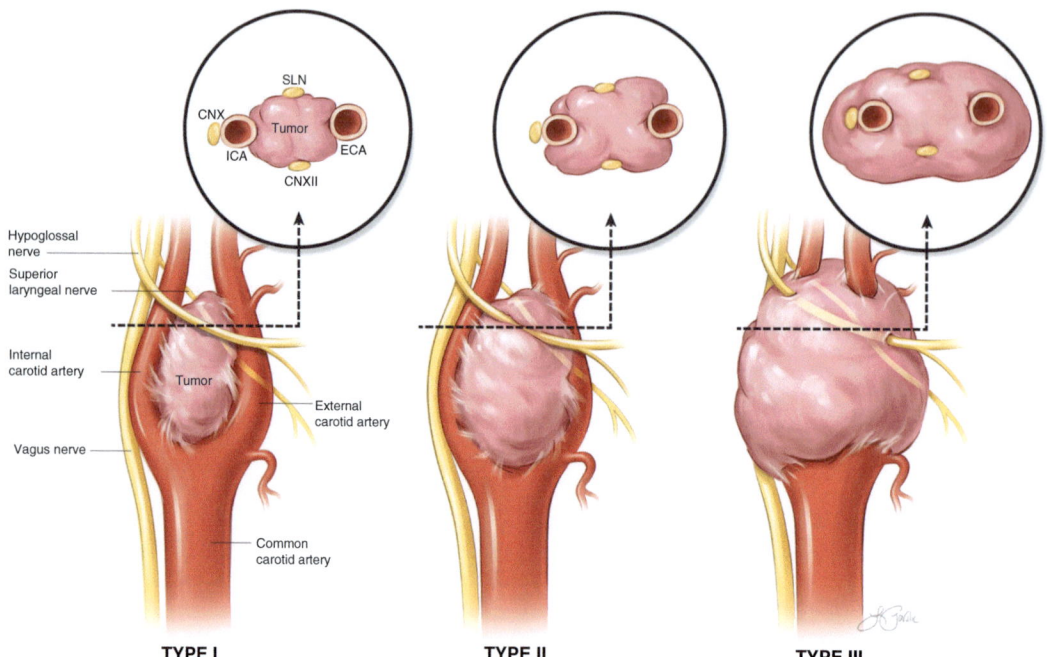

Fig. 21.3 Shamblin classification of carotid body tumors. Type I tumors are small lesions at the carotid bifurcation and can generally be removed without difficulty. Type II tumors are larger, significantly splay the carotid bifurcation, but do not circumferentially encase the carotid arter- ies. Type III tumors are large, encapsulate the internal and/or external carotid arteries, and often adhere or incorporate the adjacent cranial nerves. *CN* cranial nerve, *ECA* external carotid artery, *ICA* internal carotid artery, *SLN* superior laryngeal nerve

Operative Technique

The operative positioning and setup for carotid body tumor resection is similar in many ways to a standard carotid endarterectomy. In general, we prefer general anesthesia (although regional can be considered for smaller tumor resections), positioning in a supine or beach chair position with the head slightly extended and rotated to the left. Additional considerations specific to CBT resection include routine vein mapping, and preparation of one thigh into the operative field for potential saphenous vein harvest should be needed for reconstruction. Additionally, the choice of incision may vary depending upon the extent of the tumor. Incision choices include a curvilinear incision along the midportion of the tumor, a "hockey stick" incision along the anterior border of the SCM, and, in the case of a very high tumor, a modified radical neck T incision (Fig. 21.4).

We follow a standard approach beginning with exposure of the CCA in the lower neck and progressing cephalad. Early identification of the

vagus nerve is mandatory. Cranial nerve injuries are the most frequent complication of this operation, and the risk increases with tumor size. Identification and preservation of the hypoglossal, glossopharyngeal, and superior laryngeal nerves is also undertaken. Similarly, control of the major vascular structures, the internal, external, and common carotid arteries, is essential. The dissection plane is carried out in the subadventitial space, with liberal use of bipolar cautery. This avascular plane between the tumor and the media was described by Gordon-Taylor as the "white line." CBTs derive the majority of blood flow from the external carotid and tend to be quite vascular; thus the use of topical agents, such as thrombin or regenerated cellulose, may aid with control of raw surface bleeding. If necessary, the external carotid artery can be ligated, and this will decrease overall bleeding and facilitate dissecting the tumor off of the ICA. Another option includes heparinization and temporary clamping of the ECA origin, superior thyroid artery, lingual artery, facial artery, and distal ECA [14].

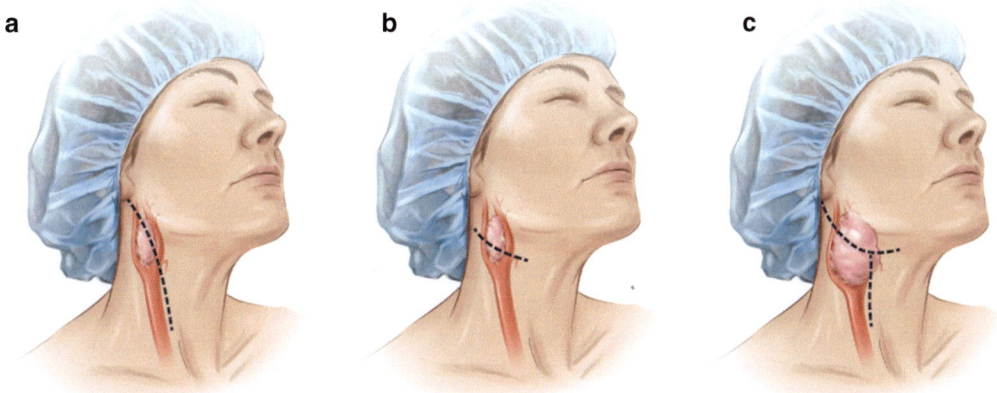

Fig. 21.4 Surgical incisions for exposure for a carotid body tumor depend on the size and/or extent of the tumor. A "hockey stick" incision along the anterior border of the sternocleidomastoid muscle (**a**) or a curvilinear incision centered on the midportion of the tumor (**b**) is advocated for Shamblin type I and II tumors. For high or large tumors, a modified radical neck T incision (**c**) can facilitate exposure

An internal to external dissection technique has also been described. This is performed by beginning the dissection from the white line of Gordon on the CCA and then dissecting the tumor free of the ICA with Mayo dissecting scissors, with the ECA the last to be dissected. The advantages of such a technique include shorter dissection time of the ICA and prevention of injury at a later time (as it is completely freed early in the course of the dissection). Furthermore, any bleeding is likely to occur during the last step (ECA dissection) at which time the course of the ICA is known and is unlikely to be injured, and the ECA can be safely ligated [15].

Finally, some have advocated for a cranial to caudal method of CBT resection [16, 17]. This approach is based upon the course of the ascending pharyngeal artery which has been proposed to be a major source of tumor blood supply. In beginning with a more cephalad dissection, the tumor is devascularized earlier in the course of the operation, and thus less blood loss occurs. Furthermore, the most "at-risk" area for nerve injury is dissected first, presumably prior to any major blood loss which could obscure the course of the cranial nerves and result in nerve injury. The advent of multiple approaches to this operation is a testament to the high attendant risk of nerve injury. It is unlikely given the relatively rare nature of this disease process that any of the above approaches will ever be rigorously compared. Thus it is up to the individual surgeon to

know his or her skill set and choose the approach most likely to limit morbidity in their patient.

High Exposure

Shamblin type II and III tumors may require more distal exposure than is feasible with standard positioning. We have found that nasotracheal intubation will gain an additional 1–2 cm of exposure. When that is insufficient, mandibular subluxation can be easily performed by a dentist, oral maxillofacial surgeon, or otolaryngologist once the patient is under anesthesia and the joint reduced prior to extubation [18]. Intraoperatively, division of the posterior belly of the digastric and, if necessary, the stylohyoid muscle (located immediately cephalad) allows for exposure of the superior border of the tumor. Occasionally, it will be necessary to elevate the parotid gland, and doing so mandates identification of the facial nerve. Although it is described, we have rarely found it necessary to excise the styloid process or resect the submandibular gland to gain distal control.

Avoiding Nerve Injury

Cranial nerve injury is the most common complication for carotid body tumor up to 24% in contemporary series [19]. Compared to surgery for atherosclerotic carotid disease, operations for CBT can be bloodier, obscuring the surgical field. Additionally, the size of the tumor may distort normal anatomic path of the nerves. Most commonly injured cranial nerves include the vagus and hypoglossal [20]. The confluence of multiple cranial nerves along the lateral border of the distal ICA (VII, IX, X, and XII) makes this area particularly treacherous and thus has spurred the development of alternate dissection techniques as described previously. A longer dissection time and need for additional exposure can put nerves at risk for retractor injury. Routine exposure of the vagus (X), hypoglossal (XII), and spinal accessory (XI) (if anticipated to be in the vicinity) is undertaken. We are cautious about deep retraction on the mandible to avoid injury to the marginal mandibular branch of the facial nerve. Posteriorly, care is taken to identify the cervical sympathetic chain to avoid resultant Horner's syndrome. Importantly, the risk of cranial nerve injury can be mitigated by resecting tumors early rather than allowing them to enlarge. For every 1 cm the tumor grows toward the skull base, the risk of cranial nerve injury is increased about 1.5 times [19].

Reconstruction

Generally, division of the ECA and its branches can be performed with limited morbidity, and there is no need for reconstruction. In fact, early division of the ECA has the potential benefit of reducing blood loss and risk of stroke. Repair of the ICA (or CCA) is more likely to be necessary with Shamblin III tumors. We have generally found that Shamblin I and II tumors do not require repair other than perhaps simple suture repair, consistent with other reports [21]. The ICA/CCA can be reconstructed with vein or prosthetic patch or interposition graft. We utilize the same principles for reconstruction as with atherosclerotic disease, including full-dose heparinization prior to manipulation of the ICA with activated clotting times >250, atraumatic vascular clamps, and shunt if required based upon stump pressure or EEG/SSEPs.

Complications

Baroreflex Failure

Baroreflex failure is a very rare but notable complication following bilateral carotid body tumor resection. It should be suspected with the development of tachycardia and hypertension 24–72 h postoperatively. Other commonly described findings include headache, emotional lability, and anxiety. Prompt identification of such a syndrome is imperative as complications can include hypertensive encephalopathy and stroke. This condition has not been described in relation to unilateral CBT resection, suggesting that contralateral preservation of the baroreceptor is adequate to maintain normal physiology.

The baroreceptors are located in the wall of the main arteries in the neck and thorax, particularly abundant in the carotid sinuses and aortic arch. A high rate of impulses (as with hypertension) from the baroreceptors inhibits the vasoconstrictor center and excites the vagal center, resulting in vasodilation and slowing of the heart rate. The opposite occurs during hypotension. Interruption of the baroreceptors results in unopposed sympathetic signals from the brainstem, leading to labile blood pressures and extreme hypertension.

Four possible manifestations may occur in the patient with baroreflex failure: hypertensive crisis, volatile hypertension, orthostatic tachycardia, and malignant vagotonia [22]. Most commonly described with sudden denervation of the baroreceptors, as caused by surgical intervention, is hypertensive crisis. This can be severe with systolic blood pressures exceeding >250 mmHg. A more frequent manifestation of baroreflex failure is the development of volatile hypertension, which develops days to weeks following the injury. Other disease processes to consider ruling out when confronted with this type of autonomic dysfunction include pheochromocytoma and autonomic neuropathy.

One series described an incidence of 20% of baroreflex failure following bilateral CBT resection, although several have postulated that the actual rate is higher [23]. Treatment is largely empiric. During a hypertensive crisis, medications with a quick onset of action and short half-life, such as nitroprusside, phentolamine, and labetalol, are preferred. For long-term treatment, clonidine has emerged as the drug of choice. Clonidine treats both the characteristic hypertension and tachycardia associated with this syndrome by stimulating alpha 2 receptors in the brainstem (preventing peripheral release of norepinephrine) and stimulating parasympathetic outflow.

Stroke, Pseudoaneurysm, and Mortality

Stroke, pseudoaneurysm, and death following CBT resection are uncommon complications. Risk factors for stroke are largely dependent upon manipulation of the ICA and include the following: reconstruction, ligation, and repair of injury [24]. Preoperative embolization does not decrease the risk of stroke, but some have advocated that early division of the ECA is effective in reducing stroke risk [25]. In a recent analysis of over 500 contemporary cases, intra- and postoperative stroke following CBT occurred in about 4% of cases, with historical rates reported between 0 and 8% [25]. Similarly, mortality has been reported to be around 1% at 30 days [25].

Pseudoaneurysm is an incredibly uncommon complication following CBT resection, with only case reports described in the literature [26, 27]. Symptoms of ICA pseudoaneurysm may present as a pulsatile lateral neck mass, a medial bulge in the pharyngeal wall, or a carotid thrill or bruit. Although multiple imaging mechanisms can be used if a pseudoaneurysm is suspected, the most efficient and lowest risk modality is duplex ultrasound. The pulse Doppler component demonstrates to and fro waveforms, while the color Doppler shows swirling of blood within the aneurysm and a communicating channel from the parent artery. Routine duplex ultrasound on follow-up would have a high sensitivity for identifying any asymptomatic pseudoaneurysms, although the complication is so rare that such a strategy cannot be advocated for all.

Review Questions

1. What is the most common presentation of carotid body tumor?
   A. Asymptomatic
   B. Cranial nerve deficit
   C. Dysphagia
   D. Hoarseness

   Answer: A

2. What should be suspected in a patient with hypertensive crisis following bilateral carotid body tumor resections?
   A. Residual paraganglioma cells
   B. Aortic coarctation
   C. Renal artery stenosis
   D. Baroreceptor failure

   Answer: D

3. Identify the correct definition of terms related to carotid body tumors.
   A. Fontaine's sign: can be displaced laterally but not vertically. Shamblin I: large, encapsulate the internal and/or external carotid arteries, and often adhere or incorporate the adjacent cranial nerves
   B. Fontaine's sign: can be displaced laterally but not vertically. Shamblin III: large, encapsulate the internal and/or external carotid arteries, and often adhere or incorporate the adjacent cranial nerves
   C. Fontaine's sign: can be displaced vertically but not laterally. Shamblin I: large, encapsulate the internal and/or external carotid arteries, and often adhere or incorporate the adjacent cranial nerves
   D. Fontaine's sign: can be displaced vertically but not laterally. Shamblin III: large, encapsulate the internal and/or external carotid arteries, and often adhere or incorporate the adjacent cranial nerves

   Answer: B

References

1. Sajid MS, Hamilton G, Baker DM, Joint Vascular Research Group. A multicenter review of carotid body tumour management. Eur J Vasc Endovasc Surg. 2007;34:127–30.

2. Kohn JS, Raftery KB, Jewell ER. Familial carotid body tumors: a closer look. J Vasc Surg. 1999;29:649–53.

3. Hallett JW, Nora JD, Hollier LH, Cherry KJ, Pairolero PC. Trends in neurovascular complications of surgical management for carotid body and cervical paragangliomas: a fifty-year experience with 153 tumors. J Vasc Surg. 1988;7:284–91.

4. Luna-Ortiz K, Rascon-Ortiz M, Villavicencio-Valencia V, Granados-Garcia M, Herrera-Gomez A. Carotid body tumors: review of a 20-year experience. Oral Oncol. 2005;41:56–61.

5. Baysal BE, Ferrell RE, Willett-Brozick JE, et al. Mutations in SDHD, a mitochondrial complex II gene, in hereditary paraganglioma. Science. 2000;287:848–51.

6. Pasini B, Stratakis CA. SDH mutations in tumorigenesis and inherited endocrine tumours: lesson from the phaeochromocytoma-paraganglioma syndromes. J Intern Med. 2009;266:19–42.

7. Boedeker CC, Neumann HPH, Maier W, Bausch B, Schipper J, Ridder GJ. Malignant head and neck paragangliomas in SDHB mutation carriers. Otolaryngol Head Neck Surg. 2007;137:126–9.

8. Jansen JC, van den Berg R, Kuiper A, van der Mey AG, Zwinderman AH, Cornelisse CJ. Estimation of growth rate in patients with head and neck paragangliomas influences the treatment proposal. Cancer. 2000;88:2811–6.

9. Westerband A, Hunter GC, Cintora I, Coulthard SW, Hinni ML, Gentile AT, Devine J, Mills JL. Current trends in the detection and management of carotid body tumors. J Vasc Surg. 1998;28:84–92.

10. Young AL, Baysal BE, Deb A, Young WF. Familial malignant catecholamine-secreting paraganglioma with prolonged survival associated with mutation in the succinate dehydrogenase B gene. J Clin Endocrinol Metab. 2002;87:4101–5.

11. Power AH, Bower TC, Kasperbauer J, Link MJ, Oderich G, Cloft H, Young WF, Gloviczki P. Impact of preoperative embolization on outcomes of carotid body tumor resections. J Vasc Surg. 2012;56:979–89.

12. LaMuraglia GM, Fabian RL, Brewster DC, Pile-Spellman J, Darling RC, Cambria RP, Abbott WM. The current surgical management of carotid body paragangliomas. J Vasc Surg. 1992;15:1038–44.

13. Kasper GC, Welling RE, Wladis AR, CaJacob DE, Grisham AD, Tomsick TA, Gluckman JL, Muck PE. A multidisciplinary approach to carotid paragangliomas. Vasc Endovasc Surg. 2007;40:467–74.

14. Spinelli F, Massara M, La Spada M, Stilo F, Barillà D, De Caridi G. A simple technique to achieve bloodless excision of carotid body tumors. J Vasc Surg. 2014;59:1462–4.

15. Rao USV, Chatterjee S, Patil AA, Nayar RC. The "INT-EX Technique": internal to external approach in carotid body tumour surgery. Indian J Surg Oncol. 2017;8:249–52.

16. Paridaans MPM, van der Bogt KEA, Jansen JC, Nyns ECA, Wolterbeek R, van Baalen JM, Hamming JF. Results from Craniocaudal carotid body tumor resection: should it be the standard surgical approach? Eur J Vasc Endovasc Surg. 2013;46:624–9.

17. van der Bogt KEA, Vrancken Peeters M-PFM, van Baalen JM, Hamming JF. Resection of carotid body tumors: results of an evolving surgical technique. Ann Surg. 2008;247:877–84.

18. Fisher DF, Clagett GP, Parker JI, Fry RE, Poor MR, Finn RA, Brink BE, Fry WJ. Mandibular subluxation for high carotid exposure. J Vasc Surg. 1984;1:727–33.

19. Kim GY, Lawrence PF, Moridzadeh RS, et al. New predictors of complications in carotid body tumor resection. J Vasc Surg. 2017;65:1673–9.

20. Davila VJ, Chang JM, Stone WM, Fowl RJ, Bower TC, Hinni ML, Money SR. Current surgical management of carotid body tumors. J Vasc Surg. 2016;64:1703–10.

21. Torrealba JI, Valdés F, Krämer AH, Mertens R, Bergoeing M, Mariné L. Management of carotid bifurcation tumors: 30-year experience. Ann Vasc Surg. 2016;34:200–5.

22. Ketch T, Biaggioni I, Robertson R, Robertson D. Four faces of baroreflex failure: hypertensive crisis, volatile hypertension, orthostatic tachycardia, and malignant vagotonia. Circulation. 2002;105:2518–23.

23. Netterville JL, Reilly KM, Robertson D, Reiber ME, Armstrong WB, Childs P. Carotid body tumors: a review of 30 patients with 46 tumors. Laryngoscope. 1995;105:115–26.

24. Gwon JG, Kwon T-W, Kim H, Cho Y-P. Risk factors for stroke during surgery for carotid body tumors. World J Surg. 2011;35:2154–8.

25. Cobb AN, Barkat A, Daungjaiboon W, Halandras P, Crisostomo P, Kuo PC, Aulivola B. Carotid body tumor resection: just as safe without preoperative embolization. Ann Vasc Surg. 2017;46:54. https://doi.org/10.1016/j.avsg.2017.06.149.

26. Ramesh A, Muthukumarassamy R, Karthikeyan VS, Rajaraman G, Mishra S. Pseudoaneurysm of internal carotid artery after carotid body tumor excision. Indian J Radiol Imaging. 2013;23:208–11.

27. Hotze TE, Smith TA, Clagett GP. Carotid artery pseudo-pseudoaneurysm after excision of carotid body tumor. J Vasc Surg. 2011;54:864.

Extracranial Carotid and Vertebral Artery Aneurysms

22

Sachinder Singh Hans

Extracranial Carotid and Vertebral Artery Aneurysms

A. Extracranial Carotid Artery Aneurysms

Aneurysms of the extracranial carotid artery are rare and account for less than 1% (0.3–0.6%) of all arterial aneurysms [1, 2]. The aneurysm is most often located at the common carotid artery and internal carotid artery junction. The mid-to-distal ICA is the second most common location of such aneurysms. Atherosclerosis is by far the most common cause, but fibromuscular dysplasia (dysplastic), trauma, prior surgical intervention, congenital deficits, infection, and irrigation can result in the formation of true carotid aneurysm or pseudoaneurysm. Sir Astley Cooper, in 1805, ligated the carotid artery in order to treat the carotid artery aneurysm; however, the patient died a few days later [1]. Dimtza reported the first successful carotid aneurysm excision in 1952, performing an end-to-end anastomosis. Winslow

et al. in 1926 reviewed the early reported cases of carotid artery aneurysms and found that among 134 patients, 82 underwent carotid ligation with operative mortality of 28%. The direct arterial repair following resection of aneurysm with end-to-end anastomosis or interposition vein graft became the standard mode of surgical treatment about five decades ago [3–7]. Surgical repair of extracranial carotid aneurysms is necessary to prevent thromboembolization and rupture of the aneurysm.

True aneurysm of the extracranial carotid artery can be fusiform or saccular. Fusiform carotid artery aneurysms are often bilateral and degenerative in etiology and are located near the carotid bifurcation [1]. Saccular aneurysms are unilateral and occur in the mid-segment of the internal carotid artery in the neck. Pseudoaneurysms result from disruption of the vessel wall, usually occurring at the site of patch grafting, secondary to infection in the prosthetic patch, arterial dissection, and or blunt/penetrating carotid artery trauma [4–8].

Clinical Presentation

Patients may present with neck mass or symptoms of TIA or stroke due to embolization. The neck mass may be mistaken for cervical lymphadenopathy, an abscess, or carotid body tumor. Large aneurysms may cause compression of the surrounding nerves and upper aerodigestive tract. Dysphasia, headache, occipital pain, and retro-orbital pain

S. S. Hans
Medical Director of Vascular and Endovascular Services, Henry Ford Macomb Hospital, Clinton Township, MI, USA

Chief of Vascular Surgery, St. John Macomb Hospital, Warren, MI, USA

Department of Surgery, Wayne State University School of Medicine, Detroit, MI, USA

© The Editor(s) (if applicable) and The Author(s) 2018
S. S. Hans (ed.), *Extracranial Carotid and Vertebral Artery Disease*,
https://doi.org/10.1007/978-3-319-91533-3_22

may occur. Patients may present with Horner's syndrome and hoarseness. Tracheal compression from ruptured carotid artery aneurysm can result in airway compromise. Rupture of carotid aneurysm in the neck is rare, but expanding hematoma in the neck may result in airway compromise secondary to compression of the trachea.

Clinical Diagnosis and Imaging Studies

On physical examination, a pulsatile mass in the neck may be palpable. In elderly patients who are thin and hypertensive, a normal pulse in the common carotid artery and subclavian artery can be confused with a common carotid artery aneurysm. In patients with mycotic aneurysms of the carotid artery, neck mass may be tender with surrounding erythema of the skin. Carotid duplex study is usually the first study performed for the diagnosis of carotid aneurysm. CT angiography of the neck or MR angiography of the neck is useful in confirming the diagnosis and planning treatment (Figs. 22.1 and 22.2). Catheter-based carotid/cerebral arteriography is often helpful in evaluating crossover intracranial circulation in

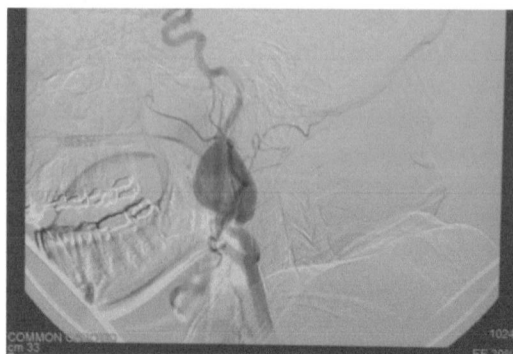

Fig. 22.2 Catheter-based arteriography showing carotid aneurysm involving ICA

the event; ICA ligation may become necessary in patients with inaccessible location of the aneurysm. However, catheter-based arteriography has a small risk of embolization with resulting TIA or stroke.

Surgical Treatment

The primary aim of treatment is resection of the aneurysm and maintaining the flow through the ICA. Aneurysm resection should be undertaken following thorough understanding of the size, location, and tortuosity of the CCA/ICA along with the presence of surrounding inflammatory response. The incision in the neck is similar to the one used for carotid endarterectomy (see Chap. 10). Internal jugular vein is mobilized after ligating and dividing all its branches, hypoglossal, vagus, and in aneurysms extending cephalad. Glossopharyngeal nerve is preserved if the dissection extends cephalad (see Chap. 11). If there is any concern of the exposure of the distal ICA and anticipating difficulty in the distal control, mandibular subluxation should be considered preoperatively. Author usually has maxillofacial or ENT surgeon who performs the procedure under nasotracheal intubation. Mobilization of the aneurysm and CCA/ICA should be careful and deliberate to prevent embolization and injury to surrounding structures including important nerves. Intraoperative shunting is rarely necessary. Author performs EEG monitoring and measurement of back pressure in the ICA as a guide to the placement of shunt (40 mmHg back pressure as cutoff for use of shunt). Heparin is

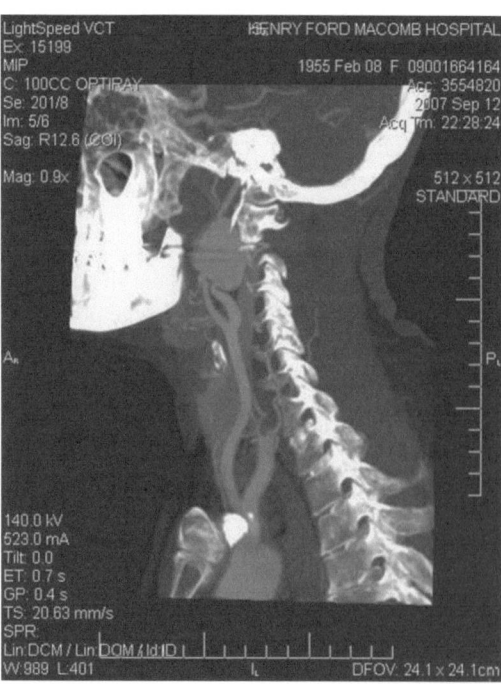

Fig. 22.1 CTA showing internal carotid artery aneurysm with tortuosity of ICA

administered intravenously by anesthesia to keep the ACT close to 300 s. Ligation of the internal carotid artery is usually not recommended unless the aneurysm is in an inaccessible location and patient has satisfactory intracerebral collateral flow.

Small aneurysms with redundant ICA can be resected and a direct end-to-end anastomosis performed with 6.0 "or 7.0" cardiovascular polypropylene suture (Ethicon: Somerville, NJ). Internal carotid artery should be spatulated so that an end-to-end (functional side-to-side) anastomosis is performed (Figs. 22.3, 22.4, and 22.5). Partial resection of the aneurysmal wall with patch angioplasty using prosthetic patch is another option available in patients with anatomically high lesions. All the thrombotic material in the aneurysm should be carefully removed in such instances. In majority of such patients, anterior wall of the aneurysm should be resected to prevent injury to nerves lying behind the aneurysm. Interposition grafting is performed using synthetic graft (Ringed PTFE, W.L. Gore Newark, DE). The PTFE interposition graft can be straight or tapered. A greater saphenous vein graft or superficial

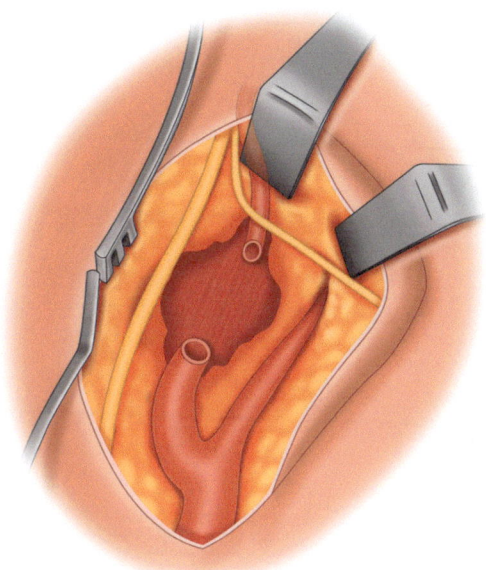

Fig. 22.4 Resection of the aneurysm

femoral artery harvested from the groin and the thigh area can also be used for conduit following resection of the aneurysm. In mycotic aneurysms involving the CCA/ICA, autogenous conduit is preferred. The most common complication of carotid aneurysm is cranial nerve injury (3–17%). The postoperative stroke-free rate varies from 80 to 87%. The stroke rate of untreated aneurysms is greater than 50%.

Endovascular Treatment

During the last decade, endovascular options have been proposed. Placement of a covered stent graft is helpful in treating patients with bleeding, rupture, and aneurysms near the base of the skull. In patients with hostile neck secondary to neck radiation, tracheostomy following laryngectomy with radical neck dissection endovascular techniques may be a better option.

Coil embolization with thrombosis of the sac has been performed with mixed results. There is risk of distal embolization. Extracranial to intracranial carotid bypass following ligation of the ICA may be indicated for carefully selected carotid aneurysms which cannot safely be approached via cervical approach. However, this procedure is rarely performed.

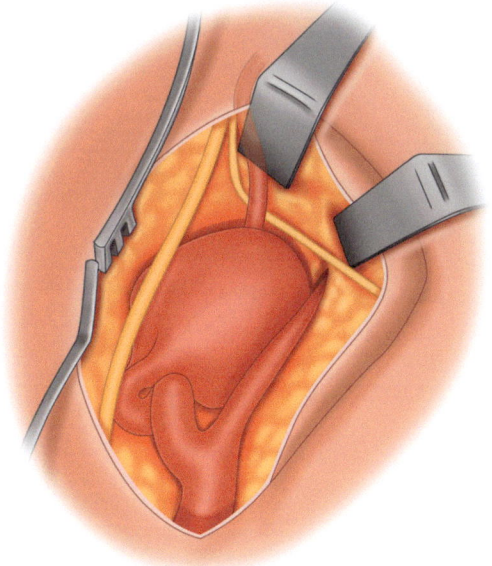

Fig. 22.3 Diagrammatic representation of the carotid artery aneurysm and surrounding XII and X nerves

Fig. 22.5 Spatulated
end-to-end anastomosis

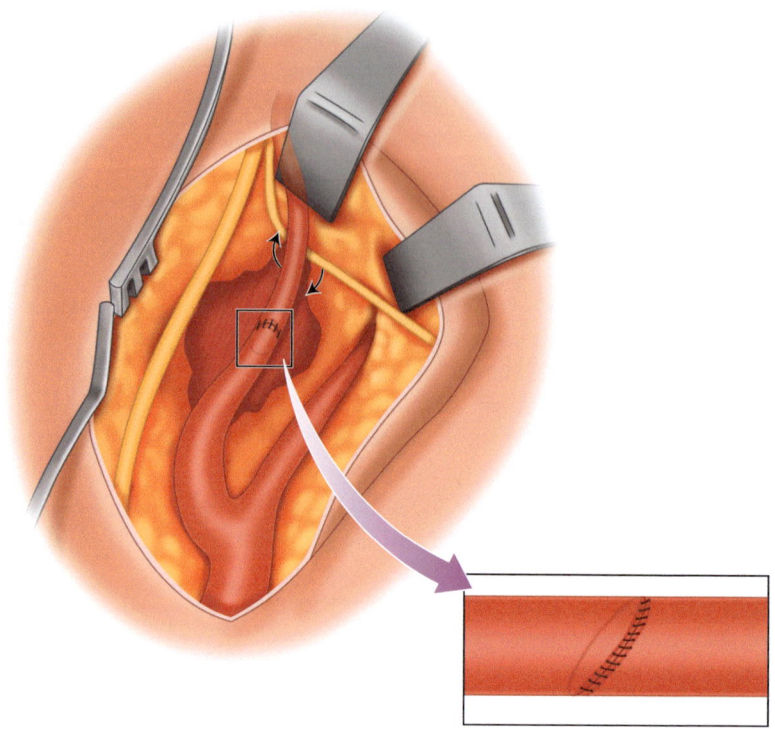

B. Extracranial Vertebral Artery Aneurysms

Extracranial vertebral artery aneurysms are rare and usually associated with trauma or dissection. Primary cervical vertebral aneurysms may result from connective tissue or hereditary disorder including Ehlers-Danlos syndrome, Marfan's disease, and neurofibromatosis [9]. Morasch et al. reported nine extracranial vertebral artery aneurysms in seven patients. Majority of the patients underwent operation in the form of vertebral bypass with saphenous vein, external carotid artery autograft, and vertebral transposition to ICA [9]. Natural history of vertebral aneurysm is not well known. Therefore, open surgical repair should be considered in large or symptomatic aneurysms. Some patients may require hybrid techniques with detachable balloons and coils. Embolization without revascularization can result in posterior circulation stroke. In patients with Ehlers-Danlos syndrome, the repair is extremely difficult due to tissue degradation, and interrupted monofilament suture using minipledgets should be used, and in spite of careful technique, the vertebral artery may require ligation.

Review Questions

1. The common cause of extracranial carotid aneurysms is:
   A. Mycotic
   B. Atherosclerosis
   C. Connective tissue disorder
   D. Cystic medial necrosis

   Answer: B

2. The most commonly used test in planning resection of extracranial carotid artery aneurysm is:
   A. Duplex ultrasound
   B. CTA
   C. MRA
   D. Transcranial Doppler

   Answer: B

3. The best method of treatment for accessible extracranial carotid aneurysm is:
   A. Resection with end-to-end anastomosis or interposition graft
   B. Coil embolization of the aneurysmal sac

C. Covered carotid stent

D. Carotid ligation

Answer: A

4. The most common postoperative complication following repair of an extracranial carotid aneurysm is:

A. Stroke

B. Neck hematoma

C. Thrombosis at the site of anastomosis

D. Cranial nerve injury

Answer: D

5. Endovascular repair is best indicated for the management of localized extracranial carotid aneurysms when:

A. The carotid aneurysm is at the bifurcation of common carotid artery

B. A saccular aneurysm is in the mid-ICA with tortuosity of the ICA

C. Aneurysm is secondary to arterial dysplasia

D. Aneurysm is in an inaccessible location in the neck or in patient with hostile neck

Answer: D

References

1. Srivastava SD, Eagleton MJ, O'Hara P, Kashyap VS, Sarac T, Clair D. Surgical repair of carotid artery aneurysms: a 10-year, single-center experience. Ann Vasc Surg. 2010;24(1):100–5.
2. Brock RC. Astley Cooper and carotid artery ligation. Guys Hosp Rep. 1968;117(3):219–24.
3. Dimtza A. Aneurysms of the carotid arteries; report of two cases. Angiology. 1956;7(3):218–27.
4. Fankhauser GT, Stone WM, Fowl RJ, O'Donnell ME, Bower TC, Meyer FB, Money SR. Surgical and medical management of extracranial carotid artery aneurysms. J Vasc Surg. 2015;61(2):389–93.
5. Zwolak RM, Whitehouse WM Jr, Knake JE, et al. Atherosclerotic extracranial carotid artery aneurysms. J Vasc Surg. 1984;1(3):415–22.
6. Painter TA, Hertzer NR, Beven EG, O'Hara PJ. Extracranial carotid aneurysms: report of six cases and review of the literature. J Vasc Surg. 1985;2(2):312–8.
7. El-Sabrout R, Cooley DA. Extracranial carotid artery aneurysms: Texas Heart Institute experience. J Vasc Surg. 2000;31(4):702–12.
8. Li Z, Chang G, Yao C, Guo L, Liu Y, Wang M, Liu D, Wang S. Endovascular stenting of extracranial carotid artery aneurysm: a systematic review. Eur J Vasc Endovasc Surg. 2011;42(4):419–26.
9. Morasch MD, Phade SV, Naughton P, Garcia-Toca M, Escobar G, Berguer R. Primary extracranial vertebral artery aneurysms. Ann Vasc Surg. 2013;27(4):418–23.

Extracranial Cerebrovascular Trauma

Emily Reardon, J. Devin B. Watson,
Melanie Hoehn, and Rajabrata Sarkar

Introduction

Injuries to the extracranial carotid and vertebral arteries continually challenge the trauma surgeons' and vascular trauma surgeons' clinical acumen and technical abilities. Additionally, the complexity of these injuries challenges\ systems of care as often multiple specialties are involved in the expeditious and coordinated mobilization of resources. The goal of this chapter is to briefly review the epidemiology, contemporary treatment algorithms, and operative strategies of these injuries. Blunt cerebrovascular injuries (BCVI) will be discussed separately from penetrating cerebrovascular injuries (PCVI).

Epidemiology

A landmark study in 2005 from Martin et al. from the National Trauma Database estimated that the incidence of carotid artery injury secondary to trauma was around 0.2% [1]. This incidence of injury included both penetrating and blunt carotid injuries with a higher proportion of blunt injuries relative to penetrating injuries (59% vs 41%) and higher rates of functional impairment at discharge in patients sustaining blunt injuries compared to penetrating injuries. The mortality rates in patients with carotid artery injuries were 26% for penetrating injuries compared to 20% for blunt injuries [1]. Given the higher functional impairment seen with blunt injury to the carotid and/or vertebral arteries, there has been increased interest in aggressively screening for BCVI with multidetector CT scanning. Contemporary studies suggest the incidence of BCVI in trauma patients is approximately 1% and increases to 2–3% in the poly-trauma patient population with higher injury severity scores [2–5]. Despite improvements in screening and recognition of BCVI, reported stroke rates still range from 4 to 14%, and mortality is 6–10% [4, 6–10].

Penetrating Cerebrovascular Injuries

Screening and Diagnosis

The systematic evaluation of the poly-trauma patient using a team-based Advanced Trauma Life Support (ATLS) protocol is critical. Expeditious evaluation and rapid maneuvers to ensure a secure

E. Reardon · M. Hoehn · R. Sarkar
Department of Surgery, Division of Vascular Surgery,
University of Maryland Medical Center, Baltimore,
MD, USA

J. D. B. Watson (✉)
Department of Surgery, David Grant Medical Center,
Travis AFB, CA, USA

© The Editor(s) (if applicable) and The Author(s) 2018
S. S. Hans (ed.), *Extracranial Carotid and Vertebral Artery Disease*,
https://doi.org/10.1007/978-3-319-91533-3_23

airway and large bore IV access should be accomplished prior to leaving the trauma resuscitation bay. Securing the airway by whatever means necessary by the most experienced clinicians in the trauma bay enables patients with either blunt or penetrating neck trauma to be more expediently triaged, imaged, and dispositioned to the operating room or hybrid suite. In most trauma centers, computed tomography angiography (CTA) of the neck and chest can be performed quickly and can vastly change the operative priorities, how and where the procedure is performed, and who will be engaged for patient treatment, e.g., standard vs hybrid OR and community hospital vs hospital with cardiac surgery capability for zone 1 injuries.

Physical examination in the trauma bay, chest X-ray, and CTA of the head and neck are usually able to localize most penetrating vascular injuries. Bodanapally et al. report an 88–94% sensitivity for identifying vertebral artery injuries and a more impressive 93–100% sensitivity for penetrating internal carotid injuries [11]. While penetrating neck injury zones are playing a less important role in the operative management of penetrating neck trauma in the modern era, we feel that the use of this terminology is still helpful when communicating with referring Emergency Departments (ED) as well as in general operative planning [12]. Zone 1 injuries represent any injury from the clavicles to the cricoid cartilage. Zone 2 injuries involve penetrating injuries from the cricoid cartilage to the angle of the mandible, while zone 3 injuries occur with neck injuries cranial to the angle of the mandible (Table 23.1).

Table 23.1 Penetrating neck injuries

Hard signs of vascular injury	Soft signs of vascular injury
Pulsatile bleeding	Stable, neck hematoma
Large, actively expanding neck hematoma	Minor bleeding or history of bleeding
Diminished distal pulse or neurological deficit	Unequal upper extremity blood pressure measurements
Bruit or thrill	

Management of Penetrating Cerebrovascular Injuries (PCVI)

Standard ATLS evaluation of the trauma patient should occur in the ED in the standard fashion. It cannot be overstated of the importance in rapidly securing the airway by any means necessary. Ideally, the most experienced anesthesia or ED provider should be performing the intubation in the trauma bay. In instances with hemodynamic instability and difficult airway, there should be little hesitation to proceed to a surgical airway in order to stabilize and expedite care. Again, without a secure airway, the patient will not be able to be transferred to the CT scanner or OR safely. There are several key exam findings that should be personally evaluated by a senior member of the operative team as these findings will dictate the location, general conduct, and order of operations of the procedure. These findings include the following:

1. Glasgow Coma Scale
2. Localizing neurologic signs including cranial nerve exam as well as ability to move all extremities
3. Brachial blood pressure evaluations of both upper extremities
4. Pulse examination of brachial and femoral vessels in both extremities

An exhaustive search for entrance and exit wounds to ascertain the missile or blade trajectory is paramount. If the patient's airway is secure and the patient is otherwise hemodynamically stable with a zone 1 penetrating neck injury, proceeding to the CT scanner prior to performing a controlled intubation in the operating room with a team poised to gain proximal control of bleeding at that time is the most prudent approach. Often the patient with zone 1 penetrating neck injuries will decompensate upon intubation and require emergent intervention after loss of vascular tone. While uncommon, any patient with a penetrating neck injury and stable airway should be frequently reevaluated for the need for definitive airway management throughout their spectrum of emergency care. A high index of suspicion for cervical spine injuries is required with any high-velocity gunshot wound or fragment injury to the neck.

Zone 1 Injuries

Zone 1 neck injuries deserve special mention. Previously, all zone 1 injuries mandated aortic arch angiogram, and often median sternotomy was used to obtain proximal control of innominate artery and left common carotid artery depending upon patient stability. Left subclavian artery injuries were previously managed with either a second or third intercostal space anterolateral thoracotomy with extension of the thoracotomy to a trap door incision with median sternotomy. Complete descriptions of these separate procedures are outside of the scope of this chapter. While these exposures remain critical to the safe treatment of zone 1 penetrating injuries, more often endovascular approaches may be used in a timely manner and can obviate the need for either median sternotomy or thoracotomy. It is our practice to treat all zone 1 injuries in a hybrid OR or on a fluoroscopy-capable OR table with immediate radiology tech support. In addition to widely prepping both necks and chest, it is our practice to prep both femoral arteries into the field as well as the right arm prepped with placement of a right brachial arterial line for right-sided penetrating neck injuries. Proceeding with a standard neck exploration for zone 1 or suspected zone 1 injuries without the contingency for immediate proximal arterial control either by open or endovascular means ends poorly. Obtaining wire access into the descending thoracic aorta can be done very quickly using a 5 Fr sheath in most trauma patients prior to proceeding with the neck exploration. Minimal time is required to obtain control of branch vessels in the advent of clinical decompensation once the wire is in the descending thoracic aorta.

In instances of zone 1 hematoma in which patients are clinically unstable, it is our practice to consult cardiothoracic surgery for assistance in managing these injuries sooner rather than later due to the time needed to mobilize cardiopulmonary bypass resources and surgeons.

Endovascular Tool Kit for Zone 1 Neck Injuries
1. Micropuncture system
2. Bentson or starter wire
3. Long marker pigtail catheter
4. Simmons, Vitek, or Judkins R4 catheter for cannulating arch vessels
5. Floppy angled glide wire (260 cm)
6. 6 Fr guide sheath
7. Percutaneous closure device
8. 10 mm angioplasty balloon for generic great vessel control

---

Zone 2 Injuries

Zone 2 injuries, in which there are hard signs of major vascular injury, while troubling are often very similar with regard to operative exposure and conduct as the elective carotid endarterectomy exposure. Principles of gaining exposure outside the area of hematoma and proceeding from areas of known, normal anatomy to abnormal anatomy are critically important. The need to identify the anterior border of the sternocleidomastoid muscle early in the procedure is critical, and is not straightforward in the presence of a large neck hematoma. Any branch vein off of the internal jugular, but most especially the facial vein, should be ligated with impunity in order to optimize broad exposure of the common and internal carotid arteries. In cases where there is significant bleeding from one of the internal jugular veins, ligation in order to obtain hemostasis and simplify exposure is warranted. Care should be taken not to haphazardly divide the omohyoid muscle as this muscle can be most helpful in providing muscle coverage for carotid artery or aerodigestive repairs, especially when mobilized from the lateral insertion point and rotated to cover the internal carotid artery or trachea. When considering the number of important cranial nerves in the vicinity of the carotid artery, resisting the urge to blindly clamp bleeding vessels in the midst of audible hemorrhage can be difficult. Having an assistance place a finger or Kittner peanut can prevent a potentially catastrophic cranial nerve injury.

Once exposure and clamping of the common, internal, and external carotid arteries are accomplished, then several questions and decision branch points converge:

1. Can this injury be safely reconstructed in the context of the patient's other injuries and physiologic status?
2. How to reconstruct the injury? Simple repair? Patch repair? Interposition graft? Conduit choice?
3. Heparinize or not to heparinize?

Key Steps for Zone 2 Neck Exploration

1. Prep the neck to knees and have the arm available for access.
2. Bump under shoulder blades if able.
3. Utilize extensile incision on anterior border of sternocleidomastoid.
4. Identification of internal jugular vein with lateral retraction and division of facial vein.
5. Proximal control of common carotid artery with identification of the vagus nerve.
6. Distal exploration of the carotid artery to the bifurcation.
7. Assessment of injury.

Adjuncts for High Zone 2/Low Zone 3 Exploration

1. Ligation of occipital artery
2. Division of digastric muscle with care taken to avoid glossopharyngeal nerve injury
3. Conversion from endotracheal tube to nasotracheal intubation or conversion to tracheostomy
4. Subluxation of the mandible
5. Placement of sheath into common carotid artery with placement of #2 Fogarty balloon past the area of injury with concomitant angiogram

Embarking upon a carotid injury repair in the setting of a severely acidotic, hypothermic, and coagulopathic patient can yield a successfully repaired blood vessel but dead patient at the conclusion of the procedure. Utilization of a temporary vascular shunt may provide both a means to perfuse the brain while providing hemostasis while other injuries and systemic resuscitation are being addressed [13].

Placement of a temporary prosthetic interposition graft as an intermediate shunt while more thorough assessment and repairs of other injuries can be performed with fewer worries of shunt dislodgement or need for anticoagulation. Placement of a small sheath into the common carotid artery with placement of an over-the-wire Fogarty balloon past the area of injury can allow for temporary hemostasis and angiogram through the sheath to determine the area of injury and potential open or endovascular options.

ICA Thrombosis

Instances where the operative exploration yields a thrombosed internal carotid artery deserve special mention. In modern practice, many patients with hemispheric defects will have some form of axial imaging performed en route to the OR. Establishing the extent of thrombosis as well as the level of internal carotid occlusion is critical to operative decision-making. Instances in which patients present with localizing hemispheric deficit and a thrombosed internal carotid artery injury, the old paradigm suggested ligation of the thrombosed artery. Our recommendation in the management of ICA thrombosis is to perform local thrombectomy to the level of the carotid siphon. If there is backbleeding present, then reconstruction of the injured ICA is performed. Management of internal carotid artery thrombosis deserves special mention. When CTA demonstrates thrombosis of the ICA extending into the intracranial portion of the ICA as well as hemispheric deficit, we generally will ligate the ICA to prevent worsening the injury with more distal embolization on reperfusion.

Concomitant Arterial and Aerodigestive Injuries

When there are both hard signs of aerodigestive and vascular injury, neck exploration to repair aerodigestive injuries is generally required. Depending on the hemodynamic stability of the patient, this particular patient population benefits the most from endovascular therapy as it can mitigate some of the infectious complications associated with open vascular repairs in contaminated fields. However, in this particular circumstance, endovascular repair is generally favored prior to neck exploration and repair of aerodigestive injuries to avoid destabilizing neck hematomas. In the presence of aerodigestive injury and vascular injuries not amenable for endovascular repair, we favor temporary vascular shunting until aerodigestive injuries can be managed with contamination controlled. The placement of the temporary shunt allows for harvesting of saphenous vein or alternative autologous conduit for repair, while other injuries are addressed. Autologous conduit for vascular reconstruction is preferred in these cases due to the potential infection of prosthetic materials.

Zone 3 Injuries

Injuries to zone 3 internal carotid arteries are fortunately rare. Often zone 3 injuries that are initially diagnosed on CTA are managed in an endovascular fashion with covered stents due to the challenge open operative repair presents. The management of non-reconstructable zone 3 injuries is managed with ligation as described earlier.

Management of Penetrating Vertebral Artery Injuries

The vertebral artery trauma from penetrating trauma is fortunately a rare occurrence. The vertebral artery is divided into four anatomic segments: V1 is the proximal vertebral artery at origin from subclavian artery, V2 is the portion within the bony cervical canal, V3 is the portion of the vessel from the exit of the bony cervical foramen to the entrance in the base of the skull, and the V4 segment is the intracranial portion of the artery.

Hemorrhage control for penetrating vertebral artery injuries is extraordinarily challenging given the location of the vertebral artery within the cervical canal or at the base of the skull. The penetrating vertebral artery injuries frequently will involve nerve roots adjacent to the vertebral artery. Hemostasis with further operative exposure of the anterior portion of the transverse process to expose the V2 segment of the vertebral artery frequently puts the patient at additional risk of hemorrhage secondary to venous injury. Definitive hemostasis using endovascular therapy is preferred to open hemorrhage control of the vertebral artery. Generally, hemostasis can be obtained with coil embolization of the proximal V1 or V2 segments of the artery with direct packing of the distal injured segment. A hybrid approach for hemostasis involving one surgical team exploring the neck while another team obtains radial or brachial artery access to gain wire access to the vertebral artery is often prudent. The stroke risk of ligation or embolization of a unilateral vertebral artery injury in the setting of a patient in hemorrhagic shock remains unknown. Repeat imaging with CTA or an arteriogram to further interrogate the posterior circulation is generally performed after vertebral artery intervention in order to screen for a hypoplastic, non-injured vertebral artery and intact posterior circulation. Additionally, the use of endovascular techniques to treat vertebral artery arteriovenous fistulae and pseudoaneurysms is preferred to open techniques due to anatomic reasons described above [14, 15].

Blunt Cerebrovascular Injuries

Screening and Diagnosis

The majority of BCVI patients present before the onset of any neurological symptoms. This time frame can range from hours up to years after injury, with the most common latency period being between 10 and 72 h [4, 16–18]. Neurologic symptoms can stem from either of two mechanisms, embolism or dissection, whereby clot formed at the site of vessel injury dislodges or results in an intimal flap leading to flow-limiting stenosis. Injury sites can also degenerate into pseudoaneurysms which serve as a nidus for embolization [19]. Early recognition enables prompt initiation of treatment and has been shown to markedly decrease the incidence of stroke [3, 6, 20, 21].

Over the past few decades, aggressive screening protocols have been formulated, aiming to identify high-risk patients for BCVI, and this has paralleled advancements in computed tomography (CT) scanning. While digital subtraction angiography (DSA) remains the reference standard for detection of BCVI, multidetector CT angiography (MDCTA) has become the screening modality of choice due to a number of factors including its speed and accessibility, noninvasive nature, relative low cost, and ability to detect associated injuries [22–25]. Screening protocols vary by institution and however are generally based on a combination of clinical and radiographic findings [2, 5, 26, 27]. Literature suggests however that up to 20% of injuries can be missed using widely accepted practice guidelines [6, 16, 28, 29]. As a result, our institution, among others, has implemented a more liberalized approach. Since 2004, taking advantage of contemporary MDCTA, patients who present to the R Adams Cowley Shock Trauma Center at the University of Maryland who are clinically judged as being high risk for significant injury undergo a "whole body" CT scan (WBCT) including a dry head CT and a single intravenous contrast-enhanced spiral scan from the circle of Willis through the pelvis. This has resulted in identification of a substantial group of patients with BCVI that would have otherwise evaded screening [30].

Management of BCVI

Ischemic strokes occur in roughly 30–40% of untreated blunt carotid injuries and 10–15% of untreated blunt vertebral injuries [19]. Treatment focuses on prevention of ischemic insult and is

guided by the pathophysiology of the disease, anatomic location, and injury classification. BCVIs most commonly occur from hyperextension, hyperflexion, or rotational forces, leading to stretching of the arterial wall in contact with bony prominences. They can involve any region of the carotid artery; however, the most vulnerable areas are at the skull base, including the distal cervical segment (C1) of the internal carotid artery (ICA) followed by the petrous (C2) and cavernous (C4) segments [22, 31, 32]. Likewise, vertebral injuries are most commonly seen in segments traversing vertebrae C2–C6 (V2), followed by V3 [22, 31, 33]. These locations make surgical intervention challenging. In 1999 Biffl et al. published a BCVI grading system that is still widely used today, known as the Denver grading scale (Table 23.2) [18]. The natural history of these injuries varies. Grade 1 and 2 injuries have a propensity to stenose, thrombose, or thromboembolize. Grade 3 (arterial pseudoaneurysm) injuries can thromboembolize or enlarge resulting in extrinsic compression, arteriovenous fistulae, or rarely free rupture. In the absence of an intact circle of Willis, grade 4 injuries result in profound distal hypoperfusion and ischemic stroke; however, they can also thromboembolize. Grade 5 injuries are usually nonsurvivable [34, 35].

Pharmacotherapy, either anticoagulation or antiplatelet agents, is recommended for the large majority of lesions, whereas operative or endovascular repair is generally reserved for symp-

Table 23.2 Modified Denver criteria for blunt cerebrovascular injury [18]

Grade	Definition	Stroke rate, % (CAI:VAI)
I	Irregularity of vessel wall or dissection with <25% luminal narrowing	3:6
II	Intraluminal thrombus, raised intimal flap, dissection or intramural hematoma with >25% luminal narrowing	14:38
III	Pseudoaneurysm	26:27
IV	Occlusion	50:28
V	Transection	100:100

CAI carotid artery injury, *VAI* vertebral artery injury

tomatic injuries, asymptomatic high-risk injuries for stroke, or worsening injury despite pharmacotherapy [36]. Controversy on the management of BCVI however still exists. Rationale for the use of pharmacotherapy is threefold; it can decrease the potential for embolization, formation of thrombus, and propagation into the cerebral vasculature [37]. However, in the setting of traumatic brain and spinal cord injuries, there is often a general reluctance to initiate pharmacotherapy due to concern for hemorrhage. Reports on the use of endovascular stents for carotid injury have been conflicting. Initial studies, in the early 2000s, demonstrating benefit were retracted due to high rates of in-stent stenosis at longer-term follow-up [7, 20]. However, several more recent studies, endorsing a more universal

administration of antiplatelet agents after stenting, have reported better outcomes [8–10]. At present, pharmacotherapy is considered so effective that use of intravascular stents is reserved for <10% BCVI population [36, 38]. The most recent evidence-based algorithm currently followed at the R Adams Cowley Shock Trauma Center at the University of Maryland is presented in Fig. 23.1. In patients who have stable carotid or vertebral artery pseudoaneurysms (grade 3 injuries), we perform serial CTA head and neck imaging at 4–6 weeks after injury and every 3 months after injury for the first year with liberalization of imaging thereafter. The goal of serial imaging is to assess for enlargement of pseudoaneurysm or distal embolization in which case intervention may be warranted.

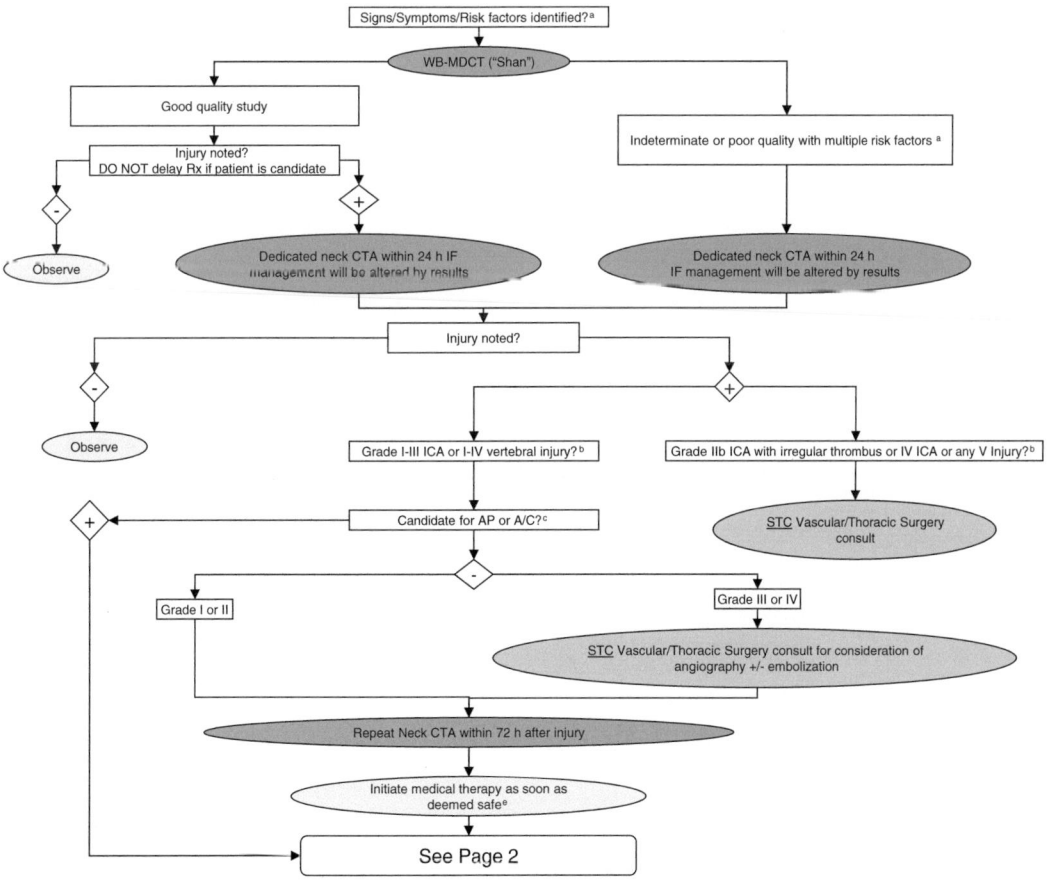

Fig. 23.1 BCVI management algorithm

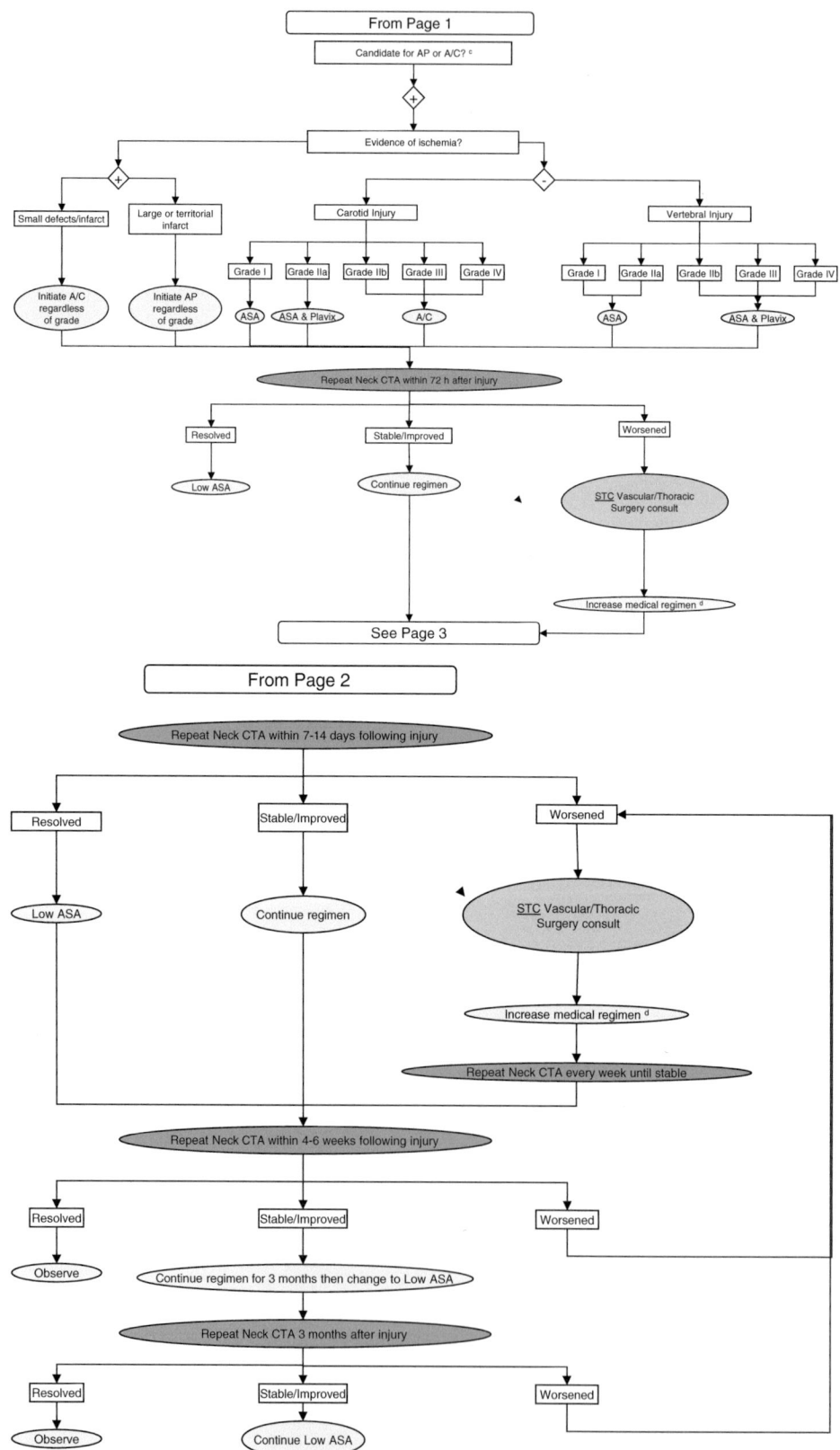

Fig. 23.1 (continued)

Signs/Symptoms/Risk Factors [a]	
Mechanism	Hanging or near-hanging
	Choking
	Direct blow to neck
	Cervical hyperextension injury
	Cervical distraction injury
Symptoms	Arterial hemorrhage or expanding neck hematoma
	Cervical bruit
	Unexplained focal neurologic deficit
	Neurologic exam inconsistent with head CT findings
	Stroke on CT scan
	Seat belt mark or neck hematoma
	Horner's syndrome
	Severe epistaxis
Associated injuries	Severe TBI (GCS<9) or DAI
	Cervical spine fractures (except isolated spinous process)
	Cervical spine dislocations
	Cervical SCI
	Basilar skull fracture (involving the carotid canal or sphenocavernous complex)
	Midface fractures (LeForte II or III, facial smash, naso-ethmoidal complex)
	Complex mandibular fractures
	Severe thoracic trauma (AIS>3)

Injury Grades [b]	
Grade I	Luminal irregularity or dissection/intramural hematoma with <25% luminal narrowing
Grade II	Dissection or intramural hematoma of ≥25% of the lumen
Grade IIa	Dissection or intramural hematoma of 25-50% of the lumen
Grade IIb	Dissection or intramural hematoma of >50% of the lumen or intimal flap
Grade III	Pseudoaneurysm
Grade IV	Vessel occlusion
Grade V	Vessel transection

Medical Therapy [c]		
Antiplatelets agents ("AP")		
Low ASA		Aspirin 81 mg qD
ASA		Aspirin 325 mg qD
Plavix		Clopidogrel 75 mg qD
Anticoagulation ("A/C")		
Unfractionated heparin		Initiate at 15U/kg/hr
		Titrate to PTT 60-80 s
Coumadin		Warfarin
		Titrate to INR 2.0-3.0
		Consider prior to D/C
Lovenox		Enoxaparin 1mg/kg q12h with anti factor Xa level checked after 4th dose to confirm dosage

Increasing Medical Regimen [d]

With worsening (increased grade, increased flow limitation, increased size of psuedoanerysm, recanalization of injuries), medical therapy should be titrated up by one or two "levels" depending on severity of worsening.

Low ASA	to	ASA (Aspirin 325 mg qD)
ASA	to	ASA & Plavix (Aspirin 325 mg qD + Clopidogrel 75 mg qD)
ASA & Plavix	to	A/C (Unfractionated heparin. Initiate 15U/kg/hr. Titrate to PTT 60-80 s)
A/C	to	High dose unfractionated heparin (Titrate to PTT 80-100 s)

Patients Who are Not Candidates for AP or A/C [e]

Typically AP agents can be started prior to A/C. Initiate therapy with "increasing medical regimen" when deemed safe as above (d) up to initial therapy as indicated in algorithm.

Fig. 23.1 (continued)

Review Questions

1. Zone 1 penetrating neck injuries refer to which area of the thoracic inlet to the base of the skull?
   A. Clavicles to the thyroid cartilage
   B. Clavicles to the cricoid cartilage
   C. Thyroid cartilage to the angle of the mandible
   D. Angle of the mandible to the base of the skull

   Answer: A

2. Division of which muscle risks glossopharyngeal nerve injury?
   A. Sternothyroid muscle
   B. Omohyoid muscle
   C. Sternocleidomastoid muscle
   D. Digastric muscle

   Answer: D

3. Which of the following adjuncts will not improve distal exposure of the internal carotid artery?
   A. Nasotracheal intubation
   B. Surgical airway—either tracheostomy or cricothyroidotomy
   C. Mandibular dislocation
   D. Mandibular subluxation

   Answer: C

4. Which blunt cerebrovascular injury carries the highest risk of stroke?
   A. Grade 2 carotid artery injury
   B. Grade 2 vertebral artery injury
   C. Grade 3 carotid artery injury
   D. Grade 3 vertebral artery injury

   Answer: B

References

1. Martin M, Mullenix P, Steele S, et al. Functional outcome after blunt and penetrating carotid artery injuries: analysis of the National Trauma Data Bank. J Trauma. 2005;59(4):860–4.
2. Franz RW, Willette PA, Wood MJ, Wright ML, Hartman JF. A systematic review and meta-analysis of diagnostic screening criteria for blunt cerebrovascular injuries. J Am Coll Surg. 2012;214(3):313–27. https://doi.org/10.1016/j.jamcollsurg.2011.11.012.
3. Miller PR, Fabian TC, Croce MA, et al. Prospective screening for blunt cerebrovascular injuries: analysis of diagnostic modalities and outcomes. Ann Surg. 2002;236(3):386–393-395. https://doi.org/10.1097/00000658-200209000-00015.
4. Biffl WL, Ray CE, Moore EE, et al. Treatment-related outcomes from blunt cerebrovascular injuries: importance of routine follow-up arteriography. Ann Surg. 2002;235(5):699–707. https://doi.org/10.1097/00000658-200205000-00012.
5. Biffl WL, Cothren CC, Moore EE, et al. Western trauma association critical decisions in trauma: screening for and treatment of blunt cerebrovascular injuries. J Trauma Inj Infect Crit Care. 2009;67(6):1150–3. https://doi.org/10.1097/TA.0b013e3181c1c1d6.
6. Stein DM, Boswell S, Sliker CW, Lui FY, Scalea TM. Blunt cerebrovascular injuries: does treatment always matter? J Trauma. 2009;66(1):132–44. https://doi.org/10.1097/TA.0b013e318142d146.
7. Cothren CC, Moore EE, Ray CE, et al. Carotid artery stents for blunt cerebrovascular injury: risks exceed benefits. Arch Surg. 2005;140(5):480–5. https://doi.org/10.1001/archsurg.140.5.480.
8. Edwards NM, Fabian TC, Claridge JA, Timmons SD, Fischer PE, Croce MA. Antithrombotic therapy and endovascular stents are effective treatment for blunt carotid injuries: results from Longterm Followup. J Am Coll Surg. 2007;204(5):1007–13. https://doi.org/10.1016/j.jamcollsurg.2006.12.041.
9. Berne JD, Reuland KR, Villarreal DH, McGovern TM, Rowe SA, Norwood SH. Internal carotid artery stenting for blunt carotid artery injuries with an associated pseudoaneurysm. J Trauma. 2008;64(2):398–405. https://doi.org/10.1097/TA.0b013e31815eb788.
10. DiCocco JM, Fabian TC, Emmett KP, et al. Optimal outcomes for patients with blunt cerebrovascular injury (BCVI): tailoring treatment to the lesion. J Am Coll Surg. 2011;212(4):549–57. https://doi.org/10.1016/j.jamcollsurg.2010.12.035.
11. Bodanapally UK, Dreizin D, Sliker CW, Boscak AR, Reddy RP. Vascular injuries to the neck after penetrating trauma: diagnostic performance of 40-and 64-MDCT angiography. Am J Roentgenol. 2015;205(4):866–72. https://doi.org/10.2214/AJR.14.14161.
12. Prichayudh S, Choadrachata-Anun J, Sriussadaporn S, et al. Selective management of penetrating neck injuries using "no zone" approach. Injury. 2015;46(9):1720–5. https://doi.org/10.1016/j.injury.2015.06.019.
13. Inaba K, Aksoy H, Seamon MJ, et al. Multicenter evaluation of temporary intravascular shunt use in vascular trauma. J Trauma Acute Care Surg. 2016;80(3):359–65. https://doi.org/10.1097/TA.0000000000000949.
14. Greer LT, Kuehn RB, Gillespie DL, et al. Contemporary management of combat-related vertebral artery injuries. J Trauma Acute Care Surg. 2013;74(3):818–24. https://doi.org/10.1097/TA.0b013e31827a08a8.
15. Mwipatayi BP, Jeffery P, Beningfield SJ, Motale P, Tunnicliffe J, Navsaria PH. Management of extracranial vertebral artery injuries. Eur J Vasc Endovasc Surg. 2004;27(2):157–62. https://doi.org/10.1016/j.ejvs.2003.11.008.
16. Cothren CC. Treatment for blunt cerebrovascular injuries. Arch Surg. 2009;144(7):685–90. https://doi.org/10.1001/archsurg.2009.111.
17. Cothren CC. Anticoagulation is the gold standard therapy for blunt carotid injuries to reduce stroke rate. Arch Surg. 2004;139(5):540. https://doi.org/10.1001/archsurg.139.5.540.
18. Biffl WL, Moore EE, Offner PJ, Brega KE, Franciose RJ, Burch JM. Blunt carotid arterial injuries: implications of a new grading scale. J Trauma. 1999;47(5):845–53. https://doi.org/10.1097/00005373-199911000-00004.
19. Fabian TC. Blunt cerebrovascular injuries: anatomic and pathologic heterogeneity create management enigmas. J Am Coll Surg. 2013;216(5):873–85. https://doi.org/10.1016/j.jamcollsurg.2012.12.053.
20. Eastman AL, Muraliraj V, Sperry JL, Minei JP. CTA-based screening reduces time to diagnosis and stroke rate in blunt cervical vascular injury. J Trauma. 2009;67(3):551–6. https://doi.org/10.1097/TA.0b013e3181b84408.
21. Fabian TC, Patton JH Jr, Croce MA, Minard G, Kudsk KA, Pritchard E. Blunt carotid injury. Importance of early diagnosis and anticoagulant therapy. Ann Surg. 1996;223(5):513–25. https://doi.org/10.1097/00000658-199605000-00007.
22. Bodanapally UK, Sliker CW. Imaging of blunt and penetrating Craniocervical arterial injuries. Semin Roentgenol. 2016;51(3):152–64. https://doi.org/10.1053/j.ro.2015.12.001.
23. Burlew CC, Biffl WL. Imaging for blunt carotid and vertebral artery injuries. Surg Clin North Am. 2011;91(1):217–31. https://doi.org/10.1016/j.suc.2010.10.004.
24. Eastman AL, Chason DP, Perez CL, McAnulty AL, Minei JP. Computed tomographic angiography for the diagnosis of blunt cervical vascular injury: is it ready for primetime? J Trauma. 2006;60(5):925–9. Discussion 929. https://doi.org/10.1097/01.ta.0000197479.28714.62.
25. Utter GH, Hollingworth W, Hallam DK, Jarvik JG, Jurkovich GJ. Sixteen-slice CT angiography in patients with suspected blunt carotid and vertebral artery injuries. J Am Coll Surg. 2006;203(6):838–48. https://doi.org/10.1016/j.jamcollsurg.2006.08.003.

26. Bromberg WJ, Collier BC, Diebel LN, et al. Blunt cerebrovascular injury practice management guidelines: the eastern Association for the Surgery of trauma. J Trauma. 2010;68(2):471–7. https://doi.org/10.1097/TA.0b013e3181cb43da.

27. Biffl WL, Moore EE, Offner PJ, et al. Optimizing screening for blunt cerebrovascular injuries. Am J Surg. 1999;178(6):517–22. https://doi.org/10.1016/S0002-9610(99)00245-7.

28. Emmett KP, Fabian TC, DiCocco JM, Zarzaur BL, Croce MA. Improving the screening criteria for blunt cerebrovascular injury: the appropriate role for computed tomography angiography. J Trauma. 2011;70(5):1058–63. https://doi.org/10.1097/TA.0b013e318213f849.

29. Geddes AE, Burlew CC, Wagenaar AE, et al. Expanded screening criteria for blunt cerebrovascular injury: a bigger impact than anticipated. Am J Surg. 2016;212(6):1167–74. https://doi.org/10.1016/j.amjsurg.2016.09.016.

30. Bruns BR, Tesoriero R, Kufera J, et al. Blunt cerebrovascular injury screening guidelines: what are we willing to miss? J Trauma Acute Care Surg. 2014;76(3):691–5. https://doi.org/10.1097/TA.0b013e3182ab1b4d.

31. Sliker CW, Mirvis SE. Imaging of blunt cerebrovascular injuries. Eur J Radiol. 2007;64(1):3–14. https://doi.org/10.1016/j.ejrad.2007.02.015.

32. McKevitt EC, Kirkpatrick AW, Vertesi L, Granger R, Simons RK. Identifying patients at risk for intracranial and extracranial blunt carotid injuries. Am J Surg. 2002;183(5):566–70. https://doi.org/10.1016/S0002-9610(02)00845-0.

33. Osborn AG. Incidence of vertebral artery thrombosis in cervical spine trauma: correlation with severity of spinal cord injury. Yearb Diagn Radiol. 2006;2006:379–81. https://doi.org/10.1016/S0098-1672(08)70494-6.

34. Laser A, Bruns BR, Kufera JA, et al. Long-term follow-up of blunt cerebrovascular injuries. J Trauma Acute Care Surg. 2016;81(6):1063–9. https://doi.org/10.1097/TA.0000000000001223.

35. Lauerman MH, Feeney T, Sliker CW, et al. Lethal now or lethal later: the natural history of grade 4 blunt cerebrovascular injury. J Trauma Acute Care Surg. 2015;78(6):1071–5. https://doi.org/10.1097/ta.0000000000000654.

36. Shahan CP, Croce MA, Fabian TC, Magnotti LJ. Impact of continuous evaluation of technology and therapy: 30 years of research reduces stroke and mortality from blunt cerebrovascular injury. J Am Coll Surg. 2017;224(4):595–9. https://doi.org/10.1016/j.jamcollsurg.2016.12.008.

37. Shahan CP, Magnotti LJ, McBeth PB, Weinberg JA, Croce MA, Fabian TC. Early antithrombotic therapy is safe and effective in patients with blunt cerebrovascular injury and solid organ injury or traumatic brain injury. J Trauma Acute Care Surg. 2016;81(1):173–7. https://doi.org/10.1097/TA.0000000000001058.

38. Burlew CC, Biffl WL, Moore EE, et al. Endovascular stenting is rarely necessary for the management of blunt cerebrovascular injuries. J Am Coll Surg. 2014;218(5):1012–7. https://doi.org/10.1016/j.jamcollsurg.2014.01.042.

Paola M. P. Seidel and Geoffrey K. Seidel

Introduction

Stroke can result in transient, subtle, or severe neurologic compromise. Thrombolytic agents, clot retrieval procedures, and other interventions help prevent or minimize permanent neurologic deficits in thousands of patients; however, despite these advances, patients remain at risk for significant impairment and subsequent functional disability. This chapter focuses on increasing the awareness of acute and post-acute rehabilitation interventions which maximize long-term functional recovery in patients that experience neurologic deficits after a cerebral vascular event.

Poststroke Rehabilitation Care in the Acute Setting

Rehabilitation of the stroke patient ideally begins within the first 24 h after recognition of a cerebral vascular event. Initiation of rehabilitation services

as soon as possible results in better functional outcomes [1]. Because stroke patients experience a high frequency of medical complications [2], delays in implementation of a coordinated rehabilitation program often lead to preventable complications resulting in permanent physical impairment and increased mortality. Poststroke rehabilitation in the acute setting begins within the first 24 h after onset. Consultation with a physician specialist in Physical Medicine and Rehabilitation (physiatrist) begins with a neurologic assessment and coordination of a multidisciplinary team approach utilizing the expertise of physical, occupational, and speech therapists, nursing, and other medical specialties to maximize functional outcome and prevent morbidity and mortality. The physiatrist plays a crucial role in the management of oral secretions, dysphagia, aspiration pneumonia, bowel and bladder dysfunction, prevention of deep vein thrombosis, skin ulceration, communication impairments, aphasia, contractures, spasticity, and emotional lability in the early period after stroke. Successful stroke rehabilitation involves customized treatment plans, coordination with multiple medical and surgical specialists, as well as appropriate education of both the patient and caregivers. The physiatrist and stroke treatment team members in conjunction with a discharge coordinator will determine the most appropriate discharge plan, to an inpatient rehabilitation center, a subacute

P. M. P. Seidel
Department of Physical Medicine and Rehabilitation, Wayne State University, Detroit, MI, USA

G. K. Seidel (✉)
Department of Physical Medicine and Rehabilitation, Wayne State University, Detroit, MI, USA

Michigan State University, Lansing, MI, USA

© The Editor(s) (if applicable) and The Author(s) 2018
S. S. Hans (ed.), *Extracranial Carotid and Vertebral Artery Disease*,
https://doi.org/10.1007/978-3-319-91533-3_24

nursing facility, or a community-based rehabilitation program.

The initiation of stroke rehabilitation begins with consultation of a physiatrist, a physician specializing in Physical Medicine and Rehabilitation. The physiatrist receives specialized training in evaluation of the central nervous system, assessment of patient functional status, and methods of optimizing neurologic and musculoskeletal recovery. A comprehensive physiatric evaluation includes a complete history and physical examination focusing on neurologic and musculoskeletal assessment. After defining the character and extent of physical and cognitive impairment, the physiatrist will develop a coordinated, multidisciplinary patient-specific rehabilitation plan. The specialized rehabilitation team is composed of a speech pathologist, physical therapist, occupational therapist, rehabilitation nurse, psychologist, therapeutic recreational therapist, and other therapists when indicated. Leading these providers, the physiatrist will also coordinate with medical and surgical subspecialists as indicated to treat comorbidities as well as facilitate transfer to an appropriate rehabilitation setting to optimize functional outcome.

The physiatrist's initial evaluation will include an assessment of swallowing function. This is a critical concern and should be performed before the patient resumes eating or drinking. The risk of silent aspiration and subsequent pneumonia is high in the acute poststroke patient, and the physiatrist will aid in determining if the patient can safely swallow and requires adaptive feeding or placement of a gastrointestinal feeding tube. The decision to allow oral intake is complicated because successful swallowing requires not only a functional swallowing mechanism but also a comprehensive evaluation of a range of motor, postural, and cognitive skills. Aspiration risk is impacted by body positioning and the use of sedative medications and further increased if the patient has a low level of arousal, poor head and/ or trunk control, reduced activity level, poor oral hygiene, or underlying gastroesophageal reflux [3]. Within the first 24 h, before the patient begins oral feeding, the physiatrist in conjunction with a speech pathologist will perform a bedside swallow evaluation to determine and grade aspiration risk. The physiatrist, speech pathologist, and rehabilitation nurse continually monitor and optimize the patient's positioning, fluid consistency, and control of oral secretions to avoid aspiration.

In patients with subtle neurologic impairments, the bedside dysphagia screen alone is sometimes inadequate to rule out aspiration [4]. Often a silent killer, aspiration pneumonia is often overlooked in patients who visually appear to be adequately managing oral secretions but possess subtle impairments of pharyngeal motility. Formal videofluoroscopic modified barium swallow studies are performed in a radiology suite with a speech pathologist utilizing barium liquid, modified to include barium paste of various consistencies and a crumbly food item like a barium-coated cookie to determine the nature of aspiration based upon food texture and consistency and to subsequently explore compensatory strategies to minimize aspiration [3]. Dysphagia evaluation may also include endoscopy, fiberoptic endoscopic swallowing evaluation, and/ or esophageal manometry when indicated. It is impractical, time-inefficient and over utilization of resources for each and every patient who experiences a stroke to have formal modified barium swallow testing. Therefore, constant vigilance and clinical observation is necessary from all stroke team members regarding aspiration risk.

When significant dysphagia is identified, different approaches to treatment are implemented to maintain critical hydration, the administration of medications and nutritional support. Management may include simple interventions such as proper positioning during feeding, altered food consistencies, or instruction on compensatory swallowing techniques. In more severe cases, the transient use of a nasogastric tube or longer-term placement of a percutaneous alimentary tube placement is appropriate. It is the authors' experience that very few patients who initially require percutaneous feeding tube placement will require this intervention long term.

The Free Water Protocol is a recent advance in the management of dysphagia. It is based upon research that has demonstrated that ingestion of small amounts of water in the presence of good oral hygiene does not result in a higher incidence of aspiration pneumonia [5]. The aspiration of small amounts of water into the lungs is reabsorbed and, if clear of oral bacteria, does not result in infection. If a patient can sit upright, use appropriate swallowing compensatory strategies, follow verbal commands, and participate in oral cleaning care, he or she may be approved to drink small amounts of water 30 min after meals. It is imperative that oral hygiene is maintained or the oral bacterial load can result in aspiration pneumonia. The implementation of this protocol has significantly reduced dehydration in a large group of stroke patients [6]. Dysphagia resolves in 98% of hemiplegic patients within 30 days [7].

The physiatrist's assessment will define and stage the patient's level of neurologic recovery to help guide physical therapists, occupational therapists, and nursing in determining which therapeutic exercises are appropriate, the judicious use of orthotics to prevent contractures, and the development of compensatory strategies that facilitate relearning basic activities of daily living, transfer skills, and ambulation. Early mobility is critical in preventing skin breakdown, optimizing bladder recovery, minimizing deconditioning, and facilitating global functional recovery.

Patients who experience CNS compromise are at high risk of pressure sores. Functional outcome can be completely compromised should the patient develop a decubitus ulcer, significantly increasing the risk of sepsis and mortality. Occupational therapists working with a rehabilitation nurse will not only implement turning protocols to help prevent skin breakdown but will assist with determining the optimal durable medical equipment needed for bed positioning, adjustment, seating, and cushioning. The team will begin to teach the patient and/or family how to increase bed mobility and the importance of regular pressure relief. The importance of patient and family education regarding pressure relief cannot be overemphasized. Patients and families must actively participate in the rehabilitative process from the start for successful outcomes to occur. Few hospital settings offer one-on-one, 24-h staffing; thus

active patient and family engagement significantly enhances rehabilitation success.

As the patients' gross motor skills begin to return, occupational therapists will work with physical therapists on teaching the patient to transfer safely, instructing family members in the use of gait belts and sliding boards, assisting in the selection of customized patient-specific wheelchair seating and propulsion features, and how to use developing spasticity to facilitate functional ambulation. Physical presentation and cognition will determine what type of gait aide will be helpful in facilitating ambulation. The team will assess each patients gait mechanics to determine the appropriate assistive device at each stage of stroke recovery. Patients may need a standard walker (rigid or foldable), hemi-walker, platform walker, wheeled walker (with or without rear gliders), rollator walker with hand brakes (with or without seat), or cane to facilitate further gait recovery while balancing fall prevention. Canes vary, including large- and small-based quad canes and single-point canes, with a variety of tips, handles, and options. Assistive gait device selection is based upon the patients' functional deficit combined with the patients' ability and willingness to use the device.

Simultaneously, occupational therapists will assist the patient with relearning basic skills such as eating, washing, dressing, and toileting. Managing bowel and bladder issues are critical at this early stage, as they often determine an individual's discharge destination. Family members, overwhelmed with the challenges of physical compromise, are often willing to assist a loved one with feeding and dressing but will be much less inclined to take home an incontinent person at discharge. Many stroke patients, even those who are primarily confined to wheelchairs, are able to remain continent with timed voiding and other interventions. Patients, whether discharged to home or to nursing facilities, are considerably less likely to suffer skin breakdown if they are successfully able to remain continent of bowel and bladder.

Simultaneously, the continued involvement of the speech pathologist following stroke will assist the entire team in diagnosing evolving language and comprehension issues. The physiatrist and speech pathologist will provide guidance in handling patients who are aphasic, disinhibited, and impulsive or display neglect of a limb or side of their body. Failure to recognize and understand that a hyper-verbal patient may appear to comprehend instructions but has significant cognitive deficits can result in safety risks. Likewise, failure to appreciate that a nonverbal individual has intact cognition can frustrate patients unnecessarily and hamper recovery.

The physiatrist and psychiatrist often work together in assessing and treating the emotional lability that often accompanies central nervous system lesions. Emotional lability is a common feature in stroke patients manifesting as despondency, defiance, anger, tearfulness, and fear. Behavioral responses directly impact a patients' ability to engage in therapy as well as interact with medical providers and family members. Management of mood disorders is complicated by preexisting depression and anxiety, grief reactions with functional loss, and maladaptive coping strategies. Selection of the appropriate classes of antidepressants, antianxiety, and medications that are most effective in addressing pseudobulbar symptoms is imperative, as some classes of pharmaceuticals will slow cognitive and motor recovery.

Acute ischemic stroke median hospital length of stay nationally has decreased to 4 days [8]. Despite increasingly shortened acute care stays, implementation of rehabilitation strategies within the first 24 h is imperative. The neurologic impairments secondary to stroke generally require a longer period of recovery, and these early interventions not only help reduce morbidity and mortality but also help predict longer-range recovery. These assessments will help determine where the patient will best receive treatment after discharge from the hospital. The physiatrist will assist the family, social worker, and discharge team toward the appropriate rehabilitation setting after the acute care hospital treatment has completed including inpatient rehabilitation centers, subacute facilities, or home with concurrent outpatient services. Early identification of functional deficits in the acute stroke patient, followed by appropriately coordinated intervention, offers even the most severely impaired stroke patients the greatest opportunity to reach maximal functional recovery and the highest quality of life after sustaining a stroke. Upon discharge from the hospital, the physiatrist will often continue to see the patient at regular intervals to assist in the coordination of poststroke care. This provides the continuity of care required to maximize neurologic functional recovery, prevent complications, and address longer-term issues such as altered sexual function, emotional adjustment to disability, community reintegration, and prognosis.

Key Management Issues in the Acute/Subacute Stroke Period

In addition to issues related to cognitive and neurologic recovery, complications resulting from immobility and poor body positioning are an important focus in the treatment and rehabilitation management of acute stroke patients. Deep vein thrombosis (DVT), pressure ulcers, and contractures are preventable, and their absence substantially improves functional outcome.

Patients immobilized by stroke are at high risk for DVT and subsequent pulmonary embolism. The best intervention to prevent DVT is early mobilization. Patients who remain immobile are understandably at increased risk; thus DVT prevention-intervention strategies are imperative in the acute poststroke period. In addition to early patient mobilization, mechanical and pharmacological DVT prophylaxis is generally indicated. While sequential compression garments in combination with anti-embolism stockings are recommended, they may also compromise insensate skin. Knee-high compression garments may roll at the top creating a tourniquet effect or sheer skin during placement or removal. Patients, families, and rehabilitation treatment team members must all be vigilant with compressive garment skin care. Sequential compression garments and compressive stockings were not found to reduce the frequency of symptomatic proximal DVT or PE [9]; thus, the continued use of these devices may be reconsidered in various stroke rehabilitation settings utilizing evidenced-based medical decision-making practices. Pharmacologic anticoagulation therapies including heparin, warfarin, and salicylate derivatives are often used to manage recurrent stroke risk and do assist in DVT prevention. Intracerebral and/or gastrointestinal bleeding is associated with anticoagulated use that deviates from optimal therapeutic ranges. Low-/ultra-low molecular weight heparin products reduced overall mortality by 12 deaths per thousand patients compared to no anticoagulation [8] and are in general considered lower-risk agents for gastrointestinal and CNS bleeding complications with similar efficacy than heparin and warfarin [10]. No DVT prophylaxis treatment process in isolation or in combination is considered 100% effective in preventing DVT in stroke patients [8].

Decubitus ulcers are a significant rehabilitation challenge, associated with poor functional outcomes and patient demise. Patients with advanced age, poor nutrition, incontinence, dehydration, and impaired circulation in conjunction with immobility are at high risk of skin breakdown and pressure sore formation. Here, good nursing care is critical to prevent this highly undesirable complication. Repositioning every 2 h in a lateral recumbent position, using proper transfer techniques that minimize sheer forces in bed and during transfers, can substantially reduce the frequency of integumentary compromise. Special attention to heels and other pressure points on paralytic limbs and keeping patients clean and dry in the perianal areas are basic but often neglected tasks. Maintaining good hydration and nutrition is also imperative to skin integrity and can be overlooked if patients are frail or remain on nothing by mouth orders for prolonged periods.

Urinary incontinence occurs in 50% of acute stroke patients, and 25% experience ongoing urinary incontinence at hospital discharge [11]. Generally, the pontine micturition center remains functional following stroke, and urinary incontinence results from a combination of immobility due to paralysis, decreased initiation, and a lack of voluntary inhibition. Fecal incontinence is also common but is generally due to the patient's mobility status as opposed to a neurogenic etiology. Regardless, both pose a risk factor for skin breakdown and are often best managed by timed voiding and maintaining low post-void residuals with catheterization where needed. A knowledgeable nurse that works cooperatively with the rehabilitation team is instrumental in obtaining good poststroke outcomes.

Motor paralysis is a core deficit in stroke. Stroke patients regain isolated muscle control in a predictable sequence as motor recovery occurs. Brunnstrom described the following motor recovery stages: flaccid, early synergic flexor/extensor group motor function, and spastic synergy dominant and isolated motor control with smooth coordinated joint motion [12]. Motor recovery speed is patient specific, and time spent in each stage is variable depending on lesion severity, CNS edema resolution rate, and other factors. The rehabilitation team evaluates the motor functional stage for each patient and caters specific therapeutic strategies to optimize functional gains (Table 24.1).

Joint contractures of upper and lower limbs occur in patients with impaired independent motor function. Because patients with poor initiation of motor movement cannot mobilize joints adequately early in the recovery process, patient and family are instructed to move the joint frequently through range of motion to prevent soft tissue contractures. If joint range of motion is maintained, then as muscle function returns, the patient can recover useful motor function at an earlier time in the recovery process. If soft tissue contractures develop, many patients may never

Table 24.1 Brunnstrom recovery stages [12–14]

Stage	Description
1	No motor function-flaccid
2	Early volitional limb synergy/spasticity
3	Volitional limb synergy with significant spasticity
4	Early isolated muscle control with less spasticity
5	Isolated motor movements dominant with minimal spasticity
6	Normal joint movements appear and spasticity resolves

regain functional use of a limb. For example, in the normal individual, the biceps muscle shortens to bend the elbow, and the opposite triceps muscle relaxes in a coordinated, controlled, smooth fashion resulting in functional elbow flexion. In stroke patients with upper extremity involvement, motor control is often not coordinated. Co-contraction of flexor and extensor muscles occurs simultaneously preventing joint range of motion. Rehabilitation team members use the Ashworth scale to rate muscle tone severity (please note there are several Ashworth scales with varying names, i.e., "modified Ashworth" and "modified, modified Ashworth," but all follow the same pattern and rate the same muscle tone phenomenon) [13, 14]. The larger the Ashworth number, the more the muscular resistance exists to joint motion. Normal muscle tone without resistance to motion is scored 0 and slight increase in muscle tone 1, while a severely hypertonic limb has a score of 4. The team employs different strategies to combat tone including passive stretching, pressure point therapy, bracing, serial casting, botulinum toxin, and oral and intrathecal pharmacologic interventions to modify tone, improve function, and limit soft tissue joint contractures.

Contractures occur within the first year on the hemiparetic side in 60% of patients, most often at the wrist and less frequently in the elbow and shoulder [15]. While passively ranging hemiparetic joints is helpful, alone, it is usually not sufficient to prevent contractures, especially of the wrist and fingers. To maximize the potential for future function, the wrist and fingers should be maintained in a neutral, anatomic position, with the wrist in pronation, the thumb in opposition, and the fingers extended. Resting hand splints help to maintain these positions. The hemiplegic shoulder should be positioned with 30° abduction and external rotation (often with a pillow) until active therapeutic intervention can be initiated. Contractures resulting from increased tone and muscle spasticity result in pain, reduced motion, and risk of further functional loss superimposed upon the existing CNS compromise. Lower extremity contractures are also common and are entirely preventable. Ankle plantar flexion contractures impact gait, increase the risk of fall, and

can prevent appropriate wheelchair positioning. Some plantar flexion contractures resolve with early weight bearing; however those patients with increased tone may require splinting to preserve proper positioning for future ambulation. Special resting splints, called PRAFOs, help to both maintain the foot in the upright position, dorsiflexed to 90° with the hip neutral to avoid external rotation contracture. This type of brace also has no contact with the heel, to prevent a heel pressure sore as the patients that use these braces are often dependent in bed mobility and cannot manage pressure relief on their own. Formal ankle foot orthoses are utilized later in the rehabilitation process when gait is possible. Effective fit and use of the ankle foot orthosis will depend upon appropriate positioning and splinting of the hemiplegic limb during the acute hospital stay. Failure to prevent contractures can result in irreversible impairments that may prevent future ambulation potential.

Patients with dense hemiplegia are at higher risk for other complications. Glenohumeral subluxation may result in traction on the brachial plexus. This, in combination with soft tissue contracture, peripheral nerve compression at vulnerable pressure points and edema superimposed upon premorbid musculoskeletal upper extremity joint injuries can initiate a pain cascade that may result in a devastating complication called shoulder-hand syndrome. This condition is exceptionally painful and difficult to treat once present. Shoulder-hand syndrome is considered a form of complex regional pain/reflex sympathetic dystrophy. This condition is not only painful but is challenging to treat and often results in permanent functional impairment beyond the initial neurologic insult. The best treatment is aggressive prevention. Early range of motion and proper attention to positioning of the hemiplegic limb usually avoid this complication. Should it occur, a number of possible therapeutic interventions including, but not limited to, cutaneous desensitization, elevation, compressive garments, anticonvulsant medications, and antidepressant medications with neuropathic pain management properties coupled with appropriate occupation therapy may be helpful in treating this condition.

The physiatrist also works closely with surgical and medicine specialists in the acute stroke period. Cardiologists are helpful in guiding exercise parameters in those with preexisting or concurrent cardiac disease to prevent excessive fatigue. They also can assist the physiatrist in identifying additional treatable risk factors that could contribute to a second stroke, such as metabolic syndrome, hypertension, coronary artery disease, and hyperlipidemia. Patient and family education in stroke prevention is part of the rehabilitation program. An endocrinologist may also be of assistance not only for diabetic management but also in more severely affected patients with intracerebral bleeding/massive edema and midline shift. These individuals occasionally develop a variety of pituitary abnormalities resulting in an array of endocrine dysfunctions, such as hypothyroidism, alterations in cortisol metabolism, and other endocrinopathies.

Hemi-neglect with or without visual field deficits is common in patients with right hemispheric strokes. Bedside visual field confrontation or lack of orientation toward the evaluator may indicate left-sided neglect or visual field deficit. Patients with profound neglect classically will not groom one side, walk into door frames, or acknowledge their hemiplegic limb; however, there is a wide range of symptoms associated with hemi-neglect that are less overt and easily missed if not specifically and carefully assessed. Insight into this deficit is variable but is often low. In the hospital setting, these patients often possess fluent communicative skills that can mask this impairment, placing the individual at high risk for falls and other accidents. Subtle instances of hemianopsia or neglect can go unnoticed if not specifically evaluated. In those with milder left hemiparesis, lack of insight into this deficit can be highly problematic should the individual start driving, using power tools, or working with other hazardous machineries.

Stroke can also result in a variety of speech and language disorders generally referred to as aphasia. The two most common are Broca's aphasia and Wernicke's aphasia. Broca's aphasia results from damage to the frontal operculum on the right side of the cerebrum, just anterior to the precentral gyrus. Patients with Broca's aphasia have difficulty with verbal and written expression but often have intact comprehension. They generally understand considerably more than would be apparent from their responses, or lack of response to questions. Wernicke's aphasia is often referred to as "fluent aphasia." In this case, damage to the first temporal gyrus results in poor cognitive function and fluent nonsensical speech. Patients with this type of aphasia often have poor carry-over and a worse long-term prognosis. Other types of aphasia include aprosodia, a condition where an individual demonstrates no emotion in the tone of their voice but can hear the emotional changes in the voices of others, or, the opposite, affective agnosia, where the individual's voice is emotionally expressive but is unable to recognize emotion in the speech of others. Conduction aphasia, affecting the arcuate fasciculus between the temporal and frontal lobes, inhibits an individual's ability to repeat phrases. Alexia and agraphia, the inability to read and/or write, result from lesions in the angular gyrus, a disconnection of the primary language area in the temporal parietal lobe and the visual cortex in the occipital lobe. As communication is instrumental in both the rehabilitation process and in functional activity, understanding and identifying the type of aphasia early in the poststroke patient will greatly shape the rehabilitation program.

The lack of central inhibition can result in increased tone and spasticity. Abnormal muscle tone may result in poor positioning leading to joint contractures, skin breakdown, and pain. Apraxia is another motor control dysfunction that limits functional independence in the stroke patient. Apraxia is the inability to perform patterned purposeful motor functions. Most of our daily activities depend upon a sequence of movements that allow us to unconsciously perform routine tasks such as walking, brushing teeth, or verbally expressing our thoughts. In patients with apraxia, they no longer have the ability to unconsciously perform ordinary coordinated actions. Therapists will assist these patients in breaking down routine tasks into smaller, sequential steps to assist the stroke patient in relearning how to synchronize their actions and language.

As neurologic recovery progresses, muscular tone will begin to increase. Although excessive muscular tone can be detrimental, it can also be beneficial to the recovering stroke patient. Spasticity in the lower extremities, for example, can be helpful to assist in ambulation. The power generated from co-contracting agonist/antagonistic muscle groups is effective in managing body weight during gait. On the other hand, severe spasticity can result in abnormal posture during gait or inhibit appropriate sitting posture, dressing, or proper positioning in a wheelchair user. This can result in skin breakdown and soft tissue contractures.

Treatment for spasticity has to be carefully considered with regard to each patient's specific needs. Baclofen is an effective oral medication utilized to treat spasticity but can be highly sedating. Dantrolene, another medication used to address increased tone, can result in muscle weakness and liver toxicity. Phenol blocks and botulinum toxin injections can focus treatment to specific nerves and muscles, respectively. Phenol is utilized only in the most severe cases because it results in ablation of neurologic function that may be irreversible. Botulinum toxin, if used judiciously, creates focal muscle weakness to facilitate coordinated muscle control.

Depression and emotional lability are common after stroke. It is important to treat these symptoms with medications least likely to interfere with neurologic recovery. Selective serotonin reuptake inhibitors (SSRIs) and tricyclic antidepressants (TCAs) are the only classes of antidepressants studied in stroke [16, 17], but their efficacy is not established [18]. In common practice, SSRIs, including sertraline and citalopram, are preferred because they have a lower side effect profile and are generally considered helpful. TCAs have anticholinergic effects at therapeutic doses and thus are utilized less frequently. It is best to avoid centrally active agents such as benzodiazepines and antipsychotic medications where possible due to alterations in level of arousal.

Recognizing and preventing complications in the poststroke patient are a critical component in maximizing functional outcome after stroke.

A well-functioning rehabilitation team working in concert with the surgical specialist can significantly decrease morbidity and mortality in the poststroke patient while facilitating functional neurologic recovery.

Neurologic and Behavioral Characteristics of Typical Strokes

It is beyond the scope of this chapter to describe each and every stroke syndrome. The most common syndromes result from compromise of the dominant arterial supply in the carotid distribution supplying the middle cerebral artery. When occluded, lack of blood flow results in distinct neurologic patterns which are specific to the affected side. These differences result in characteristic physical and cognitive impairments requiring different rehabilitation approaches.

Left hemispheric middle cerebral artery strokes are characterized by an initial depression of consciousness, head and eyes deviated to the left, right hemiplegia/hemiparesis, right hemisoma sensory loss, and right hemianopsia. If the left hemisphere is dominant (the individual is right-handed), patients typically present with global aphasia, which over time becomes more expressive in quality. As consciousness improves, these patients will generally recover receptive language but will continue to have expressive deficits. It is important to remember in the poststroke period that these individuals may well have the capacity to comprehend much of what is being said in front of them despite the appearance of being noncommunicative. In those who are right hemispheric dominant (left-handed), cognitive and language deficits may include perceptual abnormalities and neglect to a lesser degree.

In right hemispheric strokes, patients present with similar contralateral motor and sensory deficits; however visual field deficits are more significant as is left-sided neglect. Neglect was discussed earlier in this chapter. The primary difference between dominant and non-dominant side stroke syndromes is one of language and cognition. Right hemispheric stroke patients are generally verbally fluent but are often disinhibited and understand much less than their language skills suggest. This is particularly important, as these patients are at higher risk for falls because they lack insight into their own deficits.

Vertebrobasilar strokes involve the brain stem and/or the cerebellum. Brain stem strokes present with contralateral facial/hemiplegia, while cerebellar strokes present with significant motor incoordination. Principles of brain stem stroke rehabilitation are the same as middle cerebral hemispheric stroke rehabilitation. Brain stem strokes can be very small and often missed on imaging studies but present with very significant neurological and functional impairments due to the density of nerve tracts in the region. Clinicians often fail to recognize cerebellar strokes because these patients have normal cognition and motor power; however, these individuals are often at risk of falls despite the use of assistive devices. The stroke rehabilitation team employs different strategies to regain motor function in patients with cerebellar stroke.

Rehabilitation of patients with stroke must take into account the types of cognitive and language impairments present when considering therapeutic rehabilitation interventions. For example, patients with right hemispheric strokes will have less carry-over of therapeutic treatment and will require tasks to be taught sequentially involving more repetition. Discharge home will need to consider the level of impulsivity and neglect as these factors impact safety, compliance, and the level of supervision a patient will require upon leaving the hospital.

Post-Acute Care of the Stroke Patient

Stroke severity covers the entire range from complete loss of a hemisphere to mild residual deficits. The physiatrist, with information provided from the rehabilitation team, determines the level of care needed and the optimal setting to maximize rehabilitation potential. The American Heart Association has defined the structural organization of stroke rehabilitation in the United States as an acute in hospital admission where the median length of stay for ischemic stroke is 4 days and for intracerebral bleed 7 days [8]. Stroke recovery begins in various settings catered to the needs of the patient. Inpatient rehabilitation facilities are intensive multispecialty treatment settings within hospitals or in freestanding rehabilitation institutions where the median length of stay is 15 days (range 8–30 days) [8]. Skilled nursing facilities are less intensive rehabilitative settings where patients may stay up to 100 days. Other patients are discharged directly home and receive home-based therapy initially and then transition to an outpatient setting. A highly functional patient will be discharged home and participate in outpatient therapy with appropriate therapy interventions two to three times a week.

Criteria for inpatient rehabilitation admission depend upon the medical resources available within a community as well as the type of insurance coverage an individual possesses. From a clinical perspective, patients must be stable without progressive neurologic loss prior to leaving the acute care setting. The degree of medical stability acceptable for transfer to a rehabilitation unit depends upon the system where the patient is being treated. Often, patients are transferred to inpatient rehabilitation units despite multiple complicating comorbid conditions if these ailments are identified and stable on an established management plan. For example, a patient with a urinary tract infection responding to appropriate antibiotics, who can participate in therapies, would be able to transfer to a rehabilitation unit; however, the same patient who is febrile and hemodynamically unstable (possible early sepsis) would not meet admission criteria. A patient typically gets only one chance with acute intensive inpatient rehabilitation and should not be admitted to this setting if unable to benefit from an intensive 3 h a day of direct therapeutic intervention. There are circumstances where a patient will be managed in a step-down specialty facility with ventilation, alimentary, and intravenous support until the level of arousal, medical stability, and ability to participate in therapy improves. A physiatrist can clarify specific criteria within your institution.

Therapeutic Modalities in the Poststroke Patient

There are several traditional standard approaches to stroke rehabilitation. Neurodevelopmental (Bobath) techniques focus on postural control that strives to facilitate motor learning through promoting normal movements and inhibiting abnormal movements during neurologic recovery. The Brunnstrom approach, in contrast, emphasizes the synergistic recovery patterns that occur during neurologic recovery. Unlike Bobath, the Brunnstrom approach encourages the patient to use flexor/extensor synergies, rather than inhibit abnormal movements to facilitate function early in recover. Proprioceptive neuromuscular facilitation involves stimulating the Golgi tendon and muscle spindles and facilitating postural reflexes and gravity to move weakened muscles. While some therapists adhere strictly to one approach, most therapists in the United States integrate aspects of all three approaches based upon their experience to customize and optimize functional recovery in stroke patients.

Numerous interventions including but not limited to transcutaneous electrical nerve stimulation, acupuncture, rhythmic auditory cueing, robotic- and electromechanical-assisted training devices, exoskeletal wearable lower limb robotic devices, electromyographic biofeedback, virtual reality, and water-based exercises are used with varying benefit to individual patients. None of these modalities has yet been proven to consistently alter functional outcomes [8]. Classical therapeutic interventions, when used together in an integrated approach, yield the most predictable results.

Prognosis and Functional Outcome after Stroke

The Functional Independence Measure (FIM) is a good predictor of discharge functional status and disposition [19]. FIM reporting is required prior to rehabilitation unit admission and at discharge by the Centers for Medicare & Medicaid Services (CMS) for quality purposes and reimbursement.

Once a patient plateaus in therapy as reflected by the FIM, the patient will no longer be eligible for continued treatment and must be discharged from an inpatient rehabilitation unit. The team uses FIM terms in oral and written communication. The FIM measures physical mobility in the bed, transfers, sit-to-stand transitions, ambulation, dressing of upper and lower extremities, grooming, feeding, and other self-care tasks as well as other functional areas (Fig. 24.1). For example, 2 Mod I transfer means two people are required to provide moderate assist (50% body weight assist) for the transfer. Inpatient stroke rehabilitation programs yield larger FIM gains per day and a higher return to home rate than skilled nursing facilities [20, 21]. Most patients who improve to lower extremity Brunnstrom stage 3 (active flexion/extension synergy) regain the ability to walk [22]. Eighty-five percentage of stroke patients discharged from an inpatient rehabilitation unit are ambulatory at discharge [23].

Recovery rates vary with the severity of the lesion. The majority of motor recovery will occur within the first 3 months after the onset of a stroke with 54–80% independent with gait [24]. Most poststroke self-care gains in activities of daily living occur within 6 months, and 5% will still make ADL gains up to 12 months [25]. Further gains do occur, but at a much slower rate of recovery. While 80% of individuals experiencing stroke return to community-based living [8], many of these individuals will still require some level of physical or cognitive assistance for a substantial period of time after leaving the rehabilitation setting. Younger stroke patients generally have better outcomes, with approximately 55% of working-age stroke patients returning to work within 1 year [26]. Individuals that drive have a higher level of independence. Approximately 50% of stroke patients who were previously driving within the community regain the ability to drive within 1 year [27]. The patient in the photo represents an example of a severe right middle cerebral arterial hypertensive hemorrhagic stroke that occurred, while she was working as a registered nurse in a postsurgical hospital setting. She experienced dense left hemiplegia, left hemi-neglect, left homonymous hemianopsia,

FIM® Instrument

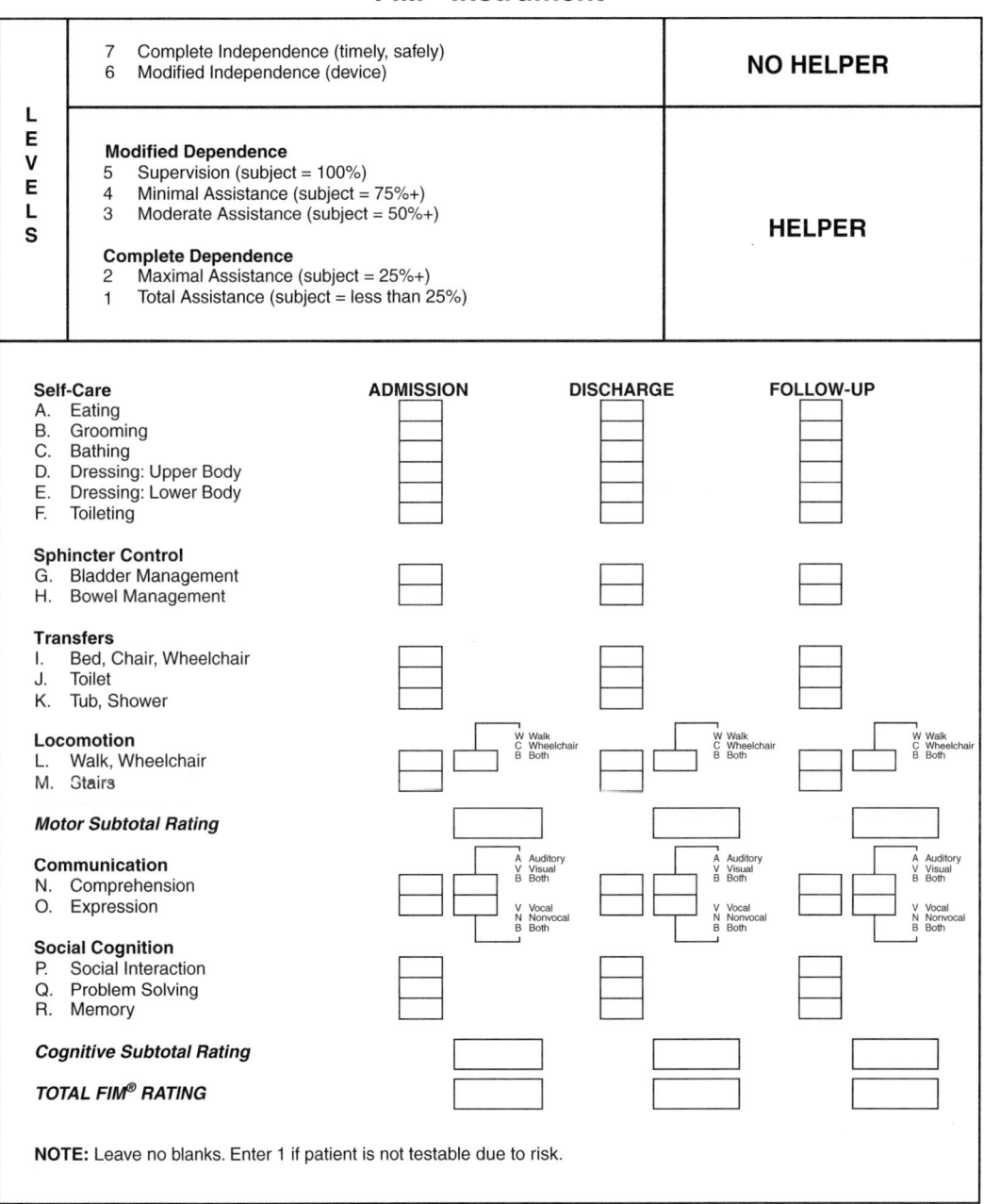

Fig. 24.1 Functional Independence Measure data form with defined level of care and functional areas assessed at admission, discharge, and follow-up. Copyright © 1997 Uniform Data System for Medical Rehabilitation, a division of UB Foundation Activities, Inc. Reprinted with permission

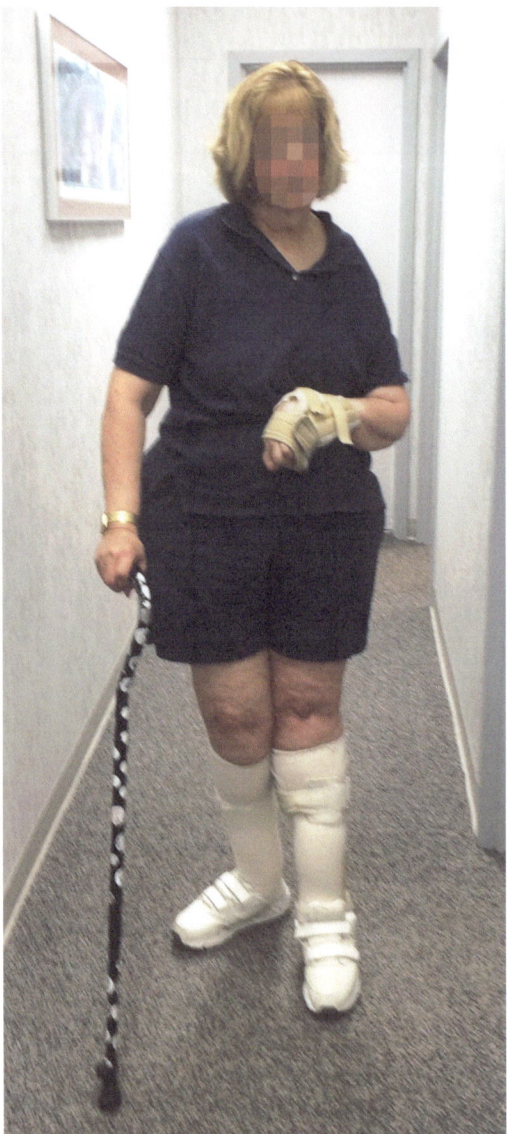

Fig. 24.2 Right hemispheric hemorrhagic stroke in the middle cerebral arterial distribution with severe post-acute stroke left hemiplegic deficits but excellent functional outcome despite ongoing left hemispasticity and gait impairment. Please see text for further discussion

panhypopituitarism with electrolyte, glycemic and other endocrine disorders, dysphagia, incontinence of bowel and bladder, significant gait, and self-care impairments. She was determined, dedicated to the rehabilitation process, was always positive and hopeful, and transitioned to home from an acute care rehabilitation facility. She had resolution of her endocrinopathies, visual field

deficit, and neglect. She returned to independent living, regained the ability to drive, and worked part time as a nurse. She has residual deficits with her left arm and leg that require an ankle foot orthosis and a wrist brace, impact gait and self-care, and require extra time for all activities of life, but she is very functional, engaged socially, and very active (Fig. 24.2).

Because stroke recovery occurs well beyond the present allowable inpatient rehabilitation period, the physiatrist generally follows these individuals as outpatients for several years assisting the stroke patient to reach their maximal functional independence at home, within the community, and vocationally.

Review Questions

1. In a well-run stroke rehabilitation program, the rehabilitation team optimally will begin their evaluation and treatment:
   A. After discharge from the hospital
   B. 24 h before anticipated transfer to an inpatient rehabilitation unit
   C. If you anticipate the patient will not be able to ambulate independently
   D. Within the first 24 h after onset of stroke symptoms

   Answer: D

2. Which of the following statements is *NOT* true regarding the Free Water Protocol?
   A. The Free Water Protocol can be performed at bedside.
   B. The Free Water Protocol acknowledges research documenting that small amounts of water aspirated into the lungs do not typically result in pneumonia.
   C. Oral hygiene is irrelevant in the risk of aspiration pneumonia.
   D. Implementation of the Free Water Protocol has significantly reduced dehydration and aspiration pneumonia in stroke patients with dysphagia.

   Answer: C

3. Stroke patients with a larger Ashworth number would likely be in what Brunnstrom stage of their rehabilitation?
   A. Flaccid stage
   B. Early synergic flexor/extensor motor function stage
   C. Spastic synergy dominant stage
   D. Isolated motor control and smooth coordinated joint motion

   Answer: C

4. Shoulder-hand syndrome, a form of complex regional pain syndrome, is a painful condition that is challenging to treat and impairs recovery. The best way to treat this condition is through:
   A. Early comprehensive aggressive prevention program initiated in the first 24 h of admission
   B. Cutaneous desensitization of the extremity
   C. Elevation of the limb
   D. Prophylactic use of gabapentin within the first 24 h of the first sign of paralysis

   Answer: A

5. After surgery, you are attempting to provide important discharge instructions to your patient. Which of the following patients may be alert and attentive but would have the most difficulty understanding your instructions?
   A. A patient with aprosodia
   B. A patient with a lesion in the frontal operculum of the right cerebrum
   C. A patient with damage to the first temporal gyrus
   D. A person with right hemiplegia

   Answer: C

6. Spasticity can adversely affect patients causing skin breakdown, abnormal posture during gait, and wheelchair seating or result in soft tissue contractures. It also can be beneficial in providing enough tone in a paralytic limb to facilitate ambulation. When selecting the appropriate medication to treat spasticity in a stroke patient, which of the following considerations is *least* relevant to the decision?
   A. Level of sedation
   B. Dose-dependent muscle weakness
   C. Liver toxicity
   D. Myonecrosis

   Answer: D

7. Emotional lability is common in post-stroke patients. Many medications used to treat agitation negatively impact neurologic recovery. Which of the following classes of medications are relatively contraindicated in stroke patients?
   A. Serotonin reuptake inhibitors
   B. Benzodiazepines
   C. Tricyclic antidepressants
   D. Anticonvulsants

   Answer: B

References

1. Miller EL, Murray L, Richards L, Zorowitz RD, Bakas T, Clark P, et al. Comprehensive overview of nursing and interdisciplinary rehabilitation care of the stroke patient: a scientific statement from the American Heart Association. Stroke. 2010;41(10):2402–48.
2. Kalra L, Yu G, Wilson K, Roots P. Medical complications during stroke rehabilitation. Stroke. 1995;26(6):990–4.
3. Langmore SE, Terpenning MS, Schork A, Chen Y, Murray JT, Lopatin D, et al. Predictors of aspiration pneumonia: how important is dysphagia? Dysphagia. 1998;13(2):69–81.
4. Singh S, Hamdy S. Dysphagia in stroke patients. Postgrad Med J. 2006;82(968):383–91.
5. Feinberg MJ, Knebl J, Tully J. Prandial aspiration and pneumonia in an elderly population followed over 3 years. Dysphagia. 1996;11(2):104–9.
6. Panther K. The free water protocol. Swallowing Swallowing Disord/Dysphagias. 2005;14:4–9.
7. Barer DH. The natural history and functional consequences of dysphagia after hemispheric stroke. J Neurol Neurosurg Psychiatry. 1989;52(2):236–41.
8. Winstein CJ, Stein J, Arena R, Bates B, Cherney LR, Cramer SC, et al. Guidelines for adult stroke rehabilitation and recovery: a guideline for healthcare professionals from the American Heart Association/American Stroke Association. Stroke. 2016;47(6):e98–e169.

9. Dennis M, Sandercock PA, Reid J, Graham C, Murray G, Venables G, et al. Effectiveness of thigh-length graduated compression stockings to reduce the risk of deep vein thrombosis after stroke (CLOTS trial 1): a multicentre, randomised controlled trial. Lancet (London, England). 2009;373(9679):1958–65.

10. Lansberg MG, O'Donnell MJ, Khatri P, Lang ES, Nguyen-Huynh MN, Schwartz NE, et al. Antithrombotic and thrombolytic therapy for ischemic stroke: antithrombotic therapy and prevention of thrombosis, 9th ed: American College of Chest Physicians Evidence-Based Clinical Practice Guidelines. Chest. 2012;141(2 Suppl):e601S–e36S.

11. Thomas LH, Cross S, Barrett J, French B, Leathley M, Sutton CJ, et al. Treatment of urinary incontinence after stroke in adults. Cochrane Database Syst Rev. 2008;1:Cd004462.

12. Brunnstrom S. Recovery stages and evaluation procedures. In: Movement therapy in hemiplegia: a neurophysical approach. New York: Harper & Row; 1970. p. 34–55.

13. Lang CE, Bland MD, Bailey RR, Schaefer SY, Birkenmeier RL. Assessment of upper extremity impairment, function, and activity after stroke: foundations for clinical decision making. J Hand Ther. 2013;26(2):104–14.

14. Velstra IM, Ballert CS, Cieza A. A systematic literature review of outcome measures for upper extremity function using the international classification of functioning, disability, and health as reference. PM & R. 2011;3(9):846–60.

15. Malhotra S, Pandyan AD, Rosewilliam S, Roffe C, Hermens H. Spasticity and contractures at the wrist after stroke: time course of development and their association with functional recovery of the upper limb. Clin Rehabil. 2011;25(2):184–91.

16. Chollet F, Acket B, Raposo N, Albucher JF, Loubinoux I, Pariente J. Use of antidepressant medications to improve outcomes after stroke. Curr Neurol Neurosci Rep. 2013;13(1):318.

17. Karaiskos D, Tzavellas E, Spengos K, Vassilopoulou S, Paparrigopoulos T. Duloxetine versus citalopram and sertraline in the treatment of poststroke depression, anxiety, and fatigue. J Neuropsychiatry Clin Neurosci. 2012;24(3):349–53.

18. Bhogal SK, Teasell R, Foley N, Speechley M. Heterocyclics and selective serotonin reuptake inhibitors in the treatment and prevention of poststroke depression. J Am Geriatr Soc. 2005;53(6):1051–7.

19. Hall KM, Cohen ME, Wright J, Call M, Werner P. Characteristics of the functional independence measure in traumatic spinal cord injury. Arch Phys Med Rehabil. 1999;80(11):1471–6.

20. Keith RA, Wilson DB, Gutierrez P. Acute and subacute rehabilitation for stroke: a comparison. Arch Phys Med Rehabil. 1995;76(6):495–500.

21. Kramer AM, Steiner JF, Schlenker RE, Eilertsen TB, Hrincevich CA, Tropea DA, et al. Outcomes and costs after hip fracture and stroke. A comparison of rehabilitation settings. JAMA. 1997;277(5):396–404.

22. Brandstater ME. Stroke rehabilitation. In: DeLisa JA, Gans BM, Walsh NE, editors. Physical medicine and rehabilitation medicine: principles and practice. 4th ed. Philadelphia: Lippincott Williams & Wilkins; 2004. p. 1654–76.

23. Feigenson JS, McDowell FH, Meese P, McCarthy ML, Greenberg SD. Factors influencing outcome and length of stay in a stroke rehabilitation unit. Part 1. Analysis of 248 unscreened patients—medical and functional prognostic indicators. Stroke. 1977;8(6):651–6.

24. Wade DT, Wood VA, Hewer RL. Recovery after stroke—the first 3 months. J Neurol Neurosurg Psychiatry. 1985;48(1):7–13.

25. Wade DT, Hewer RL. Functional abilities after stroke: measurement, natural history and prognosis. J Neurol Neurosurg Psychiatry. 1987;50(2):177–82.

26. Chan ML. Description of a return-to-work occupational therapy programme for stroke rehabilitation in Singapore. Occup Ther Int. 2008;15(2):87–99.

27. Perrier MJ, Korner-Bitensky N, Mayo NE. Patient factors associated with return to driving poststroke: findings from a multicenter cohort study. Arch Phys Med Rehabil. 2010;91(6):868–73.

Correction to: Difficult Conditions in Laparoscopic Urologic Surgery

Sachinder Singh Hans

Correction to:
S. S. Hans (ed.), *Extracranial Carotid and Vertebral Artery Disease*,
https://doi.org/10.1007/978-3-319-91533-3

Late corrections to chapters 3 and 10 have been corrected as listed below:

1. Chapter 3: Page 22, the last sentence in paragraph "Occlusive lesions of the....." has been updated as below:

   "For example, the costocervical and thyrocervical branches of the Subclavian Artery can develop collateral circulation between the external carotid and subclavian arteries."

2. Chapter 10: Page 146, reference 14 has been updated as below:

   "Calligaro KD, Dougherty MJ. Correlation of carotid artery stump pressure and neurological changes during 474 carotid endarterectomies performed in awake patients. J Vasc Surg. 2005;42:684–9."

The updated online version of these chapters can be found at
https://doi.org/10.1007/978-3-319-91533-3_3
https://doi.org/10.1007/978-3-319-91533-3_10

Index

© The Editor(s) (if applicable) and The Author(s) 2018
S. S. Hans (ed.), *Extracranial Carotid and Vertebral Artery Disease*,
https://doi.org/10.1007/978-3-319-91533-3

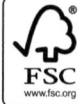

MIX
Papier aus verantwortungsvollen Quellen
Paper from responsible sources
FSC® C105338

If you have any concerns about our products,
you can contact us on
ProductSafety@springernature.com

In case Publisher is established outside the EU,
the EU authorized representative is:
Springer Nature Customer Service Center GmbH
Europaplatz 3, 69115 Heidelberg, Germany

Printed by Libri Plureos GmbH
in Hamburg, Germany